EXERCISE IN HEALTH AND DISEASE

EXERCISE IN HEALTH AND DISEASE

Edited By

FRANCIS J. NAGLE, PH.D.

Professor
Departments of Physiology and Physical Education
University of Wisconsin
Madison, Wisconsin

and

HENRY J. MONTOYE, PH.D.

Chairman and Professor of Physical Education
University of Wisconsin
Madison, Wisconsin

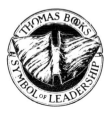

CHARLES C THOMAS • PUBLISHER

Springfield • Illinois • U.S.A.

Published and Distributed Throughout the World by

CHARLES C THOMAS • PUBLISHER

Bannerstone House

301-327 East Lawrence Avenue, Springfield, Illinois, U.S.A.

*With THOMAS BOOKS carefully attention is given to all details of manufacturing and
design. It is the Publisher's desire to present books that are satisfactory as to their physical
qualities and artistic possibilities and appropriate for their particular use. THOMAS
BOOKS will be true to those laws of quality that assure a good name and good will.*

Printed in the United States of America
CB-1

Library of Congress Cataloging in Publication Data

Main entry under title:

Exercise in health and disease.

Papers presented at a symposium sponsored by the
Departments of Physical Education and Dance and
Continuing Medical Education at the University of
Wisconsin, Madison; held June 8-9, 1979.
Bibliography: p.
Includes index.
1. Exercise—Physiological aspects—Congresses. 2.
Exercise therapy—Congresses. 3. Health—Congresses.
I. Nagle, Francis J. II. Montoye, Henry Joseph. III.
Wisconsin. University—Madison. Dept. of Physical
Education and Dance. IV. Wisconsin. University—
Madison. Dept of Continuing Medical Education.
[DNLM: 1. Exertion—Congresses. 2. Exercise
therapy—Congresses. WE103 E96 1979]
QP301.E96   612'.04   80-17826
ISBN 0-398-04120-2

CONTRIBUTORS

Michael S. Bahrke, Ph.D., Assistant Professor of Physical Education, University of Kansas, Lawrence, KS.

Frank J. Cerny, Ph.D., Associate Director, Children's Lung Center, Children's Hospital of Buffalo; Assistant Professor of Pediatrics, Department of Pediatrics, SUNY, Buffalo, NY.

Alan D. Claremont, Ph.D., Project Specialist, Department of Preventive Medicine, University of Wisconsin, Madison, WI.

Jack T. Daniels, Ph.D., Associate Professor of Physical Education, University of Texas at Austin, Austin, TX.

Jerome A. Dempsey, Ph.D., Professor of Preventive Medicine, Director Pulmonary Function Lab, University of Wisconsin, Madison, WI.

Rodney K. Dishman, Ph.D., Assistant Professor of Physical Education, Southwest Missouri State University, Springfield, MO.

John A. Faulkner, Ph.D., Professor of Physiology, Medical School, University of Michigan, Ann Arbor, MI.

Robert H. Fitts, Ph.D., Assistant Professor of Biology, Marquette University, Milwaukee, WI.

Hubert V. Forster, Ph.D., Associate Professor of Physiology, The Medical College of Wisconsin, Milwaukee, WI.

James B. Gale, Ph.D., Professor of Physical Education, Sonoma State College, Rohnert Park, CA.

Norman Gledhill, Ph.D., Assistant Professor, York University, Toronto, Ontario, Canada.

Howard J. Green, Ph.D., Associate Professor, Human Kinetics, Department of Kinesiology, University of Waterloo, Waterloo, Ontario, Canada.

James M. Hagberg, Ph.D., Director Human Applied Physiology Lab, Department of Preventive Medicine, Washington University School of Medicine, St. Louis, MO.

Edward T. Howley, Ph.D., Associate Professor, Departments of Zoology and Physical Education, University of Tennessee, Knoxville, TN.

J. Duncan MacDougall, Ph.D., Associate Professor, Departments of Physical Education and Medicine, McMaster University, Hamilton, Ontario, Canada.

Henry J. Montoye, Ph.D., Chairman and Professor of Physical Education, University of Wisconsin, Madison, WI.

William P. Morgan, Ed.D., Professor of Physical Education, University of Wisconsin, Madison, WI.

Francis J. Nagle, Ph.D., Professor, Departments of Physiology and Physical Education, University of Wisconsin, Madison, WI.

John Naughton, M.D., Professor of Medicine and Dean, Medical School, SUNY, Buffalo, NY.

Neil B. Oldridge, Ph.D., Associate Professor of Physical Education and Medicine, McMaster University, Hamilton, Ontario, Canada.

John R. Palmer, Ph.D., Dean, School of Education, University of Wisconsin, Madison, WI.

Richard A. Peterson, Ph.D., Director, Kellogg Fitness Center, Hope College, Holland, MI.

Glen Porter, Ph.D., Exercise Physiologist, Cardiopulmonary Laboratory, Gundersen Clinic, La Crosse, WI.

Michael A. Ross, Ph.D., Director of Fitness, Testing and Counseling, YMCA of Greater New York, West Side YMCA, 5 West 63rd Street, New York, NY.

Michael T. Sharratt, Ph.D., Assistant Professor, Department of Kinesiology, University of Waterloo, Waterloo, Ontario, Canada.

Everett L. Smith, Jr., Ph.D., Assistant Professor, Department of Preventive Medicine, University of Wisconsin, Madison, Madison, WI.

Karl G. Stoedefalke, Ph.D., Professor of Physical Education and Associate Dean, School of Physical Education, Penn State University, State College, University Park, PA.

W. G. Weaver, School of Physical and Health Education, Queen's University, Kingston, Canada.

PREFACE

By 1964, after fourteen years as an Applied Physiologist with the U.S. Air Force in Texas and The Civil Aeromedical Research Institute in Oklahoma City, Bruno Balke had clearly distinguished himself as a research scientist. In 1964 he accepted a professorship at the University of Wisconsin, Madison where he continued his research in exercise physiology and turned his attention to the graduate education of young people.

He saw a striking need for in-depth biological science training for students aspiring to college and university positions in exercise and sport sciences. As a colleague of Dr. Balke in 1964, I can affirm that this was the overriding consideration in motivating him to leave his post in the government service and to assume an academic position at the University of Wisconsin.

It is truly fitting then that in 1979 (June 8-9) the University of Wisconsin honors this man with the presentation of this series of scientific papers. (This Symposium was sponsored by The Department of Physical Education and Dance and The Department of Continuing Medical Education at the University of Wisconsin and was endorsed by the American College of Sports Medicine.) Aside from those papers presented by close colleagues (John Naughton, M.D., William Morgan, Ed.D., and John Faulkner, Ph.D.), all the papers were given by Dr. Balke's former graduate students, trained at Wisconsin between 1964 and 1979.

Francis J. Nagle

ACKNOWLEDGMENTS

Thanks are due many people for making this Symposium possible. First, we wish to thank Lyn Opelt of Continuing Medical Education, University of Wisconsin, for help in publicizing and organizing the Symposium on the UW campus. Also, thanks are due Mrs. Sue Munson for extensive secretarial and other assistance and to the Quinton Instrument Company for its financial support. Most of all, a debt of gratitude is owed to Bruno's colleagues and former graduate students who participated in the Symposium. These men and women came to Madison at their own expense to honor Bruno. All but a few of his students were able to attend. In some instances this meant changing vacation or other plans, and this clearly reflects the esteem the students held for their teacher.

F.J.N.
H.J.M.

WELCOMING REMARKS

John R. Palmer, Ph.D.

It is a long way from Braunschweig, Germany (where Dr. Balke was born) to the cool mountains of Colorado. Fortunately, Madison was on the route and we had Dr. Balke with us for about a decade. Perceiving physical exercise as beneficial is certainly not new but Dr. Balke was one of a handful of pioneers who began to look at exercise from a scientific, medical perspective. The move was a timely one, for the sedentary tendencies of our contemporary society are creating major health problems. Many of you devote your time and talents to this research area. The best way anyone can honor Dr. Balke is by contributing research to the field. If this symposium helps you to continue your research efforts and gives you new ideas about how to examine exercise and health, it will have accomplished its purpose. We are pleased to have you here on this special occasion.

Common Symbols

a-vO_2 diff	Arterial to venous oxygen difference
C_aO_2	Arterial O_2 content
$C_{\overline{mv}}O_2$	Mixed venous blood O_2 content
CSF	Cerebrospinal fluid
FEF	Forced expiratory flow
FEV_1	Forced expired volume in 1.0 second
GOT	Glutamic Oxaloacetic Transaminase
H^+	Hydrogen ion
MVC	Maximal voluntary contraction
N_2	Nitrogen
O_2	Oxygen
P_ACO_2	Alveolar CO_2 partial pressure
P_AO_2	Alveolar O_2 partial pressure
P_aCO_2	Arterial CO_2 partial pressure
P_aO_2	Arterial O_2 partial pressure
$P_{ET}CO_2$	End tidal partial pressure CO_2
$P_{ET}O_2$	End tidal partial pressure O_2
pH_a	Arterial pH
P_i	Inorganic phosphate
P_IO_2	Inspired O_2 partial pressure
$\dot{Q}_c$	Total capillary blood flow
$\dot{Q}$max	Maximal total blood flow
S_aO_2	Arterial O_2 saturation
V_A	Alveolar volume
$\dot{V}_A$	Alveolar minute ventilation
VC	Vital capacity
V_D	Dead space volume
$\dot{V}_D$	Minute dead space ventilation
$\dot{V}_E$	Minute ventilation
$\dot{V}O_2$	Total body O_2 consumption
$\dot{V}O_2$max	Maximal O_2 consumption
V_T	Tital volume

CONTENTS

Part 3—EXERCISE IN DISEASE PREVENTION AND
THERAPY

EXERCISE IN HEALTH
AND DISEASE

Part 1

EXERCISE AND LUNG FUNCTION IN HEALTH AND DISEASE

PRESIDING: JEROME A. DEMPSEY

Chapter 1

VENTILATORY ACCLIMATIZATION OF SEA LEVEL RESIDENTS DURING SOJOURN AT HIGH ALTITUDE*

H.V. FORSTER, J.A. DEMPSEY, AND G.E. BISGARD

VENTILATORY acclimatization of sea level residents during sojourn at high altitude is generally viewed as the increase in pulmonary and alveolar ventilation ($\dot{V}_E$, $\dot{V}_A$), which in man occurs gradually between 1 hour and 1 to 2 weeks of hypoxia (12, 19, 27). The magnitude and time course of this increase is not the same at all altitudes in a given species, nor is it the same at a given altitude in all species (27). This increase proceeds slower in man than in most species, but it is greater in man than in most species. For example, in man at 4300 m altitude, nearly 2 weeks are required before eupneic ventilation stabilizes at its elevated level, which is sufficient to increase P_AO_2 and decrease P_ACO_2 by approximately 10 mmHg (12). In contrast, the change in pony is complete after only 12 hours of hypoxia, but alveolar gases have only changed 5 to 7 mmHg from 1 hour of hypoxia (14, 24). The ventilatory changes are not, however, restricted to eupneic conditions. In this chapter we present evidence documenting the general hyperventilatory responsiveness that occurs during sojourn, and we summarize data pertaining to potential mechanisms of the change.

EVIDENCE OF GENERAL HYPERVENTILATORY RESPONSIVENESS

Data presented in Figure 1-1 were obtained on sea level residents before and during sojourn at 3100 m altitude (5). Ventilation was measured at rest and during the fifth minute of 5 or 6 intensities of treadmill exercise. At sea level, the subjects exercised

*Our studies have been supported by grants from the National Institute of Health, the American Lung Association, and from the Wisconsin Heart Association and also by funds from the A.H. Robins Co.

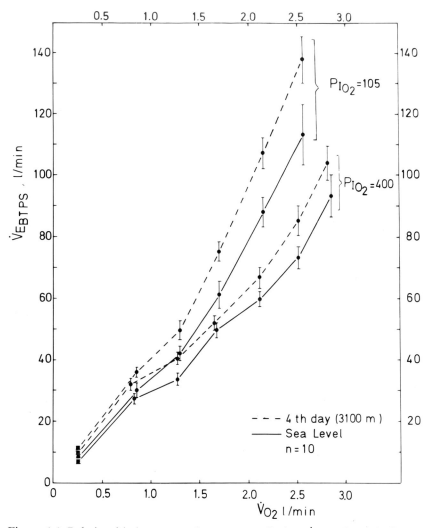

Figure 1-1. Relationship between pulmonary ventilation ($\dot{V}_E$) and metabolic rate ($\dot{V}O_2$) in 10 sea level residents during hypoxic (P_IO_2 = 105 mmHg) and hyperoxic (P_IO_2 = 400 mmHg) conditions at sea level and on the fourth day of sojourn at 3100 m altitude. Mean ($\pm$ SEM) values are plotted.

while breathing 15% O_2, and a second time while breathing 60% O_2. These percentages were chosen to provide the same inspired PO_2 as ambient hypoxia and 100% O_2 at altitude. At each $\dot{V}O_2$ and at both P_IO_2, $\dot{V}_E$ was greater at 3100 m than at sea level. The absolute difference for a given P_IO_2 increases as $\dot{V}O_2$ increases so that the percent increase becomes independent of $\dot{V}O_2$ (20–25%). Others have observed similar findings (1, 4, 20, 21, 26).

The $\dot{V}_E$ response to isocapnic hypoxia is presented in Figure 1-2 for the same 10 subjects as above (10). At both altitudes, the subjects breathe 5 different O_2-N_2 gas mixtures for 15 minutes, interspersed by 15 minutes breathing ambient air. The initial mixture in a study always provided a P_AO_2 of 250 mmHg. By appropriately adjusting the flow of 100% CO_2 into the inspired gas mixtures, we maintained $P_{ET}CO_2$ constant at the level observed at a P_AO_2 of 250 mmHg. At sea level, this iso-$P_{ET}CO_2$ was 39.0 mmHg; at 3100 m altitude it was 33.5 mmHg. At each P_AO_2, $\dot{V}_E$ was greater at altitude than at sea level. Note particularly that restoration to normal and hyperoxic P_AO_2 during sojourn caused only a minimal decrease from $\dot{V}_E$ during ambient hypoxia. In other words, the stimulus causing the increased $\dot{V}_E$ between acute and chronic hypoxia is sustained during 15 minutes of high O_2 breathing. These findings are consistent with data obtained by others (1, 4, 20, 21, 29, 31, 32, 36).

The $\dot{V}_E$ responsiveness to hyperoxic CO_2 inhalation was also

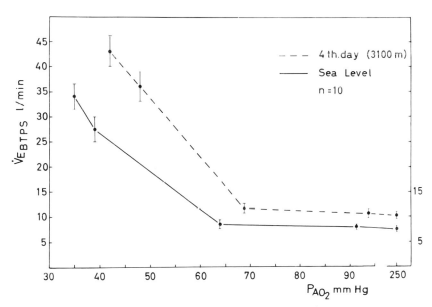

Figure 1-2. Relationship between pulmonary ventilation ($\dot{V}_E$) and alveolar oxygen tension (P_AO_2) in 10 sea level residents at sea level and on the fourth day of sojourn at 3100 m altitude. Mean (± SEM) values are plotted.

assessed in the same 10 subjects as above (10). Prepared hyperoxic gas mixtures (P_IO_2 = 280 mmHg) enriched with CO_2 (P_ICO_2 = 28 and 42 mmHg) were inhaled for 15 minutes interspersed by 15 minutes breathing ambient air. Figure 1-3 presents CO_2 response

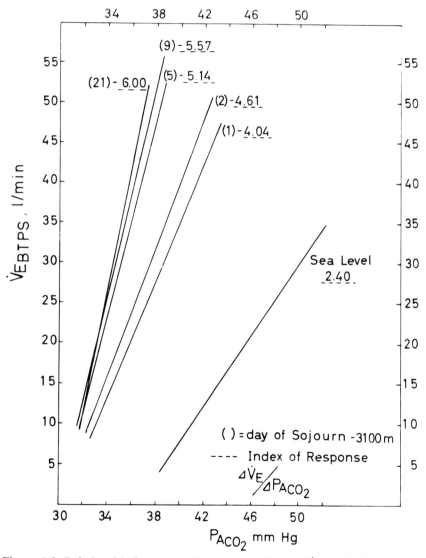

Figure 1-3. Relationship between pulmonary ventilation ($\dot{V}_E$) and alveolar carbon dioxide tension (P_ACO_2) in one sea level resident at sea level and after 1, 2, 3, 9, and 21 days of sojourn at 3100 m altitude.

curves of a representative subject during the course of the study. As shown by other investigators, during altitude sojourn $\dot{V}_E$ at any P_ACO_2 is higher at altitude than at sea level; both the slope and intercept of the response lines are altered by the sojourn (1, 3, 16–18, 23, 28, 33).

The effect of altitude sojourn on the $\dot{V}_E$ response to the pharmacologic agent doxapram HCl has been studied by the authors (11). Both bolus injections and steady state infusions were completed on 7 subjects during hyperoxic conditions at sea level and

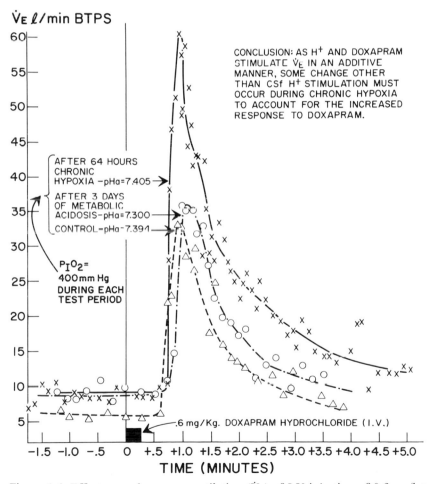

Figure 1-4. Effect on pulmonary ventilation ($\dot{V}_E$) of I.V. injection of 0.6 mg/kg doxapram hydrochloride during 3 different conditions in one subject. Each data point represents one breath ($V_t \times 60$/breath duration in sec).

after 3 days at 3400 m altitude. As shown in Figure 1-4 by the data on one subject, the $\dot{V}_E$ response to the agent was markedly greater at altitude than at sea level.

In summary, as shown in Figures 1-1 through 1-4, $\dot{V}_E$ is generally greater in sea level residents sojourning at altitude than it is at sea level. This difference is evident when comparisons are made at equivalent $\dot{V}O_2$, P_AO_2, P_ACO_2, arterial pH, and at the same dosages of doxapram HCl.

MECHANISMS OF $\dot{V}_E$ ACCLIMATIZATION DURING ALTITUDE SOJOURN

Dr. Kellogg recently summarized the rationale and supportive data of theories regarding this mechanism (19). Findings pertinent to 4 theories will be discussed.

Effect of Differences in Physical Properties of Inspired Air

It has been postulated that some aspect of the difference in physical properties of the inspired gas might contribute to the difference in $\dot{V}_E$ between sea level and high altitude. However, no data are available in support of this theory. The potential effect of these differences was studied by having 3 subjects exercise for 15 minutes at several work intensities at 3 equivalent P_IO_2, once at sea level and again during 15 minutes of hypobaria (4000 m, $P_B = 465$ mmHg). In all 3 subjects at each level of oxygenation, the relationship between $\dot{V}_E$ and $\dot{V}O_2$ was identical at both atmospheric pressures (Fig. 1-5).

Role of Plasma [H⁺]

It has been hypothesized that acclimatization occurs as renal mechanisms adjust plasma [HCO_3^-] to alleviate the alkalosis in plasma induced by the hyperventilation upon initial exposure to hypoxia (19). In essence, according to this theory, acclimatization results from a relative increase in H^+ stimulation of the arterial chemoreceptors. This hypothesis was tested by adjusting P_IO_2 during studies on 4 subjects at sea level so that P_aO_2 was the same as during the fourth day of sojourn at high altitude (5). Arterial pH was 0.03 to 0.05 more alkaline at altitude than at sea level (Fig. 1-6); hence, the difference in $\dot{V}_E$ as shown in Figure 1-1 was, in essence, the cause and not the result of the difference in arterial pH. Several other authors have observed similar findings (2, 19, 24).

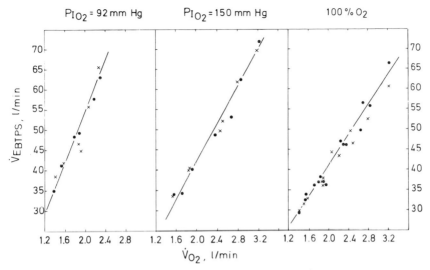

Figure 1-5. Relationship between pulmonary ventilation ($\dot{V}_E$) and metabolic rate in one subject at 3 levels of oxygenation while at an atmospheric pressure of 750 mmHg (solid circles), and again during 15 minutes at a pressure of 465 mmHg (×). Data points represent steady state values for one experiment.

Intracranial Chemoreceptor Mediation

Similar rationale provides the basis of the theory that acclimatization results because of a relative increase in H^+ stimulation at the intracranial chemoreceptor. Severinghaus et al. formulated this theory on the basis of their findings of a normal CSF pH during sojourn at high altitude (31). They assumed $[H^+]$ in CSF is in equilibrium with $[H^+]$ in cerebral interstitial fluid (ISF) and that the intracranial chemoreceptor is responsive to $[H^+]$ in its local ISF environment below the floor of the fourth cerebral ventricle. If these assumptions are correct, then CSF $[H^+]$ provides a valid index of H^+ stimulation at the intracranial chemoreceptor. Accordingly, the authors and others have subsequently studied the relationship between $\dot{V}_A$ and CSF $[H^+]$ during sojourn at high altitude.

The authors have sampled lumbar spinal fluid from 30 humans during 4 separate studies at 3100 m to 4300 m altitude (6–8, 12). In addition, at the same altitudes, CSF was withdrawn from the cisterna magna of 25 ponies (14, 24). Measurements on both species have been made at sea level, during the first hour of hypoxia, at various times during sojourn up to 45 days, and again

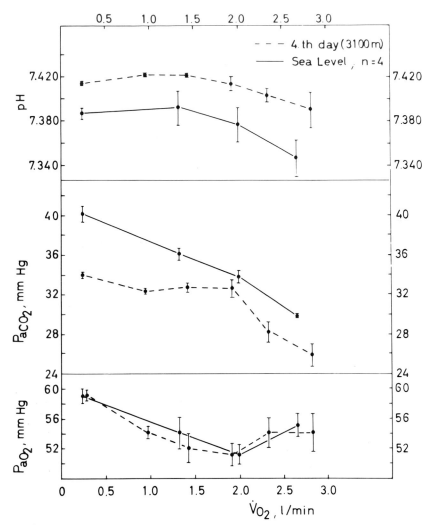

Figure 1-6. Arterial oxygen tension (P_aO_2), arterial carbon dioxide tension (P_aCO_2), and arterial pH at various metabolic rates ($\dot{V}O_2$) during 15 minutes of hypoxia at sea level and on the fourth day of sojourn at 3100 m altitude. Values plotted are the mean ($\pm$ SEM) responses of 4 sea level subjects.

after 1, 6, 12, and 24 hours of deacclimatization. Data on both species provide the same trend, that is, CSF [H$^+$] is inversely related to $\dot{V}_A$. This pattern is illustrated by the data in Figure 1-7 from a study on 6 ponies during 45 days at 3400 m altitude. In pony, $\dot{V}_A$ acclimatization is sustained for less than 10 days at altitude; hence, the status of CSF [H$^+$] was followed during the

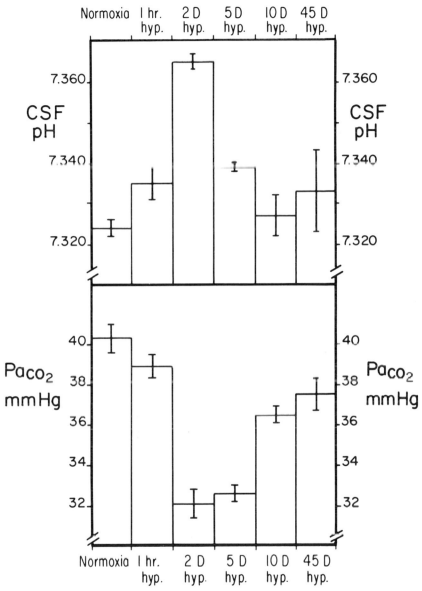

Figure 1-7. Arterial carbon dioxide tension (P_aCO_2) and cisternal CSF pH of 6 sea level ponies during normoxia at sea level, and after 1 hour (hr), 2, 5, 10, and 45 days (D) at 3400 m altitude. Mean ($\pm$ SEM) values are plotted. Note, P_aCO_2 as an index of alveolar ventilation, is inversely related to CSF pH suggesting CSF pH is the result and not the cause of changes in $\dot{V}_A$.

onset, steady state, and waning states of hyperventilation during hypoxia. In essence, CSF [H$^+$] is the result and not the cause of changes in $\dot{V}_A$ during acclimatization to and deacclimatization from high altitude. Other investigators have observations supportive of these findings (2, 22, 36).

Recent findings by Fencl (9) suggest that during altitude sojourn CSF [H$^+$] is not in equilibrium with cerebral ISF [H$^+$]. It appears an increased production of lactic acid by cerebral tissue results in an acidosis in cerebral ISF. Conceivably, [H$^+$] at the chemoreceptor could be directly related to $\dot{V}_A$ during hypoxia. In essence, then, acclimatization would be due to a metabolic acidosis of cerebral ISF, and therefore it should be independent of the carotid chemoreceptors. Accordingly, the authors surgically excised the carotid chemoreceptors in 6 ponies (14) and 7 goats (15). As shown in Figure 1-8, these goats show no acclimatization during 4 days of hypobaric hypoxia, while the ponies showed a slight but unsustained acclimatization (Fig. 1-9). The difference in $\dot{V}_A$ between normal and denervated ponies during hypoxia occurs in spite of CSF pH being 0.08 more acid in the denervated ponies (Fig. 1-10). Accordingly, even if the environment of the intracranial chemoreceptor is relatively acid during altitude sojourn, it alone is not sufficient to induce and sustain $\dot{V}_A$ acclimatization.

Change in Excitability of Medullary Respiratory Neurons

The present hypothesis is that acclimatization occurs because of an increase in excitability of respiratory neurons. This hypothesis is suggested by the general hyperventilatory responsiveness characteristic of sojourners that coincides on a temporal basis with an increasing P$_a$O$_2$ and an increasing arterial and CSF pH; thus, stimulus level at the known chemoreceptors appears to be decreasing as acclimatization proceeds. Supportive also of this theory are findings that the $\dot{V}_E$ response to doxapram HCl is not altered by acute respiratory acidosis, chronic metabolic acidosis (Fig. 1-4), nor muscular exercise but (as already discussed) the response is markedly enhanced by sojourn at altitude. Because the 3 enumerated conditions of increased input to the respiratory center had no effect on the response, it seems reasonable to conclude the increased response during sojourn was due to altered response characteristics of the respiratory center itself. Finally, presumptive support of this theory is provided by the finding that altitude

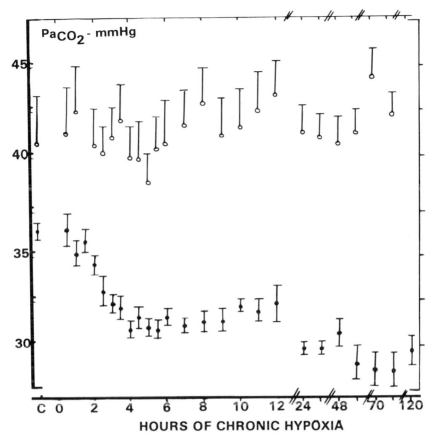

Figure 1-8. P_aCO_2 of 7 normal goats (solid circles) and 7 peripheral chemoreceptor denervated goats (open circles) during normal condition (C) at sea level and on numerous occasions during 120 hours of hypobaria that reduced P_aO_2 in both groups to 40–45 mmHg. (Mean (± SEM) values are plotted. Note, P_aCO_2, as an index of alveolar ventilation, suggests the peripheral chemoreceptors are essential for ventilatory acclimatization during chronic hypoxia.

sojourn causes changes in the spontaneous electroencephalogram (13) in visual evoked cerebral electrical activity (13) and in the electrically and mechanically elicited electromyogram (30); all of these changes are consistent with an increased excitability of the central nervous system. It should be emphasized that these findings do not prove that the respiratory center is indeed hyperexcitable at altitude; they are merely consistent with that postulate.

Another reason to favor the above theory is because two series of studies suggest a mechanism that could mediate the hyperex-

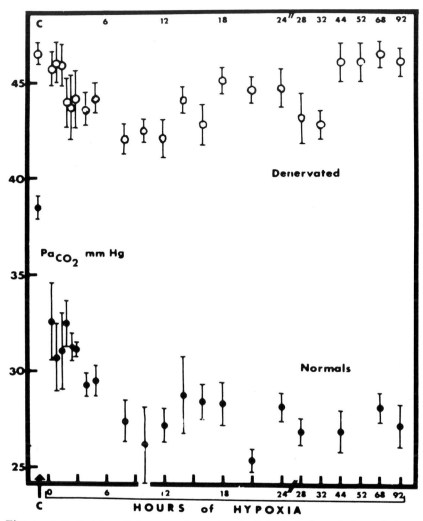

Figure 1-9. P_aCO_2 of 4 normal ponies (solid circles) and 6 peripheral chemoreceptor denervated ponies (open circles) during normal conditions at sea level and on numerous occasions during 92 hours of hypobaria that reduced P_aO_2 in both groups to 40–45 mmHg. Mean (± SEM) values are plotted.

citability. *One* series of studies by Tenney et al. has shown (1) that suprapontine structures such as the orbital frontal cortex and reticular activating system can modulate respiratory center excitability, (2) that inhibitory and facilitatory modulation are altered during chronic hypoxia, (3) that these changes probably do not coincide temporally nor are they equal at all levels of hypoxia, so

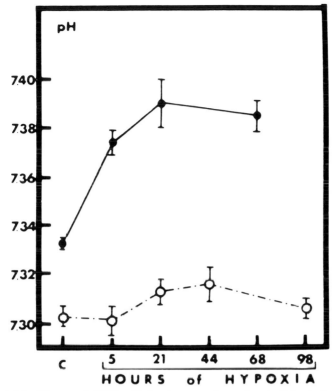

Figure 1-10. Cisternal CSF pH in 4 normal ponies (solid circles) and 6 peripheral chemoreceptor denervated ponies (open circles) during normal conditions (C) at sea level and after 5, 21, 44, 68, and 98 hours of hypobaria that reduced P_aO_2 to 40–45 mmHg in both species. Mean ($\pm$ SEM) values are plotted.

that net modulation is dependent on the algebraic sum of inhibition and facilitation, and (4) that $\dot{V}_A$ in an acclimatized animal can be restored to normal from an elevated level through surgical intervention, which eliminates suprapontine modulation (25, 34, 35). The *second* series of studies has already been alluded to, that is, findings that $\dot{V}_A$ acclimatization in ponies and goats is dependent on intact carotid chemoreceptors (14, 15). However, goats and ponies subjected to carotid body excision do hyperventilate when P_aO_2 is momentarily normalized after 2–4 days of hypoxia. Therefore, the postulate is that the two essential structures causing the hyperexcitability must be the carotid chemoreceptors and the suprapontine centers. In a normal individual sojourning at altitude, these structures provide for net facilitation, which in turn increases the respiratory center excitability. In an animal deprived of carotid bodies, suprapontine inhibition and facilitation both change during sojourn. In denervated goats, these changes coincide temporally so no acclimatization is observed. In denervated ponies, facilitation changes relatively more rapidly so that $\dot{V}_A$ is slightly above normal between 4 and 48 hours of hypoxia. However, after 48 hours the two influences have changed to the same extent so that $\dot{V}_A$ is not changed from chronic normoxia. If one restores P_aO_2 momentarily after this period of hypoxia, inhibition is rapidly alleviated while facilitation persists causing hyperventilation; thus, in both normal and denervated animals net facilitation causes $\dot{V}_A$ to be above chronic normoxic levels during the initial hours of the return to normoxia.

Although this schema of acclimatization is highly theoretical and essentially untested, all tenets (to the author's knowledge) are consistent with available findings. It, then, is unique in this respect among past and current theories; hence, it provides the best working hypothesis.

REFERENCES

1. Astrand, P.: The respiratory activity in man exposed to prolonged hypoxia. *Acta Physiol Scand, 30*:343, 1954.
2. Bureau, M. and Bouverot, P.: Blood and CSF acid-base changes and rate of ventilatory acclimatization of awake dogs to 3,550 m. *Respir Physiol, 24*:203, 1975.
3. Chiodi, H.: Respiratory adaptation to chronic high altitude hypoxia. *J Appl Physiol, 10*:81, 1957.
4. Dejours, P.; Kellogg, R.H.; and Pace, N.: Regulation of respiration and heart rate response in exercise during altitude acclimatization. *J Appl Physiol, 18*:10, 1963.
5. Dempsey, J.A.; Forster, H.V.; Birnbaum, M.L.; Reddan, W.G.; Thoden, J.; Grover, R.F.; and Rankin, J.: Control of exercise hyperpnea under varying durations of exposure to moderate hypoxia. *Respir Physiol, 16*:213, 1972.
6. Dempsey, J.A.; Forster, H.V.; and DePico, G.A.: Ventilatory acclimatization to moderate hypoxia in man: the role of spinal fluid [H+]. *J Clin Invest, 53*:1091, 1974.
7. Dempsey, J.A.; Forster, H.V.; Chosy, L.W.; Hanson, P.G.; and Reddan, W.G.: Regulation of CSF [HCO$_3^-$] during long-term hypoxic hypocapnia in man. *J Appl Physiol, 44*:175, 1978.
8. Dempsey, J.A.; Forster, H.V.; Bisgard, G.E.; Chosy, L.W.; and Hanson, P.G.: CSF [H+] as a function of changes in alveolar ventilation during

deacclimatization from chronic hypoxia. *Fed Proc, 37*:533, 1978.
9. Fencl, V.; Gabel, R.A.; and Wolfe, D.: Cerebral fluids in goats at high altitude (HA). *Fed Proc, 38*:5079, 1979.
10. Forster, H.V.; Dempsey, J.A.; Birnbaum, M.L.; Reddan, W.G.; Thoden, J.; Grover, R.F.; and Rankin, J.: Effects of chronic exposure to hypoxia on ventilatory response to CO_2 and hypoxia. *J Appl Physiol, 31*:586, 1971.
11. Forster, H.V.; Dempsey, J.A.; Vidruk, E.; and DoPico, G.: Evidence of altered regulation of ventilation during exposure to hypoxia. *Respir Physiol, 20*:379, 1974.
12. Forster, H.V.; Dempsey, J.A.; and Chosy, L.W.: Incomplete compensation of CSF [H^+] in man during acclimatization to high altitude (4300 m). *J Appl Physiol, 38*:1067, 1975.
13. Forster, H.V.; Soto R.J.; Dempsey, J.A.; and Hosko, M.J.: Effect of sojourn at 4300 m altitude on electroencephalogram and visual evoked response. *J Appl Physiol, 39*:109, 1975.
14. Forster, H.V.; Bisgard, G.E.; Rasmussen, B.; Orr, J.A.; Buss, D.D.; and Manohar, M.: Ventilatory control in peripheral chemoreceptor denervated ponies during chronic hypoxemia. *J Appl Physiol, 41*:878, 1976.
15. Forster, H.V.; Bisgard, G.E.; and Klein, J.P.: Ventilatory acclimatization during chronic hypoxia in goats: Role of carotic chemoreceptors. *Physiologist, 22*:39, 1979.
16. Kellogg, R.H.; Pace, N.; Archibald, E.R.; and Vaughan, B.E.: Respiratory response to inspired CO_2 during acclimatization to an altitude of 12,470. *J Appl Physiol, 11*:65, 1957.
17. Kellogg, R.H.: Effect of altitude on respiratory regulation. *Ann NY Acad Sci, 109*:815, 1963.
18. Kellogg, R.H.: The role of CO_2 in altitude acclimatization. In *The Regulation of Human Respiration,* edited by D.J.C. Cunningham and B.B. Loyd. Oxford, Blackwell, 1963.
19. Kellogg, R.H.: Oxygen and carbon dioxide in the regulation of respiration. *Fed Proc, 36*:1658, 1977.
20. Klausen, K.; Dill, D.B.; and Horvath, S.M.: Exercise at ambient and high oxygen pressure at high altitude and at sea level. *J Appl Physiol, 29*:456, 1970.
21. Lahiri, S.; Milledge, J.S.; Chattapadhyay, H.P.; Bhattacharyya, A.H.; and Sinha, A.K.: Respiration and heart rate of Sherpa highlanders during exercise. *J Appl Physiol, 23*:545, 1967.
22. Lahiri, S.: Acid-base in Sherpa altitude residents and lowlanders at 4,880 m. *Respir Physiol, 2*:323, 1967.
23. Michel, C.C. and Millege, J.S.: Respiratory regulation in man during acclimatization to high altitude. *J Physiol (Lond), 168*:631, 1963.
24. Orr, J.A.; Bisgard, G.E.; Forster, H.V.; Buss, D.D.; Dempsey, J.A.; and Will, J.A.: Cerebrospinal fluid alkalosis during high altitude sojourn in unanesthetized ponies. *Respir Physiol, 25*:23, 1975.
25. Ou, L.C.; St. John, W.M.; and Tenney, S.M.: The role of suprapontine structures in ventilatory acclimatization to hypoxia in cats. *Fed Proc, 37*:806, 1978.

26. Pugh, L.G.C.E.; Gill, M.B.; Lahiri, S.; Milledge, J.S.; Ward, M.P.; and West, J.B.: Muscular exercise at great altitudes. *J Appl Physiol, 19*:431, 1964.
27. Rahn, H. and Otis, A.: Man's respiratory response during and after acclimatization to high altitude. *Am J Physiol, 157*:445, 1949.
28. Reed, D.J. and Kellogg, R.H.: Effect of sleep on CO_2 stimulation of breathing in acute and chronic hypoxia. *J Appl Physiol, 15*:1135, 1960.
29. Reed, D.J. and Kellogg, R.H.: Effect of sleep on hypoxic stimulation of breathing at sea level and altitude. *J Appl Physiol, 15*:1130, 1960.
30. Schmeling, W.T.; Forster, H.V.; and Hosko, M.J.: Effect of sojourn at 3200 m altitude on spinal reflexes in young adult males. *Aviat Space Environ Med, 48*:1039, 1977.
31. Severinghaus, J.W.; Mitchell, R.A.; Richardson, B.W.; and Singer, M.M.: Respiratory control at high altitude suggesting active transport regulation of CSF pH. *J Appl Physiol, 18*:1155, 1963.
32. Severinghaus, J.W. and Crawford, R.D.: Carotid chemoreceptor role in CSF alkalosis at altitude. *Chest, 73 (Suppl)*:249, 1978.
33. Tenney, S.M.; Remmers, J.E.; and Mithoefer, J.C.: Interaction of CO_2 and hypoxic stimuli on ventilation at high altitude. *Q J Exp Physiol, 48*:192, 1963.
34. Tenney, S.M.; Scotio, P.; Ou, L.C.; Bartlett, D., Jr.; and Remmers, J.E.: Suprapontine influences on hypoxia ventilatory control. In *High Altitude Physiology: Cardiac and Respiratory Effects,* edited by R. Porter and J. Knight. Edinburgh and London, Churchill Livingstone, 1971.
35. Tenney, S.M. and Ou, L.C.: Hypoxic ventilatory response of cats at high altitude: An interpretation of "blunting." *Respir Physiol, 30*:185, 1977.
36. Weiskopf, R.B.; Gabel, R.A.; and Fencl, V.: Alkaline shift in lumbar and intracranial CSF in man after 5 days at high altitude. *J Appl Physiol, 41*:93, 1976.

Chapter 2

HYPERVENTILATION ACCOMPANYING PROLONGED STATIC CONTRACTION

M.T. SHARRATT AND M.A. BRUCE

INTRODUCTION

IT IS KNOWN that static exercise causes an increase in both systolic and diastolic blood pressure (12, 16, 23, 27). Contributing to this increase may be the influence of central nervous activity (10, 12, 21) or circulating hormones and metabolites such as catecholamines and lactic acid (13, 20). Another factor contributing to the blood pressure response is the reflex activity from exercising limbs (14, 26, 28).

Since Alam and Smirk (2) postulated a "powerful reflex originating from the ischemic working muscles," many studies have implicated the existence of a muscle receptor that responds to the accumulation of metabolic products in the working muscle. There are two lines of reasoning that support the suggestion of a muscle metabolic receptor. First, in animal and human experiments, blood pressure remains elevated throughout the postexercise period when occlusion is applied to the exercising limb (2, 26, 27, 37). Second, the injection of chemical agents in animals—for example, potassium and 2,4-dinitrophenol—simulates the blood pressure response to exercise (1, 22).

In addition to the cardiovascular responses, there is also an increase in ventilation accompanying static exercise. During the later stages of a fatiguing contraction, hyperventilation is observed (12, 30, 37). It appears unlikely that either central circulatory stimuli or central nervous activity could be major contributors to the hyperventilation (4, 22, 37). The potential involvement of a receptor in muscle that responds to the accumulation of metabolic products by increasing ventilation is controversial (22, 33, 37) and the focus of this study.

METHODS

Sixteen volunteer subjects, aged 20 to 24 years, from the University of Waterloo, were tested in this study. Eight subjects performed isometric arm contractions, sustained to exhaustion at approximately 10, 30, 50 and 70 percent of their maximum voluntary contraction (MVC). These exercise challenges are designated as levels one, two, three, and four in the following figures. The remaining subjects performed both arm and leg contractions at exercise level three, with and without occlusion of the exercising limb. In addition, these subjects performed an isometric arm contraction with occlusion of a nonexercising leg.

To perform an arm contraction, the subject was seated upright and secured by a belt around the hips. The upper arm was parallel to the body axis with an angle at the elbow as close as possible to 90 degrees. The forearm was in contact with a horizontal arm-rest at a fixed height. Angles at the shoulder and elbow were maintained constant between trials. In this position, the muscles of the shoulder, upper arm, and forearm worked in a coordinated fashion to hold weights above the ground using a simple pulley system. An assistant placed the padded grip in the subject's palm, thereby avoiding any extraneous muscle involvement. In addition, the ankles of the subject were draped over the rung of a chair in front of him to eliminate lower body activity. For a leg contraction, the subject was seated on a specially constructed bench with feet not touching the ground. Force was exerted forward at the ankle to maintain a bucket of weights off the ground using a two-wheel pulley system. Again, a 90 degree angle was maintained at the knee. No arm involvement was permitted. In all experiments, subjects were aware of the importance of continuing to work to exhaustion and were encouraged to do so throughout every trial.

Blood pressure was measured in the nonexercising arm by inflating the cuff with an automatic blood pressure unit, then determining systolic blood pressure (SBP) by auscultation. Only SBP was measured in this study to permit more frequent measurements than if diastolic had also been taken. Heart rate was monitored using a standard CM-5 lead placement connected to a Cambridge VS4. The subject breathed through a pneumotachograph (Hewlett-Packard, Model 47303A) and expired air was collected in 30 liter gas bags at specified intervals. Endtidal PCO_2 ($P_{ET}CO_2$) was monitored continuously from a Godart Capnograph (Type 17070) infrared analyser, calibrated frequently with known gas compositions. Percentage oxygen was determined using a Beckman E-2 Analyzer and percentage carbon dioxide using a Godart, Model KK, Capnograph.

Blood samples were taken from the antecubital vein of the right arm at rest and during exercise at level two. The exercise sample was taken after a marked decrease in $P_{ET}CO_2$ was noted. The subject continued to hold the weights while the sample was taken even though the arm was straightened (with assistance) during sampling. The venous blood samples were analyzed on a Radiometer BMS3 MK2-PHM71 blood microsystem for PCO_2 and pH. Bicarbonate concentrations were determined using the Severinghaus slide rule.

Two 4 by 4 latin square designs were employed in this experiment with the following dependent variables: systolic blood pressure, heart rate (HR), $P_{ET}CO_2$, minute ventilation, tidal volume, frequency of exercise, and duration of exercise. An analysis of covariance revealed whether an overall treatment difference existed for SBP, and analysis of variance was conducted for all other variables. Differences between treatment means were judged using the method of least significant difference.

RESULTS

Figure 2-1 shows the time course of SBP, HR, and $P_{ET}CO_2$ for one subject over the four different exercise levels. For example, the upper panel represents 10 percent and the lower panel 70 percent of maximal voluntary contraction to exhaustion. As noted, SBP gradually increased in all subjects throughout the period of isometric exercise for levels two, three, and four, reaching mean values of 163 mmHg, 174 mmHg, and 176 mmHg, respectively (the standard error was ±2.8 mmHg for this analysis). These values are significantly ($p < 0.05$) higher than the resting values of 114 mmHg, 116 mmHg, and 116 mmHg for each of the levels. At exercise level one, there was a small increase from 114 mmHg to 119 mmHg, and this was maintained throughout exercise. Exercise level one was terminated after 15 minutes since the subjects could have sustained the 10 percent MVC indefinitely. Duration of contraction for the other levels was 852 seconds at

TIME COURSE OF SYSTOLIC BLOOD PRESSURE, HEART RATE
AND END-TIDAL P_{CO_2} FOR ONE SUBJECT
AT VARIOUS EXERCISE LEVELS

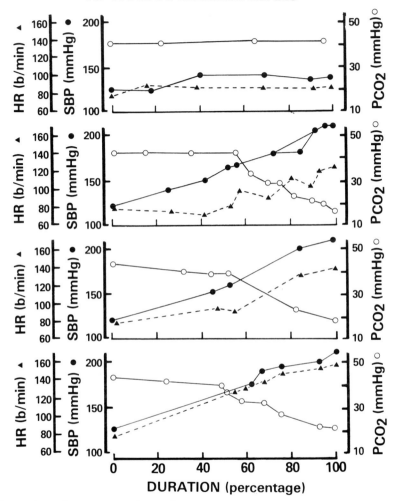

Figure 2-1. Time course of systolic blood pressure, heart rate, and end tidal P_{CO_2} for one subject at various exercise levels.

level two, 293 seconds at level three, and 167 seconds at level four. With the exception of level one, HR increased significantly ($p <$ 0.05) throughout the duration of exercise, reaching end points at 76, 106, 126, and 139 beats/min at each exercise level from one to four (SE $\pm$ 4.1 beats/min). The decreases in $P_{ET}CO_2$ started be-

SYSTOLIC BLOOD PRESSURE, HEART RATE AND END-TIDAL P_{CO_2} AT VARIOUS EXERCISE LEVELS

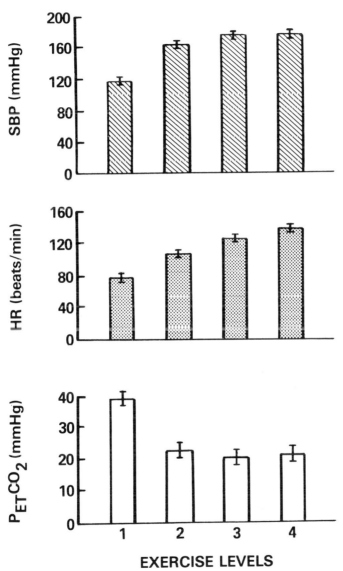

Figure 2-2. Systolic blood pressure, heart, rate, and end tidal P_{CO_2} at various exercise levels.

TABLE 2-I

VENTILATION, AT REST AND DURING EXERCISE

		Exercise Level			
		1	2	3	4
Minute Volume (LITERS/MIN)	REST	7.2 ± 1.1	9.0 ± 1.1	7.2 ± 1.1	9.0 ± 1.1
	EXERCISE	12.2 ± 5.2	36.0 ± 5.3	48.6 ± 5.2	40.7 ± 5.2
Tidal Volume (ML)	REST	434 ± 74	574 ± 74	452 ± 74	562 ± 74
	EXERCISE	445 ± 101	1179 ± 101	1467 ± 101	1239 ± 101
Frequency (BREATHS/MIN)	REST	16.5 ± 0.6	16.4 ± 0.6	15.6 ± 0.6	15.6 ± 0.6
	EXERCISE	16.4 ± 2.3	31.0 ± 2.3	34.2 ± 2.3	37.5 ± 2.3

tween 45 percent and 70 percent of the total duration of exercise and progressed until the exercise was terminated. The final $P_{ET}CO_2$ mean values of 22.5, 20.5, and 21.5 mmHg (SE ± 2.5 mmHg) at exercise levels two, three, and four were all significantly different from rest but not from each other. Thus, the observation of a similar $P_{ET}CO_2$ at exhaustion, regardless of contraction intensity, mimics the blood pressure response. It is noted in Figure 2-2 that heart rate does not follow the same pattern as SBP and $P_{ET}CO_2$ with increasing contraction intensity. Whereas SBP and $P_{ET}CO_2$ reach the same endpoint, regardless of contraction intensity, maximal heart rate appears to be proportional to exercise intensity, regardless of duration.

Although minute ventilation ($\dot{V}_E$) was almost unaffected by isometric exercise at 10 percent MVC to exhaustion, there were significant increases at every other level (Table 2-I). In fact, $\dot{V}_E$ increased about sixfold with sustained maximal voluntary contraction, and the increase seemed to be shared equally by twofold to threefold increases in tidal volume and frequency. In addition to $\dot{V}_E$, the time course of $\dot{V}CO_2$, $P_{ET}CO_2$, and the ratio $\dot{V}_E/\dot{V}CO_2$ is shown for level three in Figure 2-3. Oxygen uptake increased slightly and was maintained throughout the contraction. Although $\dot{V}_E$ and $\dot{V}CO_2$ increased throughout the duration of contraction, the ratio of $\dot{V}_E$ to $\dot{V}CO_2$ did not remain linear. For example, the ratio in the first half of the exercise was 31.5 and this increased to 50.7 at the end of exercise for this subject.

To test for the existence of a muscle metabolic receptor, occlusion studies were conducted in conjunction with the sustained maximum voluntary contraction protocol. Without occlusion at the end of exercise, SBP, HR, and $P_{ET}CO_2$ returned to near resting levels within 30 to 60 seconds. However, with occlusion of the exercising arm maintained at the end of exercise, blood pressure dropped transiently for 10–15 seconds but then remained significantly elevated at about 32 percent of the original exercise level until the occlusion was released (Fig. 2-4). When a similar protocol was used for the leg, the SBP remained elevated at 51 percent of the exercise level until the cuff was released. It is also apparent in Figure 2-4 that hyperventilation is maintained throughout occlusion since $P_{ET}CO_2$ does not change until the cuff is released. As demonstrated by an exercise test involving occlusion of the non-working leg, the presence of an occlusion cuff did not significantly

TIME COURSE OF $\dot{V}_E$, $\dot{V}CO_2$, $P_{ET}CO_2$ AND $\dot{V}_E/\dot{V}CO_2$
THROUGHOUT AN ARM CONTRACTION AT EXERCISE LEVEL 3

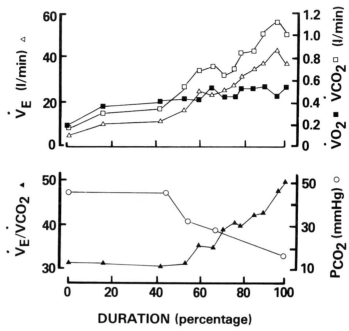

Figure 2-3. Time course of $\dot{V}_E$, $\dot{V}CO_2$, $P_{ET}CO_2$, and $\dot{V}_E/\dot{V}CO_2$ throughout an arm contraction at exercise level three.

affect the maximum SBP values attained for either arm or leg exercise. Similarly, the decreases in $P_{ET}CO_2$ at exhaustion were the same with or without the cuff. Similar maximum values were all reached even with shorter exercise duration to exhaustion with the limb occluded (Fig. 2-5); for example, the duration of arm exercise for the second group of subjects in level three was 328 seconds without occlusion and 193 seconds with occlusion ($p <$ 0.05). Previously, it was noted that the HR response to isometric exercise was different from the SBP and $P_{ET}CO_2$ response (i.e. HR is proportional to the intensity of exercise). In the occlusion studies, HR also responded differently from the other physiological variables. Whereas SBP and $P_{ET}CO_2$ remain altered in the post-exercise occlusion condition, HR tends to return toward resting levels even though the limb remains occluded.

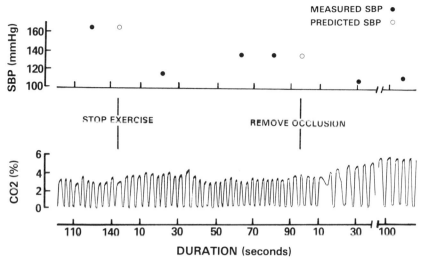

Figure 2-4. Time course of systolic blood pressure and end tital CO_2 for one subject performing an arm contraction at exercise level three with maintained occlusion.

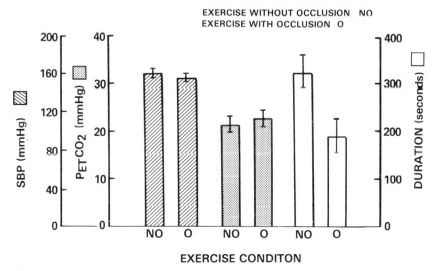

Figure 2-5. Systolic blood pressure, end tital PCO_2, and duration at exercise level three, arm exercise with and without occlusion.

DISCUSSION

The purpose of this study was to determine if there exists, in muscle, a receptor that would be activated by the accumulation of metabolic products and that would respond with an increase in both SBP and $\dot{V}_E$. In the past, studies have focused primarily on cardiovascular responses to isometric exercise and changes are well documented. In the present study, the gradual increase in SBP is consistent with previous data (5, 12, 16, 27). Also, the same maximal SBP was reached at exhaustion in levels three and four. The slightly lower maximal value for level two probably relates to the effect of blood sampling (with a temporary change in arm position) causing premature cessation of exercise. The correspondence of HR with degree of tension also confirms previous investigations, although the current values were slightly higher than expected (5, 11, 12).

This investigation also confirmed an increase in $\dot{V}_E$ during static exercise (12, 30, 37), leading to a hyperventilation in the later stages of contraction. Although the data of Wiley and Lind (37) are supported by the current findings for $P_{ET}CO_2$ and $\dot{V}_E$ values at various exercise levels, the results of Myre and Andersen (30) are not in agreement. Perhaps the sixfold increase in ventilation contributes to that discrepancy. Not only was the $\dot{V}_E$ higher than previously reported, but the duration of contraction was consistently longer than in other studies (12, 23, 30, 37). For every trial, the subject was given continuous verbal encouragement right to exhaustion. One implication of the observed hyperventilation is the dissociation of $\dot{V}_E$ and $\dot{V}CO_2$ (Fig. 2-3). Under conditions of dynamic exercise, Wasserman and his co-workers (35, 36) have reported a very positive relationship. If one assumes that the observed hyperventilation is not mediated by a hydrogen ion stimulus centrally (rather, in the muscle), then prolonged isometric exercise is one condition where the close $\dot{V}_E/\dot{V}CO_2$ relationship does not hold.

It is possible that the amount of blood flow through the muscle at each tension may be part of the mechanism to explain the commensurate rate changes for SBP and $P_{ET}CO_2$. Although blood flow tends to increase at progressively increasing tensions (16), this increase may be insufficient to meet local metabolic requirements. It is possible that the resulting accumulation of metabolites could activate a receptor within the muscle. Since SBP did not change substantially during level one, with no decrease in $P_{ET}CO_2$, it is reasonable to concur with Donald et al. (5) that blood flow was adequate for the metabolic demands of steady state work. However, with occlusion of the exercising limb, SBP and $P_{ET}CO_2$ not only reached the same end points, but these values were reached much sooner than was noted without occlusion. This observation implies that the same mechanism is involved and that onset of metabolite accumulation is potentiated by the rapid occlusion of blood flow. In support of the rate change, Coote et al. (4) have observed in anesthetized cats that occluding the arterial inflow to the exercising hindlimb increases both the magnitude and rate of rise of the pressor response.

The strongest evidence for a muscle metabolic receptor relates to the occlusion studies. Without occlusion, cardiovascular and respiratory values return to preexercise levels within 60 seconds (12, 30, 37). With occlusion, and subsequent accumulation of metabolic by-products, the cardiovascular and respiratory responses continue at elevated levels (Fig. 2-4). It has been suggested (Sargeant, 1978, personal communication) that the mechanical effect of cuffing alone can cause hyperventilation. However, the intensity of cuffing in Sargeant's study probably stimulated Group IV afferents with nociceptive properties (19) and would contribute to the hyperventilation. In the present investigation, a nonworking leg was occluded while the subject performed an arm contraction. Ventilation returned to preexercise values following contraction, whether the leg was cuffed or not.

In dynamic exercise, it has been shown that $P_{ET}CO_2$ did not decrease from normal values, even when the occlusion was maintained for 30 seconds of exercise (33). In that kind of dynamic work, with continual flushing of metabolites until occlusion, it may be that the combination of cuffing duration and intensity of exercise was inadequate to stimulate $\dot{V}_E$ by the proposed metabolic receptor. However, the results of another dynamic exercise study involving hypoxia (6) lead the authors to confirm the presence of "receptors in working muscle," sensitized by muscular hypoxia.

Heart rate returned to preexercise values following contraction, even when the occlusion cuff was on the working arm. This result is consistent with data of Wiley and Lind (37), Donald et al. (5), and McCloskey and Streatfield (27). It would appear that different mechanisms are responsible for sustained changes in SBP and HR. Further evidence of this separation of mechanisms is provided in a study on a patient with unilateral syringomyelia (24).

Before accepting the concept of a metabolic muscle receptor exclusively, one should also consider the involvement of central factors in voluntary effort. In fact, the difference between SBP and $P_{ET}CO_2$ during contraction and the levels that remained during occlusion may be attributable to central influence, as noted for SBP by McCloskey and Streatfield (27). Pain is another confounding factor and does involve a central component. However, subjects in this study reported discomfort and none complained of inordinate pain, even with occlusion. The most convincing evidence against a major role for central involvement is that SBP and $\dot{V}_E$ have been observed to increase when exercise was induced in anesthetized and decerebrate animals (4, 22, 34).

Another consideration is the involvement of metabolites in the general circulation. Base excess changes were minimal (<1 mEq/l) and do not reflect a challenge to the peripheral or central chemoreceptors. Also, circulating metabolites generally cannot be responsible for the increase in SBP or hyperventilation because the responses were noted with and without occlusion of the exercising limb. On the other hand, any decrease in base excess in venous blood during exercise does imply an elevated acidity of the muscle. In this study, a threefold increase in lactic acid was noted in the venous effluent of the working muscle, most likely reflecting a much higher level in the muscle itself (17). Consequently, the hyperventilation of static exercise may be the result of a hydrogen ion concentration operating locally. This suggestion does not exclude other metabolites that would be available to the receptor. For example, phosphate, potassium (14), or ATP (8) could be functional, and even osmolality changes cannot be dismissed as a possible "trigger" for the receptor.

If it can be assumed that a muscle metabolic receptor exists, is it necessary to postulate a new receptor, or could the observed changes in SBP and ventilation be triggered by an exaggerated response to an already existing receptor? The evidence against the primary endings of muscle spindles and golgi tendon organs appears convincing (15, 26). Rodgers (32) has suggested that secondary endings of muscle spindles may be implicated in respiratory responses, and Matthews (25) has shown that stretching spindles provoked a response in afferent fibers that was stronger in ischemic muscles than normally perfused muscles. However, a more recent study employing cold block opposed involvement of Group II afferents (34). In addition, the encapsulation of the muscle spindle might be expected to protect the endings from the local muscle environment. Group III afferents have been proposed to contribute to the SBP and ventilatory response (13, 26), but the response is not associated with muscle ischemia (31). Also, Saltin (1978, personal communication) tends to dismiss these afferents because of their primary square wave response to mechanoreceptor stimuli. One is left, almost by default, with the Group IV free nerve endings. Kalia, Senapati, Parida, and Panda (18) showed that they could still be activated after maximal stimulation of the muscle. Tibes (34) acknowledged the involvement of Group IV fibers in reflex cardiorespiratory responses, and Kniffki, Mense and Schmidt (19) identified "ergoceptive" properties of Group IV afferents responsive to chemical substances in the muscle. Thus, the sensitivity of Group IV afferent units to metabolites is well known (7, 9, 19, 29), but their role in exercise hyperpnea and hyperventilation has not yet been verified.

In conclusion, hyperventilation has been consistently demonstrated in the later stages of static voluntary contractions ($\geq 30\%$ MVC) to exhaustion. The maximal response is similar to the systolic blood pressure response; that is, a similar $P_{ET}CO_2$ is reached, regardless of the intensity of exercise. It is hypothesized that the increase in ventilation is directly related to the stimulation of a local muscle metabolic receptor. Specifically, the ventilatory response seems to be a function of the metabolic stimulation of Group IV unmyelinated free nerve endings.

REFERENCES

1. Achar, M.V.S.: Effects of injection of Locke solution with higher concentrations of potassium into the femoral artery on blood pressure in cats. *J Physiol, 198*:115, 1968.
2. Alam, M. and Smirk, F.H.: Observations in man upon a blood pressure raising reflex arising from the voluntary muscles. *J Physiol, 89*:372, 1937.
3. Berne, R.M. and Levy, M.N.: *Cardiovascular Physiology.* St. Louis, Mosby, 1977.
4. Coote, J.H.; Hilton, S.M.; and Perez-Gonzalez, J.F.: The reflex nature of the pressor response to muscular exercise. *J Physiol, 215*:789, 1971.
5. Donald, K.W.; Lind, A.R.; McNicol, G.W.; Humphreys, P.W.; Taylor, S.H.;

and Staunton, H.P.: Cardiorespiratory responses to sustained (static) contractions. *Circ Res, 20-21 Suppl. 1*:15, 1967.

6. Flenley, D.C.; Brash, H.; Clancy, L.; Cooke, N.J.; Leitch, A.G.; Middleton, W.; and Wraith, P.K.: Ventilatory response to steady-state exercise in hypoxia in humans. *J Appl Physiol, 46*:438, 1979.

7. Fock, S. and Mense, S.: Excitatory effects of 5-hydroxytryptamine, histamine and potassium ions on muscular group IV afferent units: a comparison with bradykinin. *Brain Res, 105*:459, 1976.

8. Forrester, T.: An estimate of adenosine triphosphate release unto venous effluent from exercising human forearm muscle. *J Physiol, 224*:611, 1972.

9. Franz, M. and Mense, S.: Muscle receptors with Group IV afferent fibers responding to application of bradykinin. *Brain Res, 92*:369, 1975.

10. Freyschuss, U.: Cardiovascular adjustment to somatomotor activation. *Acta Physiol Scand [Suppl], 432*:1, 1970.

11. Funderburk, C.F.; Hipskind, S.G.; Welton, R.C.; and Lind, A.R.: Development and recovery from fatigue induced by static effort at various tensions. *J Appl Physiol, 37*:392, 1974.

12. Goodwin, G.M.; McCloskey, D.I.; and Mitchell, J.H.: Cardiovascular and respiratory responses to changes in central command during isometric exercise at constant muscle tension. *J Physiol, 226*:173, 1972.

13. Huik, P.; Hudlicka, O.; Kucera, I.; and Payne, R.: Activation of muscle afferents by non-proprioceptive stimuli. *Am J Physiol, 217*:1451, 1969.

14. Haddy, F.J. and Scott, J.B.: Metabolic factors in peripheral circulatory regulation. *Fed Proc, 34*:2006, 1975.

15. Hodgson, H.J.F. and Matthews, P.B.C.: The ineffectiveness of excitation of the primary nerve endings of the muscle spindle by vibration as a respiratory stimulant in the decerebrate cat. *J Physiol, 194*:555, 1968.

16. Humphreys, P.W. and Lind, A.R.: The bloodflow through active and inactive muscles of the forearm during sustained handgrip contractions. *J Physiol, 166*:120, 1963.

17. Jorfeldt, L.; Juhlin-Dannfelt, A.; and Karlsson, J.: Lactate release in relation to tissue lactate in human skeletal muscle during exercise. *J Appl Physiol, 44*:350, 1978.

18. Kalia, M.; Senapati, J.M.; Parida, B.; and Panda, A.: Reflex increase in ventilation by muscle receptors with non-medullated fibers (C fibers). *J Appl Physiol, 32*:189, 1972.

19. Kniffki, K.-D.; Mense, S.; and Schmidt, R.F.: Responses of Group IV afferent units from skeletal muscle to stretch, contraction and chemical stimulation. *Exp Brain Res, 31*:511, 1978.

20. Kozlowski, S.; Brzezinska, Z.; Nazar, K.; Kowalski, W.; and Franczyk, M.: Plasma catecholamines during sustained isometric exercise. *Clin Sci Mol Med, 45*:723, 1973.

21. Krogh, A. and Lindhard, J.: The regulation of respiration and circulation during the initial stages of muscular work. *J Physiol, 47*:112, 1913.

22. Liang, C. and Hood, W.B.: Afferent nerve pathways in the regulation of

cardiopulmonary responses to tissue hypermetabolism. *Circ Res, 38*:209, 1976.

23. Lind, A.R.: Cardiovascular responses to static exercise (Isometrics anyone?) *Circulation, 41*:173, 1970.

24. Lind, A.R.; McNicol, G.W.; Bruce, R.A.; Macdonald, H.R.; and Donald, K.W.: The cardiovascular responses to sustained contractions of a patient with unilateral syringomyelia. *Clin Sci Mol Med, 35*:45, 1968.

25. Matthews, B.H.C.: Nerve endings in mammalian muscle. *J Physiol, 78*:1, 1933.

26. McCloskey, D.I. and Mitchell, J.H.: Reflex cardiovascular and respiratory responses originating in exercising muscle. *J Physiol, 224*:173, 1972.

27. McCloskey, D.I. and Streatfield, K.A.: Muscular reflex stimuli to the cardiovascular system during isometric contractions of muscle groups of different mass. *J Physiol, 250*:431, 1975.

28. Mitchell, J.H.; Reardon, W.C.; and McCloskey, D.I.: Reflex effects on circulation and respiration from contracting skeletal muscle. *Am J Physiol, 233*:H374, 1977.

29. Mizumura, K. and Kumazawa, T.: Reflex respiratory response induced by chemical stimulation of muscle afferents. *Brain Res, 109*:402, 1976.

30. Myre, K. and Lange-Andersen, K.: Respiratory responses to static muscular work. *Respir Physiol, 12*:77, 1971.

31. Paintal, A.S.: Functional analysis of Group III afferent fibers of mammalian muscles. *J Physiol, 152*:250, 1960.

32. Rodgers, S.H.: Ventilatory response to ventral root stimulation in the decerebrate cat. *Respir Physiol, 5*:165, 1968.

33. Rowell, L.B.; Hermansen, L.; and Blackman, J.R.: Human cardiovascular and respiratory responses to graded muscle ischaemia. *J Appl Physiol, 41*:693, 1976.

34. Tibes, U.: Reflex inputs to the cardiovascular and respiratory centers from dynamically working canine muscles. Some evidence for involvement of Group III or IV nerve fibers. *Circ Res, 41(3)*:332, 1977.

35. Wasserman, K.; Whipp, B.J.; Casaburi, R.; and Beaver, W.L.: Carbon dioxide flow and exercise hyperpnea. Cause and effect. *Am Rev Respir Dis, 115*:225, 1977.

36. Wasserman, K.; Whipp, B.J.; Casaburi, R.; Beaver, W.L.; and Brown, H.V.: CO_2 flow to the lungs and ventilatory control. In *Muscular Exercise and the Lung,* edited by J.A. Dempsey and C.E. Reed. Madison, Wis, U of Wis Pr, 1977.

37. Wiley, R.L. and Lind, A.R.: Respiratory responses to sustained static muscular contractions in humans. *Clin Sci Mol Med, 40*:221, 1971.

Chapter 3

ADAPTATION TO EXERCISE IN CHILDREN WITH CYSTIC FIBROSIS*

F.J. Cerny, T. Pullano**, and G.J.A. Cropp

A COMMON complaint of children with cystic fibrosis is a feeling of shortness of breath during exercise. This may lead to decreased activity and subsequent isolation from normal peer contact. The recognition of the general health benefits from regular exercise has led to an increase in the prescription of such exercise in many patients, including children with cystic fibrosis. For these children such a program can contribute not only to physical health but also to an increased ability to lead a more normal life-style and an improved self-image.

In efforts to determine proper exercise prescription for children with cystic fibrosis, the authors felt it was important to study first the cardiopulmonary response to exercise in groups of patients with different degrees of lung involvement. This chapter deals with the results of these studies and discusses the implications for exercise prescription in children with cystic fibrosis.

SUBJECTS

Twenty-one children with varying severity of cystic fibrosis and 17 children with no evidence of lung disease or exercise-induced bronchospasm and normal pulmonary functions were studied. Informed consent was obtained from all subjects and parents. To control for potential differences in size, subjects were matched for age, height, and weight (Table 3-I).

Classification of severity of pulmonary involvement was determined on the basis of a score derived from several pulmonary function tests. The criteria used were vital capacity (VC), forced

*Supported by NIH grant 1 RO1 AM 24066-01.
**Supported in part by March of Dimes and CF Foundation and H. Gioia CF Foundation.

TABLE 3-I
SUBJECT POPULATION

Subjects	N	Age (years)	Weight (kg)	Height (cm)
Normals	17	15.0 ± 1.2	52.1 ± 3.8	157.9 ± 2.7
CF Patients	21	15.0 ± 1.0	44.4 ± 3.4	155.2 ± 3.6

Measurements are means ± SE

expired volume in one second (FEV_1), forced expiratory flow between 25 and 75 percent of VC ($FEF_{25-75\%}$), residual volume (RV), specific airway conductance (SG_{aw} = reciprocal of airway resistance divided by lung volume), and arterial oxygen saturation (S_aO_2) as measured by ear oximetry. The maximum (worst) score for any one test was 3, thus making it possible for a patient with extremely severe disease to achieve a total score of 18. A score of <3 was considered to be normal, 3–7 as mild, 8–12 as moderate, and >12 as severe pulmonary disease. This total score correlated highly ($r = 0.91$) with the Taussig score (3), which is based on x-ray, symptoms, attitude, nutritional status, clubbing, growth rates, pulmonary functions, hospitalizations, and sputum production. We also found that the FVC, FEV_1, and $FEF_{25-75\%}$ tests correlated well ($r = .80$, 0.85, and 0.81 respectively), which would allow reasonable classification of patients with only one spirometric test (Table 3-II).

METHODS

A progressive, graded exercise test was performed on the cycle ergometer. The initial load was 0.27 (± 0.03 SE) watts/kg body weight and it was increased by 0.25 ($\pm.01$) and 0.32 ($\pm.002$) watts/kg every two minutes in the patients and normals respectively. Exercise was stopped when the subject requested it or when physiological indices such as electrocardiogram (ECG), blood pressure, or S_aO_2 indicated inappropriate adaptation to the increase in work load. This was not a maximum oxygen uptake test, but subjects were encouraged to work as hard as they were able.

During exercise, ECG, blood pressure, S_aO_2, end tidal and mixed expired O_2 and CO_2, and expired volume were monitored at each work load, using an arrangement as shown in Figure 3-1. From the expired gas concentrations and minute ventilation, oxygen consumption was calculated. Results were analyzed for significant differences using multivariate analysis (2) with a Scheffé post hoc test. To avoid comparisons with extrapolated data,

TABLE 3-II

PREEXERCISE PULMONARY FUNCTIONS IN STUDY POPULATION

Test	Normal Subjects Group 1 (n = 17)		Normal Group 2 (n = 4)			Cystic Fibrosis Patients								
						Mild Group 3 (n = 6)			Moderate Group 4 (n = 5)			Severe Group 5 (n = 6)		
	$\bar{X}$	±SE	$\bar{X}$	±SE	Diff.†	$\bar{X}$	±SE	Diff.†	$\bar{X}$	±SE	Diff.†	$\bar{X}$	±SE	Diff.†
PF Score	0.6	0.15	0.5	0.29	n.s.	5.5	0.34	$p < 0.01$	10.4	0.60	$p < 0.01$	14.8	0.54	$p < 0.01$
VC*	105	3.3	121	12.9	n.s.	96	4.4	n.s.	78	10.7	n.s.	57	5.1	$p < 0.01$
FEV_1*	97	3.4	109	8.2	n.s.	80	5.0	n.s.	52	6.3	$p < 0.01$	32	5.0	$p < 0.01$
FEF (25-75%)*	96	5.7	99	3.8	n.s.	50	2.6	$p < 0.01$	29	7.4	$p < 0.01$	13	3.7	$p < 0.01$
RV*	121	6.8	112	25.7	n.s.	196	31.5	n.s.	294	28.2	$p < 0.01$	442	54.9	$p < 0.01$

*% predicted value

†Diff. indicates statistical difference from normal subjects

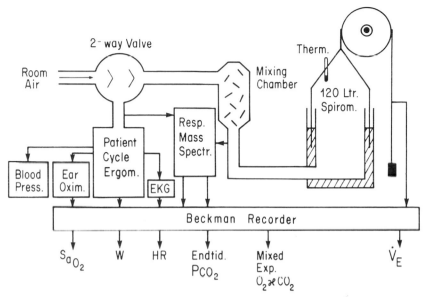

Figure 3-1. Schematic of system used for data collection.

groups were compared only as far as the mean peak work load for any group would allow. Minimum level of significance was at the $p < 0.05$ level.

RESULTS

The peak work load in normal subjects and patients with cystic fibrosis with normal pulmonary function tests was 2.9 watts/kg ($\pm$ .10 and .21 SE respectively). Although the patients with mild and moderate disease had lower peak work loads (2.7 $\pm$ 0.14 and 2.5 $\pm$ 0.28 respectively), these peak loads were not statistically different from those achieved by normal subjects. The group with severe disease had a peak work capacity of 1.4 $\pm$ 0.28, which was significantly lower than that in normals ($p < 0.01$).

The results of the cardiopulmonary adjustments during progressively increasing work loads are summarized in Table 3-III. Patients with cystic fibrosis tended to ventilate more than normal subjects at all work loads greater than 0.2 watts/kg until peak work loads were approached. In spite of the increased minute ventilation, the most severely diseased group of patients had alveolar hypoventilation, as is indicated by an increasing end tidal CO_2. This hypoventilation is also shown by progressive arterial desat-

TABLE 3-III
CARDIOPULMONARY RESPONSE TO EXERCISE†

Parameter	Group*	Load (watts/kg)				
		0.2	0.8	1.4	2.0	2.6
$\dot{V}_E$/Kg (l/min·kg⁻¹)	1	0.38 ± 0.04	0.51 ± 0.03	0.73 ± 0.04	0.99 ± 0.05	1.34 ± 0.06
	2	0.51 ± 0.08	0.64 ± 0.05	0.94 ± 0.07‡	1.20 ± 0.05‡	1.53 ± 0.07
	3	0.47 ± 0.03	0.70 ± 0.04‡	0.92 ± 0.05‡	1.27 ± 0.09‡	1.48 ± 0.08
	4	0.55 ± 0.13	0.69 ± 0.08‡	1.05 ± 0.10‡	1.47 ± 0.10‡	—
	5	0.48 ± 0.07	0.72 ± 0.08‡	1.16 ± 0.10‡	—	—
P_ECO_2 (mmHg)	1	36.5 ± 1.31	38.2 ± 1.32	39.6 ± 1.15	39.2 ± 1.22	36.0 ± 1.21
	2	37.7 ± 2.02	36.8 ± 3.74	37.7 ± 2.57	37.0 ± 2.72	36.7 ± 1.33
	3	36.0 ± 1.99	38.1 ± 1.23	35.9 ± 1.96	35.7 ± 1.32	35.8 ± 1.46
	4	36.6 ± 1.33	38.2 ± 1.24	37.7 ± 2.46	35.8 ± 1.53	—
	5	37.5 ± 1.74	43.2 ± 2.36‡	44.2 ± 2.42‡	—	—
S_aO_2 (%)	1	96.3 ± 0.26	96.2 ± 0.22	96.2 ± 0.25	96.1 ± 0.25	96.0 ± 0.24
	2	96.7 ± 0.88	96.7 ± 0.77	96.8 ± 0.76	97.2 ± 0.71	97.4 ± 0.72
	3	95.5 ± 0.56	95.5 ± 0.55	95.6 ± 0.56	95.7 ± 0.54	95.9 ± 0.57
	4	95.5 ± 0.65	95.4 ± 0.62	95.2 ± 0.62	95.1 ± 0.61	—
	5	91.0 ± 1.34‡	88.3 ± 1.42‡	83.3 ± 1.83‡	—	—
Heart Rate (per min)	1	102 ± 3.60	121 ± 4.00	141 ± 3.60	164 ± 3.50	183 ± 3.50
	2	101 ± 9.70	114 ± 6.10	139 ± 4.30	160 ± 4.80	182 ± 3.90
	3	100 ± 2.90	114 ± 2.40	134 ± 2.90	160 ± 5.00	175 ± 3.60
	4	110 ± 4.40	123 ± 4.80	146 ± 7.20	171 ± 6.10	—
	5	122 ± 3.10‡	142 ± 3.90‡	165 ± 13.00‡	—	—

*Groups as identified in Table 3-II
†mean ± SE
‡statistically different from normal

uration during exercise, with a decrease of over 14 percent in one patient.

In an apparent attempt to compensate for the decreased arterial oxygen delivery, the patients with severe disease had higher heart rates than normal subjects, and mild or moderate cystic fibrosis patients at any given work load. Peak heart rates (162 ± 9.5) were, however, significantly lower ($p < 0.05$), suggesting that exercise limitations in severe cystic fibrosis patients is not cardiovascular in origin.

DISCUSSION

These results confirm and extend the results reported by Godfrey and Mearns (1). The present authors also found higher steady state ventilation in cystic fibrosis patients. They measured increases in physiological dead space of from 125 to over 300 percent in these patients. The increase in minute ventilation is apparently adequate to compensate for wasted dead space ventilation and to maintain alveolar ventilation in all patients except those with advanced disease; in this group significant arterial desaturation and CO_2 retention occurred at work loads in excess of 0.8 watts/kg.

Both in-hospital and home exercise programs are prescribed for patients of the authors with cystic fibrosis. Before prescribing an exercise program, all patients are tested at several light to moderate work loads, while monitoring their S_aO_2 and end tidal CO_2 concentration. On the basis of the results so obtained, the possibility of potentially undesirable adaptation to exercise in unsupervised situations is avoided.

The results of this study enable us to provide exercise prescriptions to patients with cystic fibrosis with some level of confidence. A few simple pulmonary function tests and objective scoring of the patients are essential for the prescriptions. Caution is recommended in exercising patients with disease severe enough to result in a pulmonary function score of 10 or greater. Patients with disease sufficient to give rise to a score of >10 may hypoventilate during mild to moderate work loads at heart rates of 120 beats per minute. If only spirometric tests are available, a patient with FEV_1 <50 percent and/or $FEF_{25-75\%}$ <30 percent of predicted should be exercise-tested under close supervision before any exercise program is prescribed.

REFERENCES

1. Godfrey, S. and Mearns, M.: Pulmonary function and response to exercise in cystic fibrosis. *Arch Dis Child, 46*:144, 1971.
2. International Educational Services, Chicago, Illinois.
3. Taussig, L.M.; Kattwinkel, J.; Friedewald, W.T.; and diSant 'Agnese, P.A.: A new prognostic score and clinical evaluation system for cystic fibrosis. *J Pediatr, 82*:380, 1973.

Chapter 4

CHANGES IN SOMATOTYPIC AND CARDIOPULMONARY FACTORS OVER PUBERTY IN ELITE AGE-GROUP FIGURE SKATERS*

W.G. WEAVER AND J.M. THOMSON

THE PRESENT study is part of a longitudinal investigation into the physical and physiological characteristics of elite Canadian figure skaters. While there is a growing volume of data on the effects of exercise on children and adolescents (1, 4, 6, 9, 10, 21), only limited findings have been reported relating the various aspects of growth to specific sports training (9, 17, 25, 27). The longitudinal investigation was undertaken in order to develop a profile on the elite figure skaters, examining aspects of their growth and training; this presentation is limited to a comparison of skaters' physical growth in relation to their pulmonary function and exercise data, pre- to postpuberty.

The beneficial effects of physical activity on pulmonary development have been examined over the growth years, studying pre- and postpubertal children of both sexes (1, 2, 11, 17, 20, 22). Generally, it has been found that endurance training, both running (6, 13, 28) and swimming (27), does not precipitate changes in lung volumes nor pulmonary function in excess of normal, growth-related improvements. However, several investigations (1, 2, 11, 22) have reported improved pulmonary dimensions in elite swimmers, noting superior pulmonary function and exceptionally high diffusing capacities in these trained athletes.

METHODOLOGY

Twenty-seven figure skaters, aged 12 to 19 years, were divided cross-sectionally into 4 subject groups: male and female skaters

*Supported by H. & W. Canada, Fitness & Amateur Sport Directorate; Proj. No. 76-50.

into both pre- and postpubertal groupings. All skaters had trained from 6 to 13 years and were sectional or provincial champions; as well, a few skaters were Canadian Champions and three had competed in World and Olympic competitions. Anthropometric data, somatotype rating (18), and body fat determinations (31) were made on each subject; pubertal status was determined by means of hormonal assay (29, 30). Pulmonary function data included total lung capacity, determined by the helium-dilution method (17), and the standard forced vital capacity maneuver. Exercise data was determined by means of a discontinuous bicycle ergometer test with skaters performing 3 or 4 workloads, each of 5 minutes duration, at mild, then moderate, then maximal/ supramaximal intensity; Oxygen (O_2) consumption was determined by open-circuit spirometry and cardiac output (Q_c) by the steady state, nitrous oxide method (5).

RESULTS AND DISCUSSION
Physical Characteristics

The age of the prepubertal skaters was 14.3 ± 0.8 years for males and 13.1 ± 1.2 years for females, while the ages of the pubertal groups were 16.9 ± 1.4 and 15.4 ± 1.9 years respectively (see Table 4-IA). It was estimated that both males and females reached puberty 1.0 to 1.5 years later than the general age-group population (16, 23, 26) and that both pre- and postpubertal skaters were smaller and lighter (23, 24).

A comparison of both male and female skaters pre- to postpuberty showed little change in their body fat or somatotype (see Table 4-IB). Both groups possessed low body fat (15, 31) with males being 7.1 ± 0.7% prepuberty and 6.9 ± 0.5% postpuberty and the female groups 7.7 ± 0.7% and 7.3 ± 0.6% respectively. Similarly, through puberty, their somatotypes changed very little; both males and females gained in endomorphy and mesomorphy while decreasing slightly in ectomorphy (see Table 4-IB and Figure 4-1).

Pulmonary Function

In Table 4-II, the pulmonary function data for the 4 subject groups are presented; in Figures 4-2 to 4-5, their individual data are compared to normative values [i.e. predictions based upon age and size (20, 22)].

TABLE 4-I
PHYSICAL CHARACTERISTICS OF ELITE FIGURE SKATERS,
PRE- AND POSTPUBERTY*
(Mean ± 1 Standard Deviation)

A.	AGE (yrs)	HEIGHT (cm)	WEIGHT (kg)	BODY SURFACE AREA (m^2)
Males				
Prepubertal	14.3	154.9	42.3	1.4
(n = 4)	±0.8	±6.3	±1.3	±0.1
Pubertal	16.9	172.9	62.4	1.7
(n = 9)	±1.4	±4.4	±4.8	±0.1
Females				
Prepubertal	13.1	147.9	39.0	1.3
(n = 6)	±1.2	±9.6	±7.3	±0.2
Pubertal	15.4	158.5	51.2	1.5
(n = 8)	±1.9	±5.1	±5.6	±0.1

| B. | BODY FAT (%) | HEATH-CARTER SOMATOTYPE | | |
		ENDOMORPHY	MESOMORPHY	ECTOMORPHY
Males				
Prepubertal	7.1	1.4	3.4	3.8
(n = 4)	±0.7	±0.5	±0.8	±1.0
Pubertal	6.9	1.5	3.6	3.3
(n = 9)	±0.5	±0.4	±0.5	±0.6
Females				
Prepubertal	7.7	1.8	2.8	3.3
(n = 6)	±0.7	±0.5	±0.9	±1.0
Pubertal	7.3	9.4	3.4	2.8
(n = 8)	±0.6	±0.4	±0.6	±0.6

*In Table 4-IA, the age, height, weight and body surface area of the pubertal subjects (both male and female) are significantly ($p < .05$) greater when compared to the prepubertal subjects; in Table 4-IB, there are no significant differences between prepubertal and pubertal subjects.

MALE SKATERS: As shown in Table 4-II, pubertal males were superior (significant at the .05 level) to their prepubertal counterparts on all pulmonary function tests. This improvement appeared to be a function of both their accelerated growth as well as their training. For example, total lung capacity (TLC) of prepubertal males was 3.7 ± 0.6 liters with individual values closely approximating predicted; however, TLC for pubertal male skaters was 6.8 ± 0.7 liters and all individual values were greater than predicted (see Fig. 4-2). A similar trend of improved pulmonary function, relative to normative values pre- to postpuberty, was also found for functional residual capacity (FRC), vital capacity (VC), and forced expiratory volume (FEV$_{1.0}$). For prepubertal males, FRC ($\bar{x}$ = 1.7 ± 0.3 liters) values closely approximated predicted

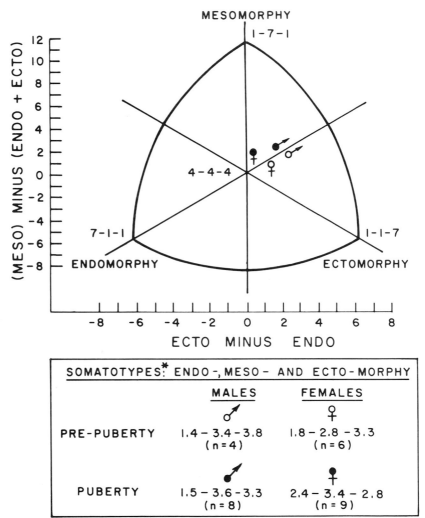

Figure 4-1. Somatotypes (see lower insert) of elite male and female figure skaters prepuberty (open circles) and postpuberty (solid circles) plotted on the Heath-Carter Somatochart (18).

TABLE 4-II
PULMONARY FUNCTION OF ELITE FIGURE SKATERS, PRE- AND POSTPUBERTY
(Mean ± 1 Standard Deviation)

SUBJECTS	TOTAL LUNG CAPACITY (liters)	VITAL CAPACITY (liters)	RESIDUAL VOLUME (liters)	INSPIRATORY CAPACITY (liters)	FUNCTIONAL RESIDUAL CAPACITY (liters)	FORCED EXPIRATORY VOLUME (1.0) (liters)	$FEV_{1.0}/VC$ (%)
Males							
Prepubertal (n = 4)	3.7 ±0.6	3.0 ±0.2	0.7 ±0.4	2.0 ±0.3	1.7 ±0.3	2.5 ±0.3	81.2 ±3.5
Pubertal (n = 7)	6.8* ±0.4	4.8* ±0.4	2.0* ±0.3	3.3* ±0.5	3.5* ±0.3	4.1* ±0.5	86.2 ±7.4
Females							
Prepubertal (n = 5)	3.8 ±0.9	2.5 ±0.5	1.3 ±0.6	1.7 ±0.3	2.1 ±0.8	2.3 ±0.5	92.1 ±3.8
Pubertal (n = 6)	4.8 ±0.7	3.2 ±0.4	1.6 ±0.5	2.1 ±0.3	2.7 ±0.6	2.7 ±0.2	86.4 ±5.7

*Pulmonary function of pubertal subjects significantly ($p < .05$) greater than prepubertal subjects.

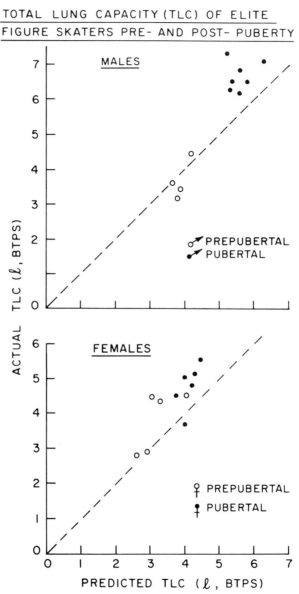

Figure 4-2. Individual values for TLC of elite male (upper portion) and female (lower portion) figure skaters prepuberty (open circles) and postpuberty (solid circles) plotted against individual predicted TLC (20) for each athlete.

FUNCTIONAL RESIDUAL CAPACITY (FRC) OF ELITE
FIGURE SKATERS PRE- AND POST- PUBERTY

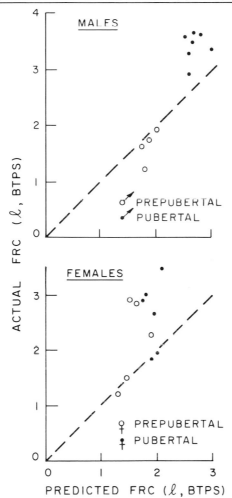

Figure 4-3. Individual values for FRC of elite male (upper portion) and female (lower portion) figure skaters prepuberty (open circles) and postpuberty (solid circles) plotted against individual predicted FRC (20) for each athlete.

while FRC values of the pubertal group ($\bar{x}$ = 3.5 ± 0.3 liters) were all greater than predicted (see Fig. 4-3). On the other hand, individual data for VC and $FEV_{1.0}$ of prepubertal males (3.0 ± 0.2 and 2.5 ± 0.3 liters, respectively) were all lower than predicted while values for their pubertal counterparts (4.8 ± 0.4 and 4.1 ± 0.5

liters, respectively) closely approximated predicted values (see Figs. 4-4 and 4-5).

FEMALE SKATERS: In contrast to the male skaters, the females tended to show only the normal, growth-related increases in pulmonary function (20, 22), comparing pre- to postpubertal data

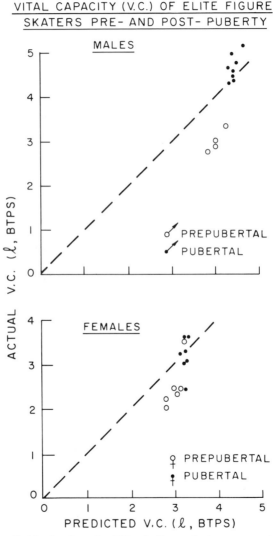

Figure 4-4. Individual values for VC of elite male (upper portion) and female (lower portion) figure skaters prepuberty (open circles) and postpuberty (solid circles) plotted against individual predicted VC (20) for each athlete.

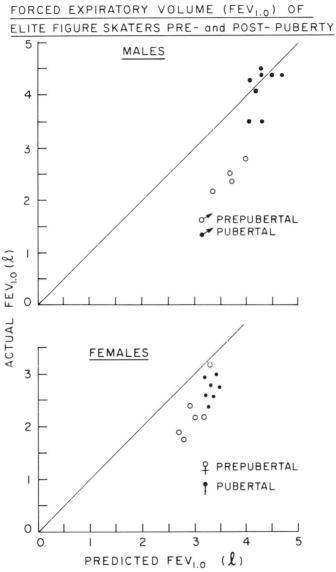

Figure 4-5. Individual values for $FEV_{1.0}$ of elite male (upper portion) and female (lower portion) figure skaters prepuberty (open circles) and postpuberty (solid circles) plotted against individual predicted $FEV_{1.0}$ (20) for each athlete.

(see Table 4-II), but with considerably more scattering of individual results. For example, pre- to postpuberty, TLC increased from 3.8 ± 0.9 to 4.8 ± 0.7 liters with most individual data approximating predicted values (see Fig. 4-2); more scatter was evident in FRC with group (mean) values increasing only slightly, pre- to postpuberty, from 2.1 ± 0.8 to 2.7 ± 0.6 liters (see Fig. 4-3). Similarly, VC and $FEV_{1.0}$ showed only small increases comparing the prepuberty females to their pubertal counterparts (2.5 ± 0.5 to 3.2 ± 0.4 liters and 2.3 ± 0.5 to 2.7 ± 0.2 liters, respectively) with most individual data closely approximating predicted values (see Figs. 4-4 and 4-5).

SUMMARY: While it appeared that there may have been a training effect, independent of normal growth factors, that enhanced pulmonary function in the male skaters, a number of factors would not support this conclusion. Only 4 male skaters were available for this group, who were small in stature relative to their age (24, 26), and who were late maturers (14, 23, 26). Furthermore, these subjects were below predicted normative values in several instances (20, 22), whereas the pubertal group on most pulmonary function tests approximated predicted values. Finally, the female skaters did not demonstrate a similar, independent effect of their training on pulmonary function over puberty, which was in agreement with earlier findings (6, 13, 27, 28).

Cardiopulmonary Response to Exercise

MAXIMAL EXERCISE: In Table 4-III, maximal O_2 consumption ($\dot{V}O_2$), minute ventilation ($\dot{V}_E$), and cardiac output ($\dot{Q}_c$) are presented. The male skaters again demonstrated the larger changes pre- to postpuberty with values being in general agreement with previous findings for this age range (7–9, 19). $\dot{V}O_2$ max increased from 2.5 ± 0.2 to 3.7 ± 0.6 l/min. While this difference was significant ($p < .05$), when their greater body size was considered, it proved a much smaller increase (i.e. 56.5 ± 10.4 to 59.3 ± 8.0 ml/kg min^{-1}). $\dot{V}_E$ max was also significantly ($p < .05$) greater in the pubertal males (105.4 ± 15.9 l/min). However, the prepubertal males only recorded a $\dot{V}_E$ max of 69.5 ± 15.6 l/min, much less than expected (9); therefore it was questionable whether this was in fact their maximal $\dot{V}_E$. As well, $\dot{Q}_c$ max for the prepubertal male skaters had to be calculated due to the lack of "maximal" data on these athletes (see footnote in Table 4-III). The postpubertal

TABLE 4-III

MAXIMAL OXYGEN CONSUMPTION, MINUTE VENTILATION AND
CARDIAC OUTPUT OF ELITE FIGURE SKATERS, PRE- AND POSTPUBERTY

(Mean ± 1 Standard Deviation)

SUBJECTS	MAXIMAL OXYGEN CONSUMPTION		MINUTE VENTILATION (l/min,BTPS)	CARDIAC OUTPUT (l/min)
	(l/min,STPD)	(ml/kg min^{-1})		
Males				
Prepubertal	2.5	56.6	69.5	(16.6)*
(n = 4)	±0.2	±10.4	±15.6	
Pubertal	3.7†	59.3	105.4†	21.1
(n = 9)	±0.6	+8.0	±15.9	±3.5
Females				
Prepubertal	2.1	50.4	72.1	15.3
(n = 6)	±0.3	±5.7	+10.8	±3.5
Pubertal	2.5	50.4	73.2	18.8
(n = 8)	±0.4	±3.5	±13.7	±3.6

*Maximal cardiac output value for prepubertal males was calculated from their submaximal regression equation ($\dot{Q} = 5.3$ $\dot{V}O_2 + 3.3$; see Fig. 4-7) at $\dot{V}O_2$max (i.e. 2.5 l/min).

†$\dot{V}O_2$max (in l/min) and $V_E$max of pubertal males significantly ($p < .01$) greater than prepubertal male subjects.

male skaters achieved a greater $\dot{Q}_c$ (21.1 ± 3.5 l/min), which agreed with previous findings for this age group (17). In contrast, comparison of the maximal cardiopulmonary responses of female skaters, pre- to postpuberty, showed little change (see Table 4-III). Although their $\dot{V}O_2$ max increased from 2.1 ± 0.3 l/min in the prepubertal females to 2.5 ± 0.4 l/min in the pubertal female skater, this difference, while in agreement with earlier findings (7, 8, 19), became negligible when their greater body size was taken into account (i.e. 50.4 ml/kg min^{-1} for both groups). Similarly, the female skaters demonstrated only small changes in both $\dot{V}_E$ max (72.1 ± 10.8 and 73.2 ± 13.7 l/min, pre- to postpuberty) and $\dot{Q}_c$ max (15.3 ± 3.5 to 18.8 ± 3.6 l/min).

SUBMAXIMAL EXERCISE: In both the male and female skaters, there was little difference between their ventilatory response to submaximal exercise, pre- and postpuberty, which was in agreement with earlier findings (1, 4, 7, 12, 17). This is illustrated in Figures 4-6 and 4-7 (presenting $\dot{V}_E$ for the male and female skaters, respectively). Over submaximal work in both the males and females, their ventilatory responses to the exercise were highly individualistic with no evidence of either a pre- to postpubertal trend nor any observable effect from their training. Similar findings were observed for cardiac output, comparing subjects pre- to postpuberty. In Figure 4-8, individual $\dot{Q}_c$ values were plotted in

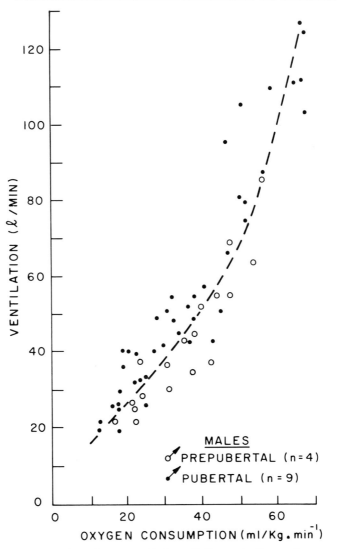

Figure 4-6. Exercise minute ventilation of elite male figure skaters prepuberty (open circles) and postpuberty (solid circles) over submaximal and maximal workloads on a progressive bicycle ergometer test.

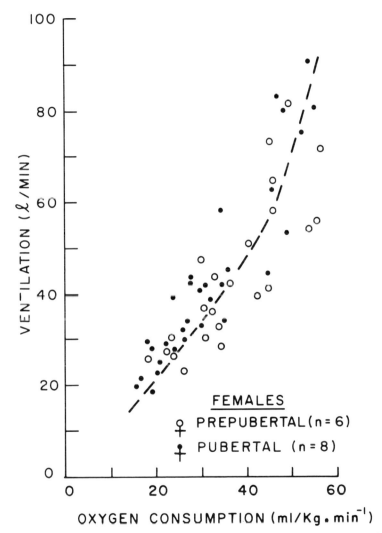

Figure 4-7. Exercise minute ventilation of elite female figure skaters prepuberty (open circles) and postpuberty (solid circles) over submaximal and maximal workloads on a progressive bicycle ergometer test.

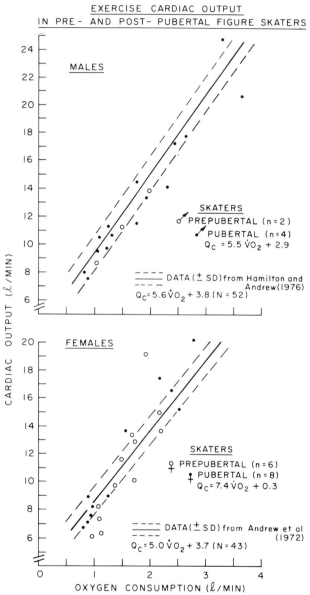

Figure 4-8. Cardiac output of elite male (upper portion) and female (lower portion) figure skaters prepuberty (open circles) and postpuberty (solid circles) over submaximal and maximal workloads on a progressive bicycle ergometer test.

relation to earlier reported data on cardiac output (1, 17), determined by means of an identical N_2O protocol. The regression line for the male skaters (see top portion of Fig. 4-8) was almost identical, with the slope being 5.5 and the Y-intercept 2.9 [compared to 5.6 and 3.8 (17), respectively]. On the other hand, the regression line for the female skaters (see bottom portion of Fig. 4-8) was found to be steeper than earlier reported data for this age group, the slope of their regression line being 7.4 [compared to 5.0 (1)]. However, this value was influenced by the maximal $\dot{Q}_c$ of 3 of the female skaters, while the majority of subjects' submaximal $\dot{Q}_c$ values fell within ±1 standard deviation of the regression line of Andrew et al. (1).

In summary, these changes in skaters' cardiopulmonary responses to both submaximal and maximal exercise appeared to be the result of normal growth. For both the pre- and postpubertal skaters, values were within the normal ranges for their age groups (3, 7, 9, 19). This was in agreement with the majority of data reported earlier (7, 12, 17, 27, 28), which has shown that, particularly over puberty, there is little independent effect of specific sports training enhancing cardiopulmonary and oxygen transport factors. With regards to the present study, this appears to hold true for the sport of figure skating.

REFERENCES

1. Andrew, G.M.; Becklake, M.R.; Guleria, J.S.; and Bates, D.V.: Heart and lung functions in swimmers and nonathletes during growth. *J Appl Physiol, 32*:245, 1972.
2. Astrand, P-O.; Engstrom, L.; Eriksson, B.O.; Karlberg, P.; Nylander, I.; Saltin, B.; and Thoren, C.: Girl swimmers. *Acta Paediatr Scand [Suppl], 147*:3, 1963.
3. Bailey, D.A.: A current view of Canadian cardiorespiratory fitness. *Can Med Assoc J, 111*:25, 1974.
4. Bar-Or, O.; Shephard, R.J.; and Allen, C.L.: Cardiac output of 10–13 year old boys and girls during submaximal work. *J Appl Physiol, 30*:219, 1971.
5. Becklake, M.R.; Varvis, C.J.; Pengelly, L.D.; Kenning, S.; MacGregor, M.; and Bates, D.V.: Measurement of pulmonary blood flow during exercise using nitrous oxide. *J Appl Physiol, 17*:579, 1966.
6. Brown, C.H.; Harrower, J.R.; and Deeter, M.F.: The effects of cross-country running on pre-adolescent girls. *Med Sci Sports, 4*:1, 1972.
7. Cumming, G.R. and Friesen, W.: Bicycle ergometer measurement of maximal oxygen uptake in children. *Can J Physiol Pharmacol, 45*:937, 1967.
8. Cunningham, D.A.; MacFarlane van Waterschoot, B.; Paterson, D.H.; Lefcoe, N.; and Sangal, S.P.: Reliability and reproducibility of maximal oxy-

gen uptake measurement in children. *Med Sci Sport, 9*:104, 1977.

9. Daniels, J. and Oldridge, N.: Changes in oxygen consumption of young boys during growth and running training. *Med Sci Sports, 3*:161, 1971.

10. Eisenmann, P.A. and Golding, L.A.: Comparison of effects of training on VO_2 max in girls and young women. *Med Sci Sports, 7*:136, 1975.

11. Engstrom, J.; Eriksson, B.O.; Karlberg, P.; Saltin, B.; and Thoren, C.: Preliminary report on the development of lung volumes in young girl swimmers. *Acta Paediatr Scand [Suppl], 217*:73, 1971.

12. Eriksson, B.O.; Grimby, G.; and Saltin, B.: Cardiac output and arterial blood gases during exercise in pubertal boys. *J Appl Physiol, 31*:348, 1971.

13. Eriksson, B.O.: Physical training, oxygen supply, and muscle metabolism in 11 to 13 year old boys. *Acta Paediatr Scand [Suppl], 61*:384, 1972.

14. Espenschade, A.S. and Eckert, H.M.: *Motor Development.* Columbus, Merrill, 1967, pp. 173-183.

15. Gledhill, N.: Fitness testing and training prescription for skaters. *Professional Circle, 10*:1, 1976.

16. Gordon, T.I.; Banister, E.W.; and Gordon, B.P.: The caloric cost of competitive figure skating. *J Sports Med Phys Fitness, 9*:98, 1969.

17. Hamilton, P. and Andrew, G.M.: Influence of growth and athletic training on heart and lung functions. *Eur J Appl Physiol, 36*:27, 1976.

18. Heath, B. and Carter, J.E.: A modified somatotype method. *Am J Phys Anthropol, 25*:37, 1967.

19. Knuttgen, H.G.: Aerobic capacity of adolescents. *J Appl Physiol, 22*:655, 1967.

20. Lyons, H.A. and Tanner, R.W.: Total lung volume and its subdivisions in children: normal standards. *J Appl Physiol, 17*:601, 1962.

21. Massicotte, D.R. and MacNab, R.B.: Cardiorespiratory adaptations to training at specified intensities in children. *Med Sci Sports, 6*:242, 1974.

22. Newman, F.; Smalley, B.F.; and Thomson, M.L.: A comparison between body size and lung function of swimmers and normal school children. *J Physiol (London), 156*:9P, 1961.

23. Ross, W.D.; Brown, S.R.; Faulkner, R.A.; and Savage, M.V.: Age of menarche of elite Canadian figure skaters and skiers. *Can J Appl Sport Sci, 1*:191, 1976.

24. Ross, W.D.; Brown, S.R.; Yu, J.W.; and Faulkner, R.A.: Somatotype of Canadian figure skaters. *J Sports Med Phys Fitness, 17*:195, 1977.

25. Sobolova, V.; Seliger, V.; Grossova, D.; Machovcova, J.; and Zelenga, V.: The influence of age and sports training in swimming on physical fitness. *Acta Paediatr Scand [Suppl], 217*:63, 1971.

26. Tanner, J.M.: *Growth at Adolescence.* London, Blackwell, 1962, pp. 30-36.

27. Vaccaro, P. and Clarke, H.: Cardiorespiratory alterations in 9-11 year old children following a season of competitive swimming. *Med Sci Sport, 10*:204, 1978.

28. Weber, G.; Kartodihardjo, W.; and Klissouras, V.: Growth and physical training with reference to heredity. *J Appl Physiol, 40*:211, 1976.

29. Winter, J.S.D. and Faiman, C.: Pituitary-gonadal relationships in male children and adolescents. *Pediatr Res, 6*:126, 1972.

30. Winter, J.S.D. and Faiman, C.: Pituitary-gonadal relations in female children and adolescents. *Pediatr Res, 7*:948, 1973.
31. Yuhasz, M.: *Physical Fitness Appraisal and Exercise Prescription.* London, Ontario, U of Western Ontario, 1976.

Chapter 5

OXYGEN TRANSPORT: A LIMITING FACTOR IN AEROBIC CAPACITY

N. GLEDHILL, A.B. FROESE, F. BUICK, AND L. SPRIET

INTRODUCTION

CONTROVERSY persists over what factor limits maximal aerobic metabolism. It has been argued by some that the oxidative capacity of muscle is far in excess of the amount of O_2 delivered during maximal aerobic exercise, and therefore, O_2 transport must be the limiting factor (14). Others have contended that under normal conditions more than enough oxygen is provided to the exercising muscle, but the oxidative machinery is taxed to its limit and cannot utilize any additional O_2 (20).

This question has been studied using a variety of experimental approaches. For example, if aerobic capacity ($\dot{V}O_2max$) is limited by O_2 transport to the working muscles, then the addition of extra muscle groups to those already eliciting a $\dot{V}O_2max$ should have no effect on $\dot{V}O_2$. Early studies reported that $\dot{V}O_2max$ during running increased when arm work was added (6, 34), but these findings were contradicted by subsequent studies (1, 5, 21, 33).

From investigations of enzyme activity in human skeletal muscle, Gollnick et al. estimated that the oxidative capacity of muscle is far in excess of the observed maximal $\dot{V}O_2$ per kg of muscle mass (14). Their calculations indicate that maximal cardiac outputs would need to be doubled in order to meet the maximal oxidizing capacity of muscle. On the other hand, Holloszy postulated that adaptations in muscle enzymes and mitochondria that result from physical conditioning could allow muscle to function at a lower PO_2 (16). This would permit an increase in aerobic capacity without any increase in O_2 transport and implies that the oxidative capacity of muscle could be a limitation to aerobic capacity.

Another approach has been to employ hyperoxic and hyperbaric environments to increase the amount of dissolved O_2 and thereby augment O_2 transport. Margaria et al. (25) reported an 8 percent increase in aerobic capacity when subjects breathed 100% O_2, and similar observations were reported by Ekblom et al. (10) and Wyndham et al. (39). Similarily, when the amount of dissolved O_2 was increased via a hyperbaric environment, Wyndham et al. (38) and Linnarsson et al. (24) reported significant increases in aerobic capacity. However, when Kaijser (20) used high atmospheric pressure to increase O_2 content, he observed no change in $\dot{V}O_2$max or in O_2 extraction from femoral venous blood. His findings are supported by Pirnay et al. (27) who found that during maximal work, femoral venous PO_2 could be lowered with beta-adrenegic blockade. Like Doll et al. (7), they concluded that since O_2 extraction in leg muscle is not maximal under normal conditions, local oxidative capacity rather than O_2 delivery limits aerobic capacity.

It is important to note, however, that there are extensive methodological problems involved in the use of hyperoxic inspirates, so the findings from such studies are suspect. Also, as Haugaard (15) pointed out, in hyperbaric environments, the effects of high gas density, high O_2 tensions, and high O_2 saturations on pulmonary ventilation and CO_2 carriage can interfere with any beneficial effect of the increased O_2 transport. Therefore, studies of hyperoxia are of dubious value in identifying the limiting factor in aerobic capacity.

The relationship between hemoglobin concentration and aerobic capacity has been studied extensively, but the results are contradictory. A number of investigators have concluded that there is a close relationship between total body hemoglobin and $\dot{V}O_2$max (17, 23, 31). Sproule et al. (32) observed very low values for maximal oxygen uptake in anemic patients in comparison with normal values for healthy subjects of comparable age. In several studies $\dot{V}O_2$max decreased when hemoglobin content was reduced (2, 22, 37). On the other hand, Rowell et al. (30) found that a 14 percent decrease in hemoglobin concentration caused no reduction in $\dot{V}O_2$max, and Vellar and Hermansen (35) concluded that hemoglobin concentration must fall below 11 g/100 ml before there is any reduction in $\dot{V}O_2$max. Further, Ekblom and Hermansen reported that although highly trained endurance athletes have the highest recorded aerobic capacities, they have abnormally low hemoglobin levels (9).

Recently, attention has been focused on the effect of an increased hemoglobin concentration on aerobic capacity. This can be accomplished by accelerating erythropoesis through acclimation to hypoxia or by the infusion of whole blood or packed red cells. Generally speaking, attempts to increase the sea level $\dot{V}O_2$max by acclimating athletes to altitude have been unsuccessful because the athletes had a lower exercise capacity during the altitude sojourn and, as a result, detrained. Thus, although the O_2 carrying capacity increased, maximal cardiac output decreased. The net effect was no change in $\dot{V}O_2$max upon return to sea level (3). However, in a recent study that employed untrained subjects, Horstman et al. reported an increased $\dot{V}O_2$max following altitude acclimation and return to sea level (19). The discrepancy is possibly due to the fact that the untrained subjects were not in training prior to or during the altitude sojourn, and therefore they did not detrain at altitude.

Several investigators have attempted to study experimentally induced erythrocythemia using autologous reinfusion of red blood cells. Robinson et al. (29) observed no change in $\dot{V}O_2$max when erythrocythemia was induced with 1000 ml of blood and similar findings were reported by Frye and Ruhling (12) following the reinfusion of one unit of blood. On the other hand, in two studies in which 800 ml of whole blood were reinfused, Ekblom et al. reported increases in $\dot{V}O_2$max of 5 and 8 percent (8, 11). A similar improvement in $\dot{V}O_2$max was observed by Robertson et al. (28) when erythrocythemia was induced with 4 units of packed red cells. However, many of these investigations failed to significantly elevate hemoglobin concentration because the blood was reinfused at a time when control levels of hemoglobin had not yet been reestablished, and/or the blood was stored by refrigeration, a technique in which storage time is limited to 3 weeks and red cell loss is substantial. Additional weaknesses in these studies include failure to control for subject and experimenter bias, and failure to rule out improvements due to training as a possible explanation for the observed increase in $\dot{V}O_2$max following erythrocythemia.

RECENT DATA

A recent investigation in the authors' laboratory of the time course of hematological changes following the removal and autologous reinfusion of 1000 ml of blood determined that, following removal, it takes 5 to 6 weeks to reestablish normocythemia (13). Blood was stored as washed frozen cells because this technique offered the advantage of unlimited storage time with minimal cell loss. Reinfusion of freeze-preserved cells 6 weeks after removal resulted in a significant increase in hemoglobin concentration and O_2 carrying capacity (13).

In a subsequent study employing a double blind crossover design, the aerobic capacity of eleven highly trained runners was studied before phlebotomy (C_1); following restoration of normocythemia (C_2); after a sham reinfusion of 50 ml of saline (Sham); following autologous reinfusion of approximately 900 ml of freeze-preserved blood; and upon reestablishment of control hematology levels after erythrocythemia (C_3) (4). Care was taken to avoid the weaknesses noted in previous studies of induced erythrocythemia. Use of the freeze-preservation technique for red cell storage maximized the subsequent erythrocythemia. By using subjects who were accustomed to exhaustive treadmill work and who possessed a high level of aerobic fitness, a potential training effect from the numerous exercise tests was avoided. Also, the possibility of subject and experimenter bias due to a psychological influence was eliminated by using the double blind design.

No hematological differences were observed among C_1, C_2, Sham, and C_3, but following reinfusion, there was a significant increase in Hb (hemoglobin) concentration, both at rest (15.1 to 16.3 gm $\cdot$ 100 ml^{-1}) and during exercise (15.7 to 16.7 g $\cdot$ 100 ml^{-1}). The sham reinfusion had no effect on aerobic capacity, but surprisingly, aerobic capacity increased in the erythrocythemic condition (Table 5-I). $\dot{V}O_2$max was significantly increased 24 hours postreinfusion (5.11 to 5.37 l $\cdot$ min^{-1}) and 7 days postreinfusion (5.33 l $\cdot$ min^{-1}).

Following reinfusion, the O_2 carrying capacity during exercise was increased by 1.38 ml $\cdot$ 100 ml^{-1}. Assuming that $\dot{Q}$max did not change from normocythemia to erythrocythemia, one can calcu-

TABLE 5-I

EXERCISE HEMATOLOGY AND AEROBIC CAPACITY FOLLOWING
AUTOLOGOUS REINFUSION OF 1000 ml OF BLOOD ($\bar{x} \pm$ SE; n = 11)

	Control		Postreinfusion			
			24 hours		7 days	
Hb gm $\cdot$ 100 ml^{-1}	15.7	0.2	16.7	0.3	16.6	0.2
Hct %	46.4	0.5	48.4	0.4	48.6	0.6
$\dot{V}O_2$max l $\cdot$ min^{-1}	5.11	0.2	5.37	0.2	5.33	0.2

late that approximately 400 ml·min^{-1} of additional O_2 would have been made available to the working muscles. However, $\dot{V}O_2$max only increased by 260 ml·min^{-1}. This suggests two possibilities. Conceivably, $\dot{Q}$max actually decreased slightly during erythrocythemia so that the O_2 supply was really only augmented by 260 ml·min^{-1}. This would suggest that O_2 delivery is the limiting factor in maximal aerobic performance. Alternatively, if $\dot{Q}$max did remain constant such that O_2 delivery truly increased by 400 ml·min^{-1}, it could be inferred that peripheral metabolism had reached its capacity with only 260 ml·min^{-1} of additional O_2. This would imply that O_2 transport is the limiting factor under normal conditions, but the metabolic capacity of the muscles to utilize O_2 is only slightly in excess of the ability of the transport system to deliver O_2.

A fall in $\dot{Q}$max subsequent to erythrocythemia and the associated increase in viscosity has been reported previously in animals (26, 36). Cardiac output was not measured in the authors' initial investigation of induced erythrocythemia. However, a follow-up study that includes measurement of arterial O_2 content and $\dot{Q}$max via dye dilution is being conducted currently. Once again, the subjects are highly conditioned endurance runners, but this time a total of 1500 ml of blood was removed over a 5 week period. The blood was stored via the high glycerol freezing technique and, when normocythemia had been reestablished, it was returned to the donors over a period of 10 to 12 days in three 500 ml reinfusions.

Results from the subjects completed to date confirm the previous finding that erythrocythemia results in an increased aerobic capacity (Table 5-II). During exercise, following the reinfusion of a total of 1000 and 1500 ml of blood, Hb concentration increased from 16.0 to 17.2 and 17.6 gm·100 ml^{-1} respectively. The corresponding $\dot{V}O_2$max values were 5.04, 5.24, and 5.38 l·min^{-1}. Surprisingly, preliminary results indicate that $\dot{Q}$max also increased with erythrocythemia. Thus, systemic O_2 transport was augmented by an amount substantially greater than the corresponding increases in aerobic capacity.

These findings indicate that although aerobic capacity is limited by systemic O_2 transport, this limitation is relatively minor. The very large discrepancy between the amount of O_2 transported and used strongly suggests that the limitation is at the muscle level.

TABLE 5-II

EXERCISE HEMATOLOGY, SYSTEMIC O_2 TRANSPORT, AND
AEROBIC CAPACITY FOLLOWING AUTOLOGOUS REINFUSION
OF 1000 ml AND 1500 ml OF BLOOD ($\bar{x} \pm$ SE; n = 4)

	Control	Postreinfusion 1000 ml	1500 ml
Hb gm·100 ml^{-1}	16.0 0.2	17.2 0.1	17.6 0.1
Hct %	45.6 0.3	49.2 0.3	50.5 0.2
CaO$_2$ ml·100 ml^{-1}	20.0 0.6	21.3 0.2	22.0 0.4
$\dot{V}O_2$max l·min^{-1}	5.04 0.21	5.24 0.22	5.38 0.25

This limitation could be in the metabolic capacity of the muscle. On the other hand, it could be due to changes in regional blood flow or in the regional distribution of that flow within the working muscle subsequent to erythrocythemia. Recent observations by Horstman et al. using an in-situ muscle preparation support the latter hypothesis (18).

Unfortunately, we are still left with an incomplete picture. However, the next phase of study is to examine the above possibilities by measuring the O_2 transport and a-vO$_2$ difference of maximally exercising muscle following induced erythrocythemia. Perhaps then a more definitive statement concerning which factor limits aerobic capacity can be made.

REFERENCES

1. Astrand, P.O. and Saltin, B.: Maximal oxygen uptake and heart rate in various types of muscular activity. *J Appl Physiol, 10*:977, 1961.
2. Balke, B.; Grills, G.P.; Konecci, E.B.; and Luft, U.C.: Work capacity after blood donation. *J Appl Physiol, 7*:231, 1954.
3. Balke, B. et al.: Training for maximum performance at altitude. In *Exercise at Altitude*, edited by R. Margaria. New York, Excerpta Medica, 179, 1967.
4. Buick, F.J.; Gledhill, N.; Froese, A.B.; Spriet, L.; and Meyers, E.C.: Effect of induced erythrocythemia on aerobic work capacity. *J Appl Physiol: Respirat Environ Exercise Physiol, 48*:636, 1980.
5. Buskirk, E. and Taylor, H.L.: Maximal oxygen intake and its relation to body composition with specific reference to chronic physical activity and obesity. *J Appl Physiol, 11*:72, 1957.
6. Christensen, E.H. and Hogberg, P.: Physiology of skiing. *Arbeitsphysiologie, 14*:292, 1950.
7. Doll, E.; Keul, J; and Maiwald, C.: Oxygen tension and acid-base equilibria in venous blood of working muscle. *Am J Physiol, 215*:23, 1968.
8. Ekblom, B.; Goldbarg, A.N.; and Gullbring, B.: Response to exercise after blood loss and reinfusion. *J Appl Physiol, 33*:175, 1972.
9. Ekblom, B. and Hermansen, L.: Cardiac output in athletes. *J Appl Physiol, 25*:619, 1968.

10. Ekblom, B.; Huot, R.; Stein, E.M.; and Thorstensson, A.T.: Effect of changes in arterial oxygen content on circulation and physical performance. *J Appl Physiol, 39*:71, 1975.

11. Ekblom B.; Wilson, G.; and Astrand, P.-O.: Central circulation during exercise after venesection and reinfusion of red blood cells. *J Appl Physiol, 40*:379, 1976.

12. Frye, A.J. and Ruhling, R.O.: RBC reinfusion, exercise, hemoconcentration, $\dot{V}O_2$. (Abstract). *Med Sci Sports, 9*:69, 1977.

13. Gledhill, N.; Buick, F.J.; Froese, A.B.; Spriet, L.; and Meyers, E.C.: An optimal method of storing blood for blood boosting. (Abstract). *Med Sci Sports, 10*:40, 1978.

14. Gollnick, P.D. et al.: Enzyme activity and fiber composition in skeletal muscle of untrained and trained men. *J Appl Physiol, 33(3)*:312, 1972.

15. Haugaard, N.: Cellular mechanisms of oxygen toxicity. *Physiol Rev, 48*:311, 1968.

16. Holloszy, J.O.: Biochemical adaptations to exercise. In *Reviews in Exercise and Sports Science*, edited by J.H. Wilmore. New York, Acad Pr, 45, 1973.

17. Holmgren, A. and Astrand, P.O.: DL and the dimensions and functional capacities of the oxygen transport system in humans. *J Appl Physiol, 21*:1463, 1966.

18. Horstman, D.M.; Gleser, M.; and Delehunt, J.: Effects of altering O_2 delivery on $\dot{V}O_2$ of isolated working muscle. *Am J Physiol, 230*:327, 1976.

19. Horstman, D. et al.: The influence of polycythemia induced by four-week sojourn at 4300 meters, on sea level work capacity. In *Exercise Physiology*, edited by F. Landry and W.R. Orban. New York, Symposia Special, 533, 1978.

20. Kaijser, L.: Limiting factors for aerobic muscle performance: The influence of varying oxygen pressure and temperature. *Acta Physiol Scand [Suppl], 78*:346, 1970.

21. Kamon, E. and Pandolf, K.B.: Maximal aerobic power during ladder-mill climbing, uphill running and cycling. *J Appl Physiol, 32*:467, 1972.

22. Karpovich, P.V. and Millman, N.: Athletes as blood donors. *Res Q, 13*:166, 1942.

23. Kjellberg, S.R.; Rudhe, U.; and Sjostrand, T.: Increase of amount of hemoglobin and blood volume in connection with physical training. *Acta Physiol Scand, 19*:146, 1949.

24. Linnarsson, D.; Karlsson, J.; Fagraeus, L.; and Saltin, B.: Muscle metabolites and oxygen deficit with exercise in hypoxia and hyperoxia. *J Appl Physiol, 36*:399, 1974.

25. Margaria, R.; Cerretelli, P.; Marchi, S.; and Rossi, L.: Maximum exercise in oxygen. *Int Z Angew Physiol, 18*:465, 1961.

26. Murray, J.F.; Gold, P.; and Johnson Jr., B.L.: The circulatory effects of hematocrit variations in normovolemic and hypervolemic dogs. *J Clin Invest, 42*:1150, 1963.

27. Pirnay, F.; Lamy, M.; and Dijardin, J.: Analysis of femoral venous blood during maximum muscular exercise. *J Appl Physiol, 3*:289, 1972.

28. Robertson, R.; Gilcher, R.; Metz, K.; Bahnson, H.; Allison, T.; Skrinar, G.;

Abbot, A.; and Becker, R.: Effect of red blood cell reinfusion on physical working capacity and perceived exertion at normal and reduced oxygen pressure. (Abstract). *Med Sci Sports, 10*:49, 1978.

29. Robinson, B.F.; Epstein, S.E.; Kahler, R.L.; and Braunwald, E.: Circulatory effects of acute expansion of blood volume: Studies during maximal exercise and at rest. *Circ Res, 19*:26, 1966.
30. Rowell, L.B.; Taylor, H.L.; and Wang, Y.: Limitations to prediction of maximal oxygen intake. *J Appl Physiol, 19*:919, 1964.
31. Sjostrand, T.: Volume and distribution of blood and their significance in regulation circulation. *Physiol Rev, 33*:202, 1953.
32. Sproule, B.J.; Mitchell, J.H.; and Miller, W.F.: Cardiopulmonary physiological responses to heavy exercise in patients with anemia. *J Clin Invest, 39*:378, 1960.
33. Stenberg, J.; Astrand, P.O.; and Ekblom, B.: Hemodynamic response to work with different muscle groups, sitting and supine. *J Appl Physiol, 22*:61, 1967.
34. Taylor, H.L.; Buskirk, E.; and Henschel, A.: Maximal oxygen intake as an objective measure of cardio-respiratory performance. *J Appl Physiol, 8*:73, 1955.
35. Vellar, O.D. and Hermansen, L.: Physical performance and hematological parameters with special reference to hemoglobin and maximal oxygen uptake. *Acta Med Scand [Supp. 522], 190*:1, 1971.
36. Weisse, A.B.; Regan, T.J.; Nadami, M.; and Hellems, H.K.: Late circulatory adjustments to acute normovolemic polycythemia. *Am J Physiol, 211*:1413, 1966.
37. Woodson, R.D.; Willis, R.E.; and Lenfant, C.: Effect of acute and established anemia on O_2 transport at rest, submaximal and maximal work. *J Appl Physiol, 44*:36, 1978.
38. Wyndham, C.H.; Kok, R.; Strydom, N.B.; Robers, G.G.; and Zwi, S.: Physiological effects of acute changes in altitude in a deep mine. *J Appl Physiol, 30*:232, 1971.
39. Wyndham, C.H.; Strydom, N.B.; van Rensburg, A.J.; and Rogers, G.G.: Effects on maximal oxygen intake of acute changes in altitude in a deep mine. *J Appl Physiol, 29*:552, 1970.

Chapter 6

FAILURE OF PULMONARY OXYGEN TRANSPORT IN ENDURANCE ATHLETES*

J.A. DEMPSEY, O. SANYER, P. HANSON, AND A. CLAREMONT

THE RESPONSE of the healthy pulmonary system to the demands of steady state muscular exercise is commonly regarded as near optimal. That is, ventilation is regulated both precisely and efficiently and O_2 exchange is such that arterial PO_2 is maintained at resting levels despite increased demands for tissue O_2 consumption, precipitous reductions in mixed venous O_2 content returning to the lung, and reduced time for equilibrium of alveolar gas with desaturated red cells in the pulmonary capillary. This well-established ability to maintain arterial PO_2 and HbO_2 saturation is shown in Figure 6-1 for conditions of moderately heavy steady state treadmill running. This response is typical for these conditions. That is, an initial hyperventilation and thus high alveolar PO_2 (P_AO_2) occurs at the onset of exercise, probably secondary to extraneous or anticipatory-type cortical stimuli. Thereafter, $\dot{V}_A$ falls and remains fairly closely matched to the concomitantly rising $\dot{V}O_2$; thus P_AO_2 is reduced and remains fairly constant or may even rise a few torr (mmHg) as hyperventilation occurs with time of exercise. The alveolar-to-arterial PO_2 difference may increase 2 to 3 times (> rest) in this type of exercise, but arterial PO_2 remains constant and HbO_2 saturation will fall at most 2–3 percent secondary to an acidotic and/or temperature-induced rightward shift in the HbO_2 dissociation curve. Several factors contribute to this homeostasis of arterial O_2 content during exercise by their control of alveolar-capillary equilibrium and of ventilation to perfusion distribution in the lung. These mechanisms have been discussed in detail elsewhere (1).

*This work was supported by NIH Grant 15469 and Career Development Award HL-00149, U.S. Army R. and D.C. contract and the University of Wisconsin Graduate School. We are especially grateful to the athletes for their participation, and are indebted to Kathy Henderson and Mary Lutz for their assistance with the blood gas analyses.

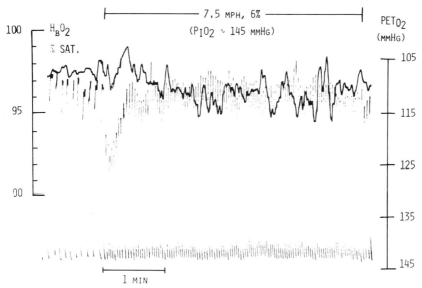

Figure 6-1. Effects of moderate treadmill running (at steady state $\dot{V}O_2$ of 3.3 l/min) on alveolar PO_2 ($P_{ET}O_2$) and arterial %HbO_2 saturation (S_aO_2). The latter was measured with an ear oximeter and lags behind the change in $P_{ET}O_2$ ~ 8–12 seconds during exercise. S_aO_2 fell a minimum of 2 percent from resting values secondary to a slight metabolic acidosis and 0.5°C rise in core temperature.

There are exceptions to this response. Recently, significant reductions have been found in arterial PO_2 during very heavy, short-term treadmill running in endurance athletes. These reductions in P_aO_2 ranged from 15 to 35 mmHg and occurred only in maximum or near-maximum exercise of 2 to 4 minutes duration. Not all runners showed this significant desaturation (i.e. 12 of 17 to date) and in most cases those who hyperventilated the least in heavy work showed the most arterial HbO_2 desaturation. Others have also reported significant desaturation in short term heavy work of various types (2, 4, 5). An example of exercise desaturation is shown in Figures 6-2 and 6-3, which contain data on the same runner as in Figure 6-1, but at heavier work loads. Note that with both the high speed and high grade types of work, at the initiation of exercise, hyperventilation and high alveolar PO_2 (120–125 mmHg) occur and %HbO_2 saturation is maintained at resting levels. However, as $\dot{V}_A$ falls and P_AO_2 is reduced (to ~ 115 mmHg), S_aO_2 falls precipitously. With time, the rate of HbO_2 desaturation is reduced somewhat as progressive hyperventilation raises the mean alveolar PO_2 close to 120 mmHg, but S_aO_2 still remains substantially (6–8%) below resting levels. These measurements of S_aO_2 using the ear oximeter have been confirmed by serial sampling of arterial blood over the time-course of several work loads. In the examples shown in Figures 6-2 and 6-3, arterial PO_2 fell from the low 90s at rest to the mid-50s at end exercise.

The principal cause of the arterial HbO_2 desaturation probably resides in an inadequate level of alveolar PO_2 achieved during heavy exercise. This reasoning is based on two types of findings: (a) the level of HbO_2 desaturation was closely correlated with the level of alveolar hyperventilation achieved, i.e. those with a <3–4 mmHg drop in P_aCO_2 and therefore minimal rise in P_AO_2 desaturated the most; and (b) during the time-course of heavy exercise (Figs. 6-2, 6-3), a maintained S_aO_2 is observed when alveolar PO_2 is high at the initiation of exercise and a marked desaturation as alveolar PO_2 fell within the ensuing seconds of continued exercise.

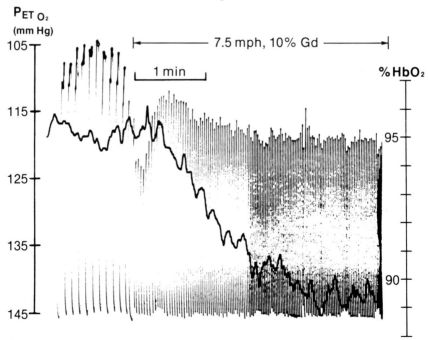

Figure 6-2. Effects of heavy exercise ($\dot{V}O_2 \sim 4$ l/min) on $P_{ET}O_2$ and S_aO_2. $P_IO_2 \sim$ 145 mmHg (ambient air). At end exercise, arterial PO_2 was 58 mmHg, pH was 7.37, and P_aCO_2 was 38 mmHg. Note that the steepest rate of desaturation coincided with a reduction in alveolar PO_2 following the hyperventilation at the initiation of exercise.

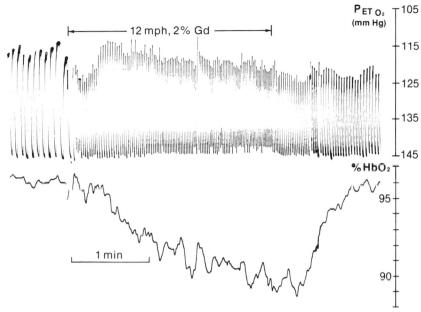

Figure 6-3. Effects of near maximum exercise ($\dot{V}O_2 \sim 4.6$ l/min) on $P_{ET}O_2$ and S_aO_2. $P_IO_2 \sim 145$ mmHg. At end exercise, arterial PO_2 was 59 mmHg, pH was 7.30, and P_aCO_2 was 37 mmHg.

These data, of course, are only correlative and do not prove a cause:effect relationship. Accordingly, the authors sought to control alveolar PO_2 experimentally during exercise by varying, very slightly, the inspired PO_2. The aim was to hold alveolar PO_2 throughout the exercise at a level which approximated that obtained during the first few seconds of air-breathing exercise when S_aO_2 was maintained at resting levels. An example of this is shown in Figure 6-4, where inspired $\%O_2$ was increased <1.5 percent and P_IO_2 raised from 145 to 155. With alveolar PO_2 held near 125 mmHg, no effect was observed of maximum work on P_aO_2 and an $\sim2\%$ fall in S_aO_2 secondary only to an acid pH_a and increased core temperature. Contrast this with Figure 6-2 where, at the same workload and $\dot{V}O_2$, an alveolar PO_2 of 115 to 120 mmHg was insufficient to prevent a progressive arterial desaturation. Further, if inspired and alveolar PO_2 (simulating 7500 to 8000 feet altitude) is reduced, it may be readily seen (Fig. 6-5) that a marked, progressive hyperventilation with alveolar PO_2 of ~95 mmHg was insufficient to prevent a steep and marked arterial desaturation to a P_aO_2, which approximated 45 mmHg.

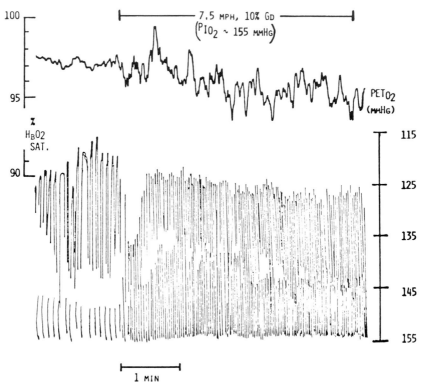

Figure 6-4. Effects of elevating inspired PO_2 ($F_IO_2 \sim 22.3\%$) and thus alveolar PO_2 on S_aO_2 during heavy exercise. S_aO_2 fell 2–2.5 percent secondary only to a reduced pH_a and increased core temperature. Contrast these minimal effects on S_aO_2 (at alveolar $PO_2 \sim 125$ mmHg) to those seen at identical workload but at alveolar $PO_2 \sim 115$ to 120 mmHg in Figure 6-2.

The level of alveolar PO_2 per se is not crucial. To the contrary, when the demand for O_2 consumption is not too heavy and thus the level of mixed venous HbO_2 desaturation and reduced O_2 content is not too severe, a ventilatory response that elicits an alveolar PO_2 of only 110 mmHg is quite sufficient for completion of pulmonary gas exchange and maintenance of arterial PO_2 (see Fig. 6-1). Hence, a high alveolar PO_2 ($>$ 120–125 mmHg) becomes crucial to homeostasis of arterial PO_2 and HbO_2 when combined with extreme metabolic demands and greatly desaturated mixed venous O_2 content.

There are three implications of these findings. First, these data point most strongly to a diffusion limitation at the alveolar-capillary level as the cause of arterial desaturation and as the

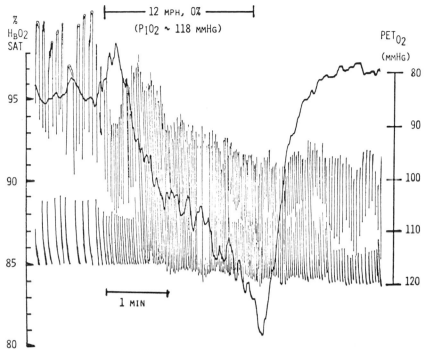

Figure 6-5. Effects of reducing inspired PO_2 ($F_IO_2 \sim 19\%$) and thus alveolar PO_2 on S_aO_2 during exercise. Contrast the magnitude and rate of HbO_2 desaturation in this condition (alveolar $PO_2 \sim 95$ mmHg) with that at an identical workload (in Fig. 6-3) but at alveolar $PO_2 \sim 120$ mmHg.

explanation for the observed effects of experimentally manipulating alveolar PO_2. A high alveolar PO_2 provides a steep alveolar to capillary diffusion gradient, which in turn increases the rate of alveolar-capillary O_2 equilibrium. This very rapid rate of equilibrium may be crucial under extreme exercise conditions where pulmonary blood flow is high and red cell transit times may be extremely short—at least in some regions of the lung. The data is also compatible with the explanation that the desaturation of heavy exercise is caused by an inadequate ventilatory response, and thus an increase in overall ventilation:perfusion ($V_A:Q_c$), which is insufficient to remove some of the "lower" $V_A:Q_c$ ratios that will contribute significantly to arterial hypoxemia in the face of low $C_{\bar{v}}O_2$ (3). Separating these two factors in the intact lung presents a formidable problem.

Second, this work clearly demonstrates that the hyperventilation of heavy exercise (and its attending physiologic cost) is necessary for adequate gas exchange and arterial blood gas homeostasis, i.e. not just for compensating the attendant metabolic acidosis by releasing carbonic acid but for maintaining arterial PO_2 by permitting a high level of alveolar oxygenation.

Finally, the observed desaturation of heavy exercise may have implications for the runner's performance capability. In most instances, where arterial PO_2 fell only 15 to 20 mmHg or less, there would only be a very small effect on arterial O_2 content and thus on systemic O_2 delivery. Actually, this situation may be the optimal one for the runner in that the physiologic cost of extreme hyperventilation (including the possibility of respiratory muscle fatigue) is avoided—and all that it "costs" him is a drop in PO_2 and a little more acidosis with no sacrifice of systemic O_2 transport. However, in many of the runners, $\%HbO_2$ was reduced >7–8 percent and one might then expect a significant effect on tissue metabolism. For example, in cases such as those shown in Figures 6-2, 6-3, and 6-5, it is imperative that the time course of change in whole-body $\dot{V}O_2$ be determined. A substantial lowering of $\dot{V}O_2$ with time is predicted as arterial O_2 content fell beyond the point where the a-vO_2 difference across the working muscle reached a maximum. The lesson from Figure 6-5 would appear to be that runners prone to even mild arterial O_2 desaturation at sea level would experience substantially more of the same at even moderately high altitudes. The same response might well prevail—with negative consequences for performance—even in those runners who do not desaturate at sea level.

Dr. Balke has always stressed in his teaching and writings the importance of breathing and breathing pattern in the performance of endurance running events. These data outlined here merely confirm his logic and practical observations.

REFERENCES

1. Dempsey, J.A.; Vidruk, E.H.; and Mastenbrook, S.M.: Pulmonary control systems in exercise. *Fed. Proc, 39*: 1498, 1980.
2. Bjurstedt, H. and Wigesty, O.: Dynamics of arterial O_2 tension in response to sinusoidal work load in man. *Acta Physiol Scand, 82*:236, 1971.
3. Gledhill, N.; Froese, A.B.; and Dempsey, J.A.: Ventilation to perfusion distribution during exercise in health. In *Muscular Exercise and the Lung*, edited by J.A. Dempsey and C.E. Reed. Madison, U of Wisc Pr, 1977.

4. Rowell, L.B.; Taylor, H.L.; Wang, Y.; and Carlson, W.B.: Saturation of arterial blood with O_2 during maximal exercise. *J Appl Physiol, 19*:284, 1964.
5. Young, I.H. and Woolcock, A.J.: Changes in the arterial blood gas tensions during unsteady-state exercise. *J Appl Physiol, 44*:936, 1978.

Part 2

EXERCISE AND METABOLISM

PRESIDING: FRANCIS J. NAGLE

Chapter 7

THE USE OF ELECTRON MICROSCOPY IN THE INVESTIGATION OF EXERCISE-RELATED MUSCLE FAILURE*

J.B. GALE

INTRODUCTION

Overview

THE STUDY of muscular fatigue has entertained many investigators. Possible "causes" of fatigue include neural transmission failure, excitation-contraction coupling loss, depletion of substrate (only glycogen and not lipids), changes in cellular pH, electrolytes, and water, and an increased concentration of metabolic inhibitors, e.g. lactic acid.

Numerous authors have reported that exhaustion following long duration work is related to the depletion of heart (10), skeletal muscle (12, 22), and/or liver (8) glycogen. If the skeletal muscle blood flow remains adequate (although it may not, as will be discussed later), there is little else to explain why lipids cannot sustain the activity. One possibility is that depletion of carbohydrates might reduce the synthesis of Kreb's cycle intermediates, e.g. oxaloacetate (OAA), which could be replenished by the carboxylation of pyruvate in skeletal muscle. Low pyruvate levels would therefore limit such replacement and subsequently "turn off" the metabolism of acetyl Co-A derived from β-oxidation. Similarly, plasma levels of mitochondrial GOT have been elevated after exhaustive exercise (78), and a loss of this enzyme from the mitochondria might limit OAA production from aspartate.

That the contractility of heart muscle is somehow associated with exhaustion may be derived from the work of Ekelund et al.

*The studies described were funded in part by the Heart Association of the Redwood Empire, Sigma Xi, NSF-Institutional Grants for Science, and Sonoma State University Faculty Development grants.

79

(30) and Saltin (88). Both have reported that exercise-induced exhaustion is accompanied by an increase in end diastolic volume and a concommitant increase in heart rate (HR), in an attempt to maintain cardiac output. (A reduced venous return due to hypohydration and its related decrease in plasma volume might have been suspected had the end diastolic volume also decreased, rather than having become elevated.) Barnard et al. (10) have also suggested, from indirect evidence, that the same phenomenon is related to fatigue in rats; HRs remained steady during long duration running and then increased about 5 percent just as the animals became exhausted. Unfortunately, cardiac outputs were not measured during these studies, although they may have fallen.

While such a probable, slightly reduced cardiac output might explain fatigue at the skeletal muscle level, it does not answer the question for the heart. Again, a decrease in cellular glycogen content does not completely explain the decrease in cellular contractility if the heart could continue to metabolize free fatty acid (FFA) or ketones. Insufficient coronary flow cannot be a primary factor as the steady state HR can be tolerated for long periods. It is the decrease in myocardial contractility that must precede the still higher HR, just before exhaustion is experienced. (Of course, at this point, decreased coronary flow may then be associated with reduced diastole.) Furthermore, the cause(s) for the reduced contractility has not been adequately described.

The failure that results from long duration activity may be precipitated by a reduction in the capacity of heart and skeletal muscle mitochondria to metabolize. Reports of fatigue-related decreases in contractility (69), *in vitro* decreases in mitochondrial capacity to oxidize fats (4, 29) and carbohydrates (29), reduced phosphorylative efficiency—as evidenced by a decrease in the ADP:0 ratio (18), the slow rate of muscle recovery noted by Wilson and Stainsby (112), and changes in apparent mitochondrial ultrastructure (37)—all support the hypothesis that exhaustion is probably related to a breakdown in the ability of mitochondria to function normally. Proof for this hypothesis, however, will not be easily forthcoming since *in vitro* homogenate preparations drastically disturb the endogenous environment and make it exceedingly difficult to directly study organelle construction at the molecular level. Such changes will probably have to be inferred from other information obtained using techniques that are very rapid and only slightly perturbing to cells.

CHANGES IN HEART AND SKELETAL MUSCLE FOLLOWING EXHAUSTIVE EXERCISE—PHYSICAL AND BIOCHEMICAL STUDIES

Contractile Properties

Although the studies of Ekelund et al. (30) and Saltin (88) offer indirect evidence of reduced myocardial contractility, it is the report of Maher et al. (69) which provides the strongest evidence that a decrease in the force of contraction is related to exhaustion. These investigators removed trabecular muscles from the left ventricles of sedentary, exercised, and exhausted rats. Peak isometric tension and velocity of shortening *in vitro* were both reduced in the exhausted group; no changes were found in the exercised but not exhausted group. Only the muscles from exhausted rats failed to respond to the inotropic effect of norepinephrine (NE).

Metabolic Properties

CARBOHYDRATE METABOLISM: As mentioned earlier, the depletion of endogenous muscle glycogen is associated with exhaustion produced by certain work intensities and durations. Costill's (22), Bergstrom's (12), and Hultman's (55) studies are representative of many studies in which glycogen depletion has been measured using either histochemical (PAS stain) or biochemical assay techniques. Glycogen depletion, or near depletion, is the contemporary *sine qua non* of skeletal muscle exhaustion. Barnard et al. (10) and Poland et al. (83, 84) have also reported similar large decreases in heart glycogen content with exhaustive exercise.

Dohm and colleagues (28, 29) have studied the effects of exhaustive exercise of both untrained and trained rats on several metabolic functions. Whole tissue (heart and skeletal muscle) homogenate glucose metabolism was unaffected by exhaustion. In trained, exhausted rats they did, however, find a decreased ability of the mitochondrial fractions to oxidize pyruvate-malate and succinate in both heart and skeletal muscle; there were no significant changes in untrained rats. (The differences between trained and untrained might be due, at least in part, to the differences in intensities and durations of exercise they would tolerate.) On the other hand Terjung et al. (102, 103) exhausted trained rats and were unable to detect reductions in metabolic capacity or control associated with exhaustion. It is very important to note that these metabolic studies were performed on homogenates under ideal conditions.

In summary, it is accepted that glycogen stores are depleted by long duration exhaustive exercise, but it is difficult to accept the contemporary concept that glycogen depletion per se is the sole cause of muscle failure. The effects of exhaustive exercise on metabolism *in vitro* are unclear, and *in vivo* changes are unknown.

LIPID METABOLISM: The ability to metabolize fats may be reduced by exhaustive exercise. Dohm et al. (29) also examined palmitate oxidation in the same study discussed above and found that palmitate oxidation of whole tissue homogenates was reduced in skeletal (-27%) and heart (-70%) muscle of untrained rats and in skeletal (-27%) and heart (-22%) muscle of trained rats. Askew et al. (4) reported both a decreased palmityl carnitine oxidation and a reduced mitochondrial yield (to be discussed below) in skeletal muscle of exhausted rats. Arcos (3) reported a total depletion of β-hydroxybutyric dehydrogenase when rats were swum to exhaustion, and Schmidt (89) has found increased concentrations of β-hydroxybutyrate in men following long duration work.

The limiting step in this FFA and ketone metabolism cannot be deduced from the data. Whether it is due to a decrease in citric acid cycle activity (28) or in the carnitine transferase systems is not yet an answerable question. Oram et al. (79) have reported that, at least for long chains, fatty acid metabolism in perfused hearts was limited by acylcarnitine transfer across the inner mitochondrial membrane. Askew et al. (5) attempted to increase carnitine levels, by feeding a diet high in carnitine; there was no effect on adipose fatty acid turnover during exercise. However, these authors did not examine the effects of the high carnitine diet on endurance performances or turnover at exhaustion.

It is interesting to note that perfusion of ischemic hearts with an FFA, palmitate-albumin, resulted in less mitochondrial swelling than that which occurred in glucose-perfused ischemic hearts (24). However, electron dense opacities replaced normal intramitochondrial granules. This may be evidence that, in a stressed heart, molecular changes in mitochondrial membranes do occur and that these changes affect (or are affected by) substrate uptake. Whether FFAs are toxic during exercise-induced failure is unknown, but if this is so it may be an explanation for exhaustion when lipids are the only substrates available. This deserves particular attention in the light of data from deLeiris et al. (24), which showed that when glucose was added to the palmitate-albumin perfusate there was a great reduction in the dense opacities.

Mitochondrial Yield

Several investigators have questioned the effect of exhaustive exercise on the ability of mitochondria to withstand fractionation processes, and the results are equivocal. Still, the fragility of mitochondria *in vitro* is a key issue in the author's research. Dohm et al. (28, 29) reported the skeletal muscle mitochondrial yield was decreased by exhaustive exercise of trained but not untrained rats. Askew (4) also reported a slightly decreased yield from exhausted skeletal muscle. Although the difference was not significant, yields from hearts of both trained and untrained, exhausted rats were lower than from resting animals.

Two well-designed studies by Terjung and his associates (102, 103) compared mitochondrial protein yield, respiratory capacities of both whole muscle homogenates and mitochondrial fractions, enzyme leakage, P:O ratios, and respiratory control index; they found no differences between resting and exhausted animals. Brooks et al. (18) had also reported no exhaustion-related damage to mitochondria as indicated by the inability of mitochondria to oxidize exogenous NADH, but they did find a loosened coupling of oxidative phosphorylation.

The equivocal results of studies by Askew et al. (4) and Dohm et al. (29), who found a decreased yield, and Terjung et al. (102, 103) may be due to the method of preparing the mitochondrial fraction. In both studies in which yield was reduced, the tissue was homogenized according to procedures described by Ernster and Nordenbrand (33), which included use of a medium containing 100 mM KCl, 50 mM Tris-HCl, 1 mM Na ATP, 5 mM $MgCl_2$, and 1 mM EDTA. Terjung and his associates used a medium containing 250 mM sucrose, 10 mM Tris-HCl, and 2 mM EDTA. Both labs adjusted pH to 7.4. As will be discussed later, Mg^{2+} and Ca^{2+} ions included during fixation procedures greatly affect mitochondrial ultrastructure; osmolality, to a lesser degree, also influences apparent morphology. Unfortunately, however, the protective effect of divalent cations on mitochondria from exhausted animals and their disruptive effect on mitochondria from resting animals (36) are unexpected in light of the differences in mitochondrial yields discussed above.

CHANGES IN HEART AND SKELETAL MUSCLE FOLLOWING EXHAUSTIVE EXERCISE— ULTRASTRUCTURAL STUDIES

Exercise

Parallel to the biochemical studies of exhaustion-induced decrements in metabolic capacities of muscle mitochondria, other laboratories were examining ultrastructural damage in the electron microscope. Laguens and his co-workers (64) swam untrained dogs ". . . until they became exhausted and sank into the water." Heart mitochondria were swollen and had reduced matrix density. Some had apparently fused to neighboring mitochondria, had partial vacuoles, or had disrupted cristae. Many studies followed Laguens et al.'s first report, and ultrastructural changes related to exhaustion were reported both in heart mitochondria (1, 3, 9, 23, 60, 63, 101) and in skeletal muscle mitochondria (2, 17, 37, 42, 95).

The generalized disruption of mitochondria and myofibrils was great in the micrographs of Gollnick and King (42) and King and Gollnick (60) in both skeletal and heart muscle, respectively. The disruption reported by Akuzawa et al. (2), Arcos et al. (3), Senger (95), and Taylor et al. (101) was similar. The ultrastructural disruption demonstrated in micrographs published by the other investigators (1, 9, 23, 63) was more focal and not as severe. The possible causes of this disruption and the probable reasons for differences are discussed below.

Related, Nonexercise, Causes of Mitochondrial Disruption

Certain pathological conditions also produce mitochondrial disruption similar to exercise-reported alterations, especially in heart muscle (113). Sixty minutes of ischemia irreversibly decreased matrical density and disorganized cristae (57). The metabolic function of these ischemia-exposed mitochondria was also impaired. Jurkowitz et al. (58) have discussed changes in the internal milieu of ischemic heart and reported that Na^+, P_i, lactate, and H^+ all increased, and each is known to be a mitochondrial swelling agent.

Raczniak et al. (85) have induced progressive heart failure by injecting monocrotaline pyrvole, thereby producing pulmonary heart disease. These investigators reported a reduced ADP:O ratio, diminished respiratory control index, and lower mitochondrial O_2 uptake. They concluded ". . . that mitochondria are one of the causative factors of heart failure."

Hearts perfused with deficient perfusates also evidenced mitochondrial alterations. Anoxia resulted in the leakage of enzymes but no apparent ultrastructural damage. However, reperfusion with a normoxic perfusate produced mitochondrial swelling and irregularities (50). Substrate-free perfusate reduced the ability of both mitochondria and sarcoplasmic reticulum to accumulate Ca^{2+}. The absence of Ca^{2+} itself produced mitochondrial damage, and reperfusion resulted in even greater disruption (14, 117) as did Ca^{2+} following hypoxia (82), perhaps due to Ca^{2+} activation of phospholipase-A (110) or due to its direct action on the mitochondrial membrane.

Hearse et al. (50) have compared biochemical data with ultrastructural studies of anoxic perfusion of arrested hearts. They have found that glucose protected glycogen, ATP, and CP levels and also protected against enzyme leakage and ultrastructural change in rats. This raises the possibility that in extended exercise low blood glucose levels [Huston et al. (56) reported reduced blood glucose associated with exhaustive exercise] may eventually be associated with reduced myocardial glycogen, which, in turn, leads to a reduced ATP concentration. Low ATP may lead to a conformational change in membrane proteins and a reduced water bonding (67). It could be that the increased intracellular free water alters the osmotic pressure and that in the more hypotonic milieu mitochondria are more susceptible to osmotic swelling, particularly during fixation.

Although a comparison of exercise and pathologically induced changes in ultrastructure cannot yet be made, Wollenberger (113) has initiated such a comparison, which may be fruitful. Dhalla (25) has emphasized the reaction of Ca^{2+} with membrane components in heart failure; the interaction of exercise and Ca^{2+} ions, which will be described below, may link exhaustion-related failure and ischemia-related failure.

CURRENT STUDIES

Exhaustion-Related Mitochondrial Disruption— A Meaningful Artifact

The author has investigated the conditions that might produce the greatest amount of exhaustion-associated mitochondrial disruption (38). Both trained and untrained rats were run to exhaustion. Rats, trained for 84 days, were examined after exhaustive runs that varied from 32 m/min for 195 min to 80 m/min for 9 min or they were killed after exercise of a duration less than that necessary to produce exhaustion. Untrained rats were also run to exhaustion or exercised at less than exhausting durations in a manner similar to that for trained rats.

Gastrocnemius and soleus muscles were removed immediately after exercise (from sodium pentobarbital anesthetized rats) and small sections were fixed in cacodylate buffered glutaraldehyde and post-fixed in osmium. Micrographs were quantitatively evaluated (111). There was no evidence of mitochondrial volume changes associated with exhaustive exercise. Mitochondria remained electron dense, cristae were preserved, and membranes were intact. The ultrastructure of mitochondria from both trained and untrained rats subjected to moderate and exhaustive exercise over a wide range of exercise intensity and duration combinations was unchanged.

While most investigations of the effects of exhaustive exercise upon mitochondrial structure did reveal disruption, several laboratories, in agreement with the findings discussed above, reported that there was no or little change in morphology. Tomanek and Banister (104) refined the fixation techniques from their earlier study, in which they reported mitochondrial disruption (9), and reported that mitochondrial disruption did not occur when they perfused the heart with fixative rather than immersing the tissue in fixative. Similarly, nondisrupted mitochondria were found by Maher et al. (69) following *in vitro* exhaustion of trabecular muscle, and by Cvorkov, Banister, and Liskop (23), although the later investigators did report (slight) swelling until their rats had been trained for three days. Bowers and his associates (17) reported both mitochondrial disruption in some animals and no disruption in others, depending on the fixation procedures.

Real changes in mitochondrial membranes may be related to these equivocal results observed when different methodologies are used. In light of the finding of exhaustion-related "increased susceptibility to swelling" reported by Sembrowich et al. (94) and similar findings in the author's laboratory (to be discussed later), it may be that the differences in technique that produce different results may be the key to understanding the effects of exhaustion on mitochondria and/or the role that mitochondrial change plays in the exhaustion process.

Relation between Method of Fixation and Morphology

The greatest amounts of swelling associated with exhaustive exercise were, with one exception (101), found in muscle fixed only with osmium (2, 42, 60). Arcos (3) reported similar disruption with chronic training (a program that was more like daily bouts of exhaustive exercise) and also used osmium as the primary fixative.

Banister et al. (9) and Cvorkov et al. (23) reported some focal swelling associated with exhaustive exercise, but their micrographs showed much less disruption than the studies mentioned above. Banister et al. and Cvorkov et al. both used glutaraldehyde as the primary fixative and postfixed in osmium. All of the studies that reported no effect of exhaustive exercise used glutaraldehyde as the primary fixative (17, 37, 69, 104).

There have been only 3 reports of severe disruption when glutaraldehyde was the primary fixative following exercise. In 2 of these, the animals were untrained and subjected to near drowning (64, 95). Taylor (101) ran guinea pigs to exhaustion. Senger weighted his rats sufficiently to produce exhaustion in only about 10 minutes while Laguens et al.'s dogs swam for 40 to 90 minutes. The source of these equivocal results is unknown, but it is conceivable that hypoxia or general sympathetic responses may have been more dominant than the effects of exercise alone. The author has since attempted to replicate Taylor et al.'s results and found no mitochondrial disruption in either trained or untrained guinea pigs when glutaraldehyde was the primary fixative (unpublished data). Taylor and his associates used a very low concentration of cacodylate buffer, only 1% (0.047 M), and few (N = 2) animals. The disagreement cannot be accounted for, but at this time, it is doubtful that there is a species-related difference in response to fixation and/or exhaustion such as might have been expected from other reported species-related differences. For example, Nayler et al. (76, 77) have reported differences in mitochondrial Ca^{2+} uptake kinetics between rats and guinea pigs, Seabra-Gomes (93) reported differences in response to hypoxia, and Saito (87) found differences in mitochondrial respiratory function during heart failure.

The author has examined the effects of both primary glutaraldehyde (cacodylate buffered) and primary osmium (veronal acetate buffered) fixations on adjacent sections of both heart and
skeletal muscles from rats at rest, moderately exercised, and exercised to exhaustion (37). While muscle from resting or moderately
exercised rats appeared similar and normal when either primary
fixative was used, great differences between the fixations were
observed when the muscles were excised from exhausted rats.
Muscle fixed in glutaraldehyde appeared no different from resting, but adjacent samples from the same exhausted rat fixed in
osmium were severely disrupted. Mitochondria were swollen and
electron lucid, cristae decreased in number, and in some instances
both inner and outer membranes were disrupted. There was also
swelling of the sarcoplasmic reticulum and tearing of myofibrils.
Unlike some reports of only focal damage (42), the disruption was
found in every portion of tissue examined, deep fiber, perinu-
clear, and subsarcolemmal. Mitochondrial disruption associated
with exhaustive exercise was artifactual and related to the method
of fixation. Significantly, both sarcolemma and nuclear membranes were not disrupted.

That the buffer might also affect fixation was later considered.
Those who used osmium as the primary fixative (3, 42, 60, 63)
used either veronal acetate or phosphate buffers. Investigators,
including the author, who used glutaraldehyde (9, 17, 23, 37, 69,
104) used either cacodylate or phosphate buffers. No pattern that
would implicate buffers, alone, as a swelling agent was found.

Although it seemed apparent that mitochondrial swelling associated with exhaustive exercise was probably artifactual and not
an *in vivo* occurrence, a more thorough investigation of the interaction between exercised state and fixatives and buffers was
initiated because this approach might be a means of exploring *in
situ* exhaustion-related changes in components within mitochondrial membranes. Such reasoning is consistent with the data of
Fortes (34) who reported that glutaraldehyde reacted differently
with mitochondrial suspensions depending upon their metabolic
state. Fortes has suggested that this reaction could be used as a
"probe of metabolism-linked changes in the mitochondrial proteins." Either different states of ionization or conformation of the
membrane proteins, which may have been associated with different metabolic states, were thought to have affected the reaction

with glutaraldehyde. Packer et al. (80) have demonstrated that conformational changes related to metabolism do occur.

ELECTRON MICROSCOPY

General Comparison of Fixatives and Buffers

That the method of fixation can affect apparent ultrastructure has been well documented (35, 53, 72, 86, 106, 114), and in fact, it is fixation artifact that has contributed to the controversy over the structure of membranes, e.g. Sjostrand (98) versus Vendenheuvel (108). Hayat (48) and Sjostrand (97) have both written detailed reviews in their texts that provide some summaries and explanations for the differences in observed ultrastructure. However, the exact sites of interaction of fixatives and the buffering media with membrane components, as well as the conformation and arrangement of these components, are yet unknown. No one other than Fortes (34) has considered the possibility that these reactions may also be affected by metabolic states.

Osmium tetroxide is an oxidizing agent that fixes tissues by cross-linking, but it also reacts without cross-linking and may result in loss of some components. Bahr (7), in a momentous study, examined the reactivity of osmium with many compounds and found it especially reactive with double bonds and sulfhydryl groups. In general, osmium is a lipid fixative, cross-linking unsaturated double bonds (61). However, it is important to note that osmium also reacts strongly with amino acids in peptides and may result in the loss of proteins (73). Prolonged immersion may also produce structural damage (74). Luftig et al. (68) and Sjostrand (98) have reviewed this area and demonstrated that osmium fixation may greatly affect the appearance of membranes, including mitochondrial membranes. Osmium denatures and/or removes both integral and peripheral proteins. These reactions may depend upon the conformational state of the proteins affected by strenuous exercise, although contemporary methodology precludes direct proof.

Glutaraldehyde, a 5 carbon dialdehyde-reducing agent, forms intermolecular and intramolecular cross-links with proteins, especially free amino groups as well as sulfhydryls and phenolic and imadazole rings. It is less reactive with lipids than is osmium. Its use for electron microscopy has been encouraged because it penetrates more rapidly than osmium, and its concentration and duration of tissue exposure (86) are not as critical. In small concentrations glutaraldehyde, in comparison to osmium, does not alter the function of proteins (81, 107), and, therefore is useful for histochemical work in electron microscopy (49, 86). More importantly, glutaraldehyde's failure to denature proteins or to induce changes in the mitochondrial inner membrane (44) may be a clue to understanding the basic changes related to osmium-exhaustion mitochondrial swelling and glutaraldehyde-exhaustion nonswelling.

Buffers may also affect the apparent morphology of tissue prepared for electron microscopy. Trump and Ericsson (106) found, in hepatic tissue, that mitochondrial contour, matrical density, and the presence of intercristal space all varied when osmium was used with each of 7 different buffers or distilled water. Wood and Luft (114) also examined apparent morphology when several buffers were each used with osmium; they too reported that differences in apparent mitochondrial morphology were related to the buffers. These investigators also modified the molarity of the fixatives by adding either salts or nonionic substances. Of great interest to the author's investigation was their finding of a "specific ion effect" greater than the effects of tonicity alone. The author has studied the effects of several divalent cations and found that morphology is greatly affected (36). This will be discussed later.

Effects of Fixatives and Buffers on Resting and Exhausted Muscles

In order to better understand the phenomenon of differential fixation artifact, a series of fixative-buffer combinations has been performed. Adjacent samples of muscle from each rat were fixed, using at least 2 of the selected methods, and all procedures were carried out in parallel. The schedule for fixations on both resting and exhausted rats is presented in Table 7-I.

Buffer selection was based on several considerations. Cacodylate has been used previously, with glutaraldehyde, in studies that have reported no mitochondrial alteration with exhaustive exercise (17, 37, 69, 104). It has not been used with osmium in exercise studies. Collidine was selected because its pK of 7.4 (11) makes it an excellent buffer in the physiologic pH range. Phosphate buffered glutaraldehyde was used by Banister et al. (9) and by Cvorkov et al. (23) who both reported some swelling in untrained rats.

TABLE 7-I

SCHEDULE OF FIXATIVE AND BUFFER COMBINATIONS INVESTIGATED

Buffers	Fixatives*	
	Osium	Gluteraldehyde
Cacodylate	S	S H
Collidine	S	S
Millonig's Phosphate	S	S
Veronal Acetate	S H	
Veronal Acetate w/Ringers	S H	

*Primary fixatives. Glutaraldehyde fixation was always followed by osmium postfixation; osmium was used alone.

S = Soleus

H = Heart

Laguens et al. (63) used both phosphate or veronal acetate buffered osmium and reported swelling. Gollnick and King (42) and King and Gollnick (60) used veronal acetate buffered osmium and demonstrated extreme mitochondrial disruption.

Strict adherence to procedures was maintained. All fixatives were adjusted to pH 7.38 to 7.42. Glutaraldehyde fixatives were carried out in the cold (0–3°C) for 2 hours and then postfixed for 1 hour in osmium, using the same buffer as used with the particular glutaraldehyde buffer fixation. Osmium fixations were carried out in the cold for 1 hour. Samples were dehydrated in graded ethanol series and propylene oxide and embedded in Epon®. Sections were cut, placed on copper grids, and stained with lead citrate and uranyl acetate. Examination was made with a Zeiss EM9A electron microscope.

Primary fixation of resting muscles with glutaraldehyde or osmium both resulted, with slight variations, in normal appearing mitochondria. All glutaraldehyde fixations in each buffer were similar. When osmium was buffered with cacodylate, s-collidine, and Millonig's phosphate the mitochondria were less electron dense when compared to the glutaraldehyde fixations and veronal acetate buffered osmium.

There were no ultrastructural changes following exhaustive exercise when glutaraldehyde was used, but regardless of the buffer, every osmium fixation of exhausted muscle was associated with mitochondrial disruption. Osmolality may have been a factor. While each of the glutaraldehyde fixatives was estimated to be about 500 mOsmol, the osmium fixatives were between 240 and 260 mOsmol (71). Therefore, both skeletal and heart muscles from resting and exhausted rats were subsequently fixed in a Ringer's-veronal acetate buffered osmium solution whose osmolality was about 340 mOsmol (48). The Ringer's contained Na^+, K^+, Ca^{2+}, and Cl^- ions.

A very surprising combination of results was found. Resting muscle mitochondria (which, heretofore, were electron dense and unswollen) were now electron lucid and swollen. Conversely, mitochondria in exhausted muscles were now electron dense and not disrupted.

Role of Ca^{2+} Ions in Electron Microscopy

One ingredient in the Ringer's solution, Ca^{2+}, deserved closer scrutiny. It is biologically active and "reacts" with mitochondria, sarcoplasmic reticulum, and contractile proteins in muscle. Although Ca^{2+} has been identified as a swelling agent *in vitro* (13), it has also been used in electron microscopy to improve membrane fixation (41, 48), perhaps by cross-linking phosphate groups of phospholipids and reducing the movement of membrane proteins. In fact, Hardonk et al. (45) have reported that Ca^{2+} ions alone prevented diffusion of some membrane enzymes.

Ca^{2+} has been used by other investigators who reported that exhaustive exercise did not affect mitochondrial ultrastructure. Terjung et al. (103) had published a micrograph of heart tissue from an exhausted rat that showed no disruption and was in agreement with their biochemical data. They used phosphate-pyrophosphate buffered osmium as the primary fixative, but they had added Ca^{2+} to their fixative (R.L. Terjung, personal communication Dec., 1973).

Although one laboratory has reported that Ca^{2+} also interacts with glutaraldehyde to produce mitochondrial swelling in exhausted skeletal muscle (17) the author's data (unpublished) and that of others who examined heart muscle (52, 104) suggest that mitochondrial morphology is unaffected by Ca^{2+} when glutaraldehyde is the primary fixative.

Experimental Results of the Effects of Ca^{2+} Ions on Morphology

In order to better understand the role that Ca^{2+} exerts on apparent ultrastructure, heart and skeletal muscles were prepared from exhausted, moderately exercised, and rested rats in 4 different 1% osmium fixatives: veronal acetate, veronal acetate with Ringer's (containing 1.13 mM Ca^{2+}), veronal acetate with Ca^{2+} free

TABLE 7-II

THE EFFECT OF VARIABLE Ca²⁺ CONCENTRATION ON
MITOCHONDRIAL ULTRASTRUCTURE*

	Veronal	Veronal w/Ringer's	Veronal w/Ringer's w/o Ca²⁺	Veronal 3 mM Ca²⁺
Exhausted	+	0	+0	0+
Moderately exercised	0	0+ (H) 0 (S)	0	+
Resting	0	0+	0	+ (H) +0 (S)

*Except where noted descriptions are for both heart and soleus muscles.
S = Soleus
H = Heart
+ = Disruption
0 = No Disruption
+>+0>0+>0

Ringer's, and veronal acetate with 3 mM Ca^{2+}. In each of the animals used, adjacent samples were prepared simultaneously in each of the 4 fixatives. Ringer's without Ca^{2+} was prepared by substituting Na^+ to maintain iso-osmolarity. Two exhausted rats were also prepared using a 1 mM Ca^{2+}-veronal acetate as well as the 3 mM Ca^{2+} concentration used throughout this series. The results of this investigation are reported in Table 7-II. Micrographs of both resting (Fig. 7-1), and exhausted (Fig. 7-2), muscles demonstrate the differences in fixation.

Ca^{2+} exerted a considerable effect upon the ultrastructure of mitochondria both from exhausted and moderately exercised or rested rats. Veronal acetate buffered osmium alone was associated with extreme disruption of mitochondria in both heart and skeletal muscle of exhausted animals. The addition of 3 mM Ca^{2+} preserved the ultrastructure, almost to resting associated levels; 1 mM Ca^{2+} also demonstrated the same effect but to a lesser degree, i.e. the effect of Ca^{2+} was concentration dependent, at least for the two concentrations investigated. Ringer's with Ca^{2+} was characterized by good fixation and more matrix material than with 3 mM Ca^{2+} alone. Removal of the Ca^{2+} from the Ringer's resulted in the apparent loss of cristae, but a moderate level of matrix material remained.

However, a paradox existed. Ca^{2+} prevented swelling in *in vitro* fixation of tissues normally exhibiting gross swelling, while its presence in fixatives used on rested or only moderately exercised animals resulted in mitochondrial swelling. Swelling was not ap-

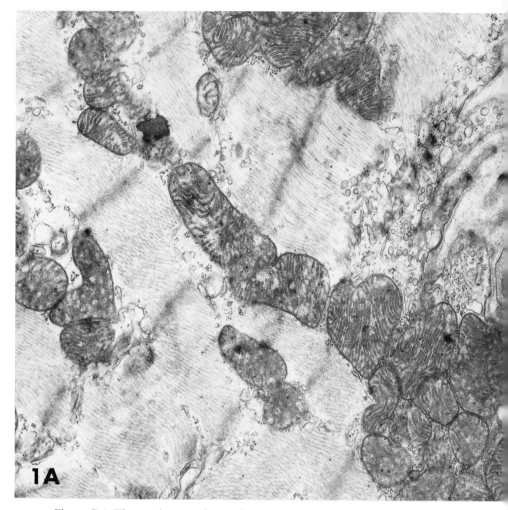

Figure 7-1. These micrographs are from adjacent sections of the apex of the left ventricle of a rat killed *at rest*. All samples were fixed in 1% OsO_4 and buffered in various solutions. ×17,500.
A. Buffered in veronal acetate.

parent in Ca^{2+} free fixatives of resting or moderately exercised tissues.

Slight differences between heart and skeletal muscle were noted. This should not be viewed with surprise. Mitochondria vary between species, organs, and even locations within a single organ (54, 59, 75). Perhaps these differences in response may eventually prove useful in understanding this phenomenon.

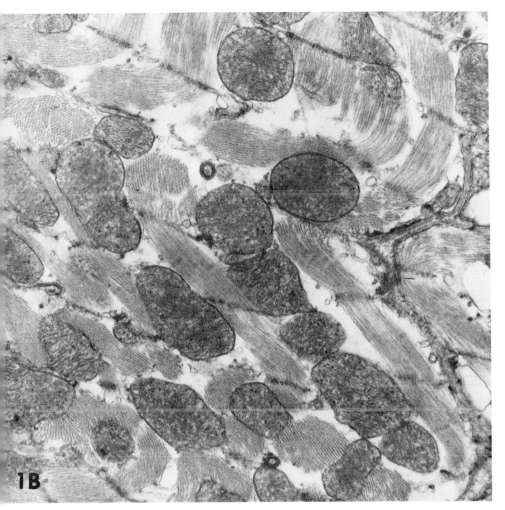

Figure 7-1*B*. Buffered in veronal acetate and Ringer's without Ca^{2+}.

ROLE OF OTHER DIVALENT CATIONS AND Ca^{2+} ION UPTAKE

Inhibition on Ultrastructure

Preliminary data on the effects of substituting other divalent cations for Ca^{2+} ions has been reported (36); 3 mM concentrations of Mg^{2+}, Sr^{2+}, Ba^{2+}, and Mn^{2+}, as well as Ca^{2+}, have been used in 1% Os, vernonal acetate buffered fixatives. Simultaneous fixations in each of these solutions (as well as veronal acetate, 0.1% ruthenium

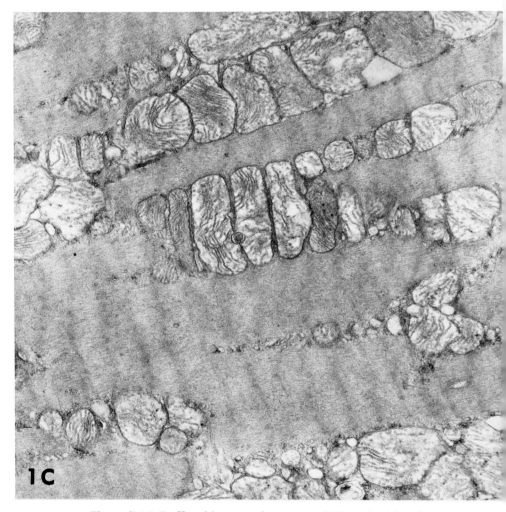

Figure 7-1C. Buffered in veronal acetate and Ringer's with Ca^{2+}.

red, and ruthenium red plus Ca^{2+}) were carried out on exhausted and resting rats. These data revealed qualitative differences in mitochondrial ultrastructure.

Assuming that both mitochondrial disruption in resting animals and maintenance of structure in exhausted animals are the result of cation binding, the (tentative) relative binding strengths are given below:

Rest $Ca^{2+} > Mg^{2+} = Ba^{2+} > Sr^{2+} > Mn^{2+}$

Exhaustion $Ba^{2+} > Mn^{2+} > Mg^{2+} > Ca^{2+} > Sr^{2+}$

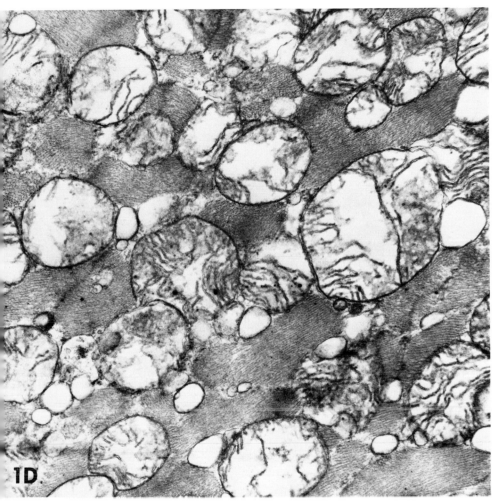

Figure 7-1*D*. Buffered in veronal acetate with 3 mM Ca^{2+}.

Calcium produced the greatest disruption at rest. This is in agreement with the data of Parr et al. (82) who reported that Ca^{2+} caused greater mitochondrial damage in heart muscle, following hypoxia, than did Ba^{2+}, Mn^{2+}, or Sr^{2+}. However, Ca^{2+} was not as effective as Ba^{2+}, Mn^{2+}, or Mg^{2+} in preventing the disruption normally observed in the osmium fixed, exhausted muscles.

The effects of Mn^{2+} are quite uncertain. It probably reacted with osmium, even though the osmium was added to the buffer just before the tissues were prepared (the fixative turned gray

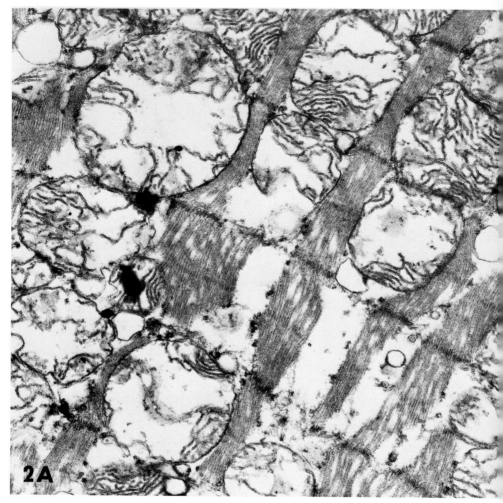

Figure 7-2. These micrographs are from adjacent sections of the apex of the left ventricle of a rat killed immediately *after exhaustive exercise.* All samples were fixed in 1% OsO_4 and buffered in various solutions. ×17,500.
A. Buffered in veronal acetate.

before tissue was added).

Hauser et al. (47) have reviewed the literature dealing with the affinity of several divalent cations to both phospholipid and protein components of membranes. They have reported the following relative affinities:

Phospholipid $Ca^{2+} > Mg^{2+} > Sr^{2+} > Ba^{2+}$
Proteins $Ca^{2+} > Sr^{2+} > Ba^{2+} > Mg^{2+}$

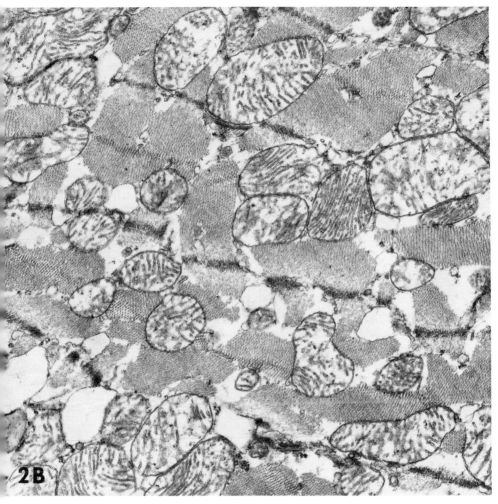

Figure 7-2B. Buffered in veronal acetate and Ringer's without Ca^{2+}.

The relative effect of the ions the author has used for resting muscles most closely matches the relative affinity of these divalent cations for phospholipids, although Ba^{2+} and Sr^{2+} are out of order. Of course, judging relative degrees of fixation is certainly a poor measure of affinity, but it may be a starting place.

The inclusion of ruthenium red with Ca^{2+} did affect the ultrastructure. At rest, Ca^{2+} no longer produced disruption. However, ruthenium red, alone, was now associated with disruption. No rat presumed to be exhausted demonstrated mitochondrial disrup-

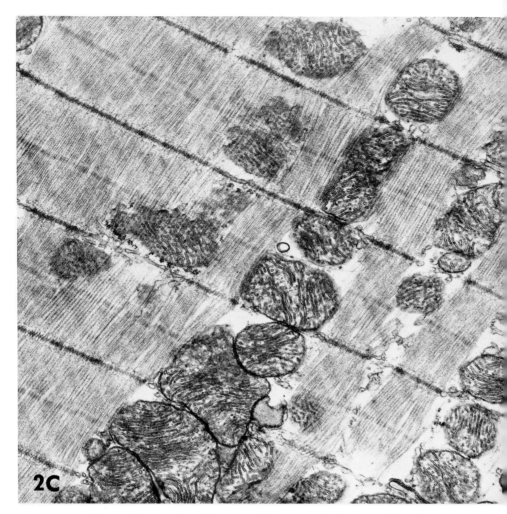

Figure 7-2C. Buffered in veronal acetate and Ringer's with Ca^{2+}.

tion with the standard veronal acetate buffered osmium without
cations, and therefore an evaluation of the effects of ruthenium
red with Ca^{2+} associated with exhaustion could not be made.
Ruthenium red, alone, produced variable effects between adjacent fibers in a rat thought to be exhausted that did not show
osmium-related disruption.

Ruthenium red is an excellent compound to use in further
studies. It is a mucopolysaccharide stain that is compatible with
electron microscopy. Quite importantly, it is also an inhibitor of

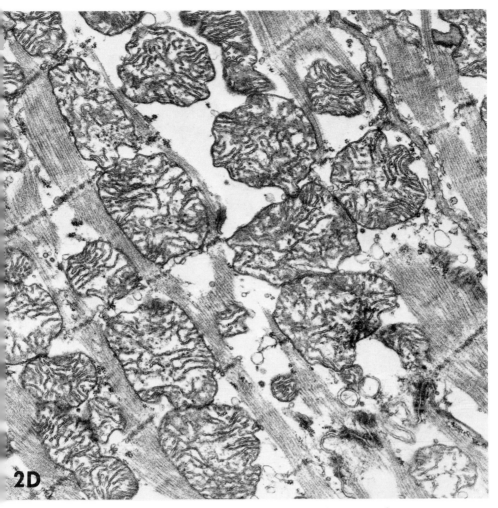

Figure 7-2*D*. Buffered in veronal acetate with 3 mM Ca^{2+}.

mitochondrial Ca^{2+} uptake (109). Parr et al. (82) found that ruthenium red provided complete protection against Ca^{2+} disruption of mitochondrial phosphorylation following hypoxia, in homogenate preparations. Ruthenium red may bind on or near cytochrome c (Schwerzman, 1976), which has been implicated as a possible carrier of Ca^{2+} across the inner membrane (70).

Cytochrome c binds Ca^{2+} only in the reduced state. Margoliash (70) and Lehninger et al. (66) have reported that mitochondrial Ca^{2+} uptake occurs in the presence of NADH and the cation is released when the pyridine nucleotide is oxidized. Although no connection can be made at this time, it seems promising to look to integral proteins that, if they were to change conformation and/or oxidation-reduction states, might affect metabolism by regulating Ca^{2+} concentrations in cellular compartments. That these, or similar, changes might be reflected in apparent ultrastructural changes in different fixation milieu is the major thrust of the author's studies.

Ca^{2+} Responses with Mitochondria

The relationship of Ca^{2+} and mitochondria has been studied extensively; Kretsinger (62) has reviewed more recent research relating to Ca^{2+} binding proteins. Ca^{2+} uptake and/or binding, as well as release, may (most simplistically) serve to regulate the intramitochondrial and/or the cytoplasmic milieu (31). There have been many reported investigations of mitochondrial Ca^{2+} uptake (which have identified high and low affinity sites and measured the kinetics of these reactions); the reason(s) for Ca^{2+} uptake is (are) still not firmly established. However, Ca^{2+} is known to inhibit [e.g. isocitrate dehydrogenase (in the mitochondrial matrix) (118)] and to stimulate [e.g. phosphorylase (in the extramitochondrial spaces) and mitochondrial membrane bound enzymes such as α-glycerol phosphate dehydrogenase, pyruvate dehydrogenase phosphate phosphatase, and pyruvate dehydrogenase (62)], as well as allowing the oxidation of extramitochondrial NADH (40).

In vitro Ca^{2+} uptake may be affected by exercise. Bonner and his colleagues (16) have recently reported that *in vitro* heart mitochondrial Ca^{2+} uptake was reduced by short duration exhaustive exercise that preceded homogenation, but the reduction was significant only in trained rats. Bonner et al. (16) and Sordahl et al. (100) have also reported that training has produced a reduction in resting mitochondrial Ca^{2+} content in *in vivo* and *in vitro*, respectively. Conversely, electron micrographs of exhausted skeletal muscle have shown swollen mitochondria with dense granules presumed to be Ca^{2+} (43). It was proposed that the mitochondria had trapped the Ca^{2+} that the sarcoplasmic reticulum could no longer sequester. This is in agreement with Hashimoto et al. (46) who reported large reductions in sarcoplasmic reticulum Ca^{2+} uptake following long duration exhaustive exercise.

A related role for Ca^{2+} uptake by mitochondria in heart tissue has most recently been suggested. Carafoli (19) and Carafoli et al. (21) have hypothesized that mitochondria, in conjunction with the sarcoplasmic reticulum, regulate the Ca^{2+} concentration in the excitation-contraction cycle of heart muscle.

The mechanism for either Ca^{2+} maintenance of ultrastructure in exhausted tissue or its disruptive effect in nonexhausted tissue cannot be clearly predicted. At this time, a most simple explanation might be that critical anionic sites on membrane proteins (metabolic or structural?; integral or peripheral?) become exposed, perhaps by a pH-induced (115) or [ATP] reduction-induced (67) protein conformation alteration. Of course, Ca^{2+} binding to phospholipids (91) or glycoproteins (20) cannot be excluded, but Dohm et al. (27) have concluded that changes in phospholipid composition were not responsible for exhaustion-related changes in skeletal muscle mitochondrial structure and function. However, there could be mitochondrial changes related to phospholipid changes not reflected in alterations in composition; the issue is not resolved.

Binding by some divalent ions may in some way hold the membrane together, perhaps by simply reducing the net negative charge (*cf.* 32). A more complex hypothesis would include an osmium-Ca^{2+}-tissue interaction, e.g. it has been reported that osmium lowers the isoelectric point (105), and if this occurs, there might be an exposure of more negative sites for Ca^{2+} to bind. In these models, there must be both sites that, when attached to a Ca^{2+}, either promote maintenance (exhaustive state) or cause disruption (nonexhaustive state) of mitochondrial ultrastructure; Ca^{2+} binding sites may only be exposed during certain conditions. An incomplete explanation for this latter idea evolves from the work of Leblanc and Clausen (65). They found that Ca^{2+} displacement of Mg^{2+} induced structural changes in heart mitochondrial membranes, and this displacement was prevented by ADP. At rest when [ADP] is low Mg^{2+} would be more vulnerable to displacement than during exercise when [ADP] is higher. (However, this only explains a possible mechanism for Ca^{2+} disruption at rest but does not explain Ca^{2+} maintenance of ultrastructure with exhaustion.)

Yarom et al. (116) have shown that endogenous Ca^{2+} was, indeed, affected by the fixative used in preparation of dog heart. Using microprobe techniques these investigators found that Ca^{2+}

retention was greater with osmium fixation than with glutaraldehyde fixation. In a related study, glutaraldehyde fixation of
skeletal muscle has been shown to result in gross ionic mobility
and even extraction of ions, including Ca^{2+}, in the trough liquid
during sectioning (99). Therefore, the hypothesis that osmium
affects Ca^{2+} binding sites seems quite tenable, even though the
mechanism is unknown.

SIMILARITIES BETWEEN EXHAUSTION, FAILURE, AND DISEASE

The work described may also be related to pathological heart
failure. Dhalla (25, 26) has pointed out that heart failure cannot
always be explained by defects in ATP production or utilization,
and that membrane systems are primarily affected by several factors known to be related to heart malfunction. Intracellular Ca^{2+}
deficiency and overload both produced adverse effects on contractility, metabolism, and ultrastructure (117) and mitochrondrial
Ca^{2+} uptake was greater in failing hearts (90). Ca^{2+} sensitivity in
fixation is an important factor common to both heart disease and
exercise.

The similarity between pathogen-induced changes on
mitochondrial membranes and the author's studies is intriguing.
Astrom et al. (6) examined the effects of viral and mycoplasma
infections on skeletal muscle mitochondria. She and her colleagues performed parallel fixations with both glutaraldehyde
and osmium as the primary fixatives. Mitochondrial disruption
was found in infected patients when the muscle was fixed with
osmium, but there was none when glutaraldehyde was used. No
alterations in ultrastructure were found in biopsies from healthy
subjects, and only the mitochondria were affected by the method
of fixation.

SUMMARY

Artifactual disruption of heart and skeletal muscle mitochondria is associated with metabolic status, osmium fixation, and the
presence of divalent cations. It appears that components of the
inner and cristae membranes and/or the endogenous milieu
undergo changes during exhaustive exercise that allow this disruption to occur, and it is likely that these are, or result in, conformational changes of membrane proteins.

Because these changes are quite transient and susceptible to the *in vitro* environment, the exact nature of these changes is difficult to discern. Biochemical techniques alone will not be sufficient because of the homogenization and fractionating procedures that occur in a favorable supernatant, whereas contemporary EM chemical fixation techniques allow rapid *in situ* stabilization. These techniques, albeit imperfect, coupled with frozen section, freeze fracture, etc., may eventually provide sufficient evidence to describe changes at the molecular level that are related to heart and/or skeletal muscle failure. Yet, optimism must be tempered by the realization that the development of a testable model surely awaits a much more certain description of the construction of the mitochondrial membranes themselves.

REFERENCES

1. Aldinger, E.E. and R.S. Sohal: Effects of digitoxin on the ultrastructural myocardial changes in the rat subjected to chronic exercise. *Am J Cardiol, 26*:369, 1970.

2. Akuzawa, M. and M. Hataya: Ultrastructural alterations in skeletal muscle fibers of rats after exercise. *Jpn J Vet Sci, 40*:425, 1978.

3. Arcos, J.C.; R.S. Sohal; S.C. Sun; M.F. Argus; and G.E. Burch: Changes in ultrastructure and respiratory control in mitochondria of rat heart hypertrophied by exercise. *Exp Mol Pathol, 8*:49, 1968.

4. Askew, E.W.; G.L. Dohm; and R.L. Huston: Fatty acid and ketone body metabolism in the rat: response to diet and exercise. *J Nutr, 105*:1422, 1975.

5. Askew, E.W.; A.L. Hecker; and W.R. Wise, Jr.: Dietary carnitine and adipose tissue turnover rate in exercise trained rats. *J Nutr, 107*:132, 1977.

6. Astrom, E.; G. Friman; and L. Pilstrom: Effects of viral and mycoplasma infections on the ultrastructure of human skeletal muscle. *Scand J Infect Dis, 7*:273, 1975.

7. Bahr, G.F.: Osmium tetroxide and ruthenium tetroxide and their reactions with biologically important substances. Electron stains III. *Exp Cell Res, 7*:457, 1954.

8. Baldwin, K.M., J.S. Reitman, R.L. Terjung, W.W. Winder, and J.O. Holloszy: Substrate depletion in different types of muscle and in liver during prolonged running. *Am J Physiol, 225*:1045, 1973.

9. Banister, E.W.; R.J. Tomanek; and N. Cvorkov: Ultrastructural modifications in rat heart: responses to exercise and training. *Am J Physiol, 220*:1935, 1971.

10. Barnard, R.J. and A.T. Thorstensson: Effect of exhaustive exercise on the rat. In *Metabolic Adaptation to Prolonged Physical Exercise*, edited by H. Howald and J.R. Poortmans. Basel, Switzerland, Birkhauser Verlag, 1975.

11. Bennett, H.S. and J.H. Luft: S-collidine as a basis for buffering fixatives. *J Biophys Biochem Cytol, 6*:113, 1959.
12. Bergstrom, J.; G. Guarnieri; and E. Hultman: Changes in muscle water and electrolytes during exercise. In *Limiting Factors of Physical Performance*, edited by J. Keul. Stuttgart, Georg Thieme Publishers, 1973.
13. Blondin, G.A. and D.E. Green: The mechanism of mitochondrial swelling. *Proc Natl Acad Sci USA, 58*:612, 1967.
14. Boink, A.B.T.J.; T.J.C. Ruigrok; A.H.J. Mass; and A.N.E. Zimmerman: Changes in high-energy phosphate compounds of isolated rat hearts during Ca^{2+}-free perfusion and reperfusion with Ca^{2+}. *J Mol Cell Cardiol, 8*:973, 1970.
15. Bonner, H.W.; C.K. Buffington; and S.W. Leslie: Influence of exercise training and exhaustion on $^{45}Ca^{++}$ content of skeletal muscle mitochondria and fragmented sarcoplasmic reticulum. *Res Commun Chem Pathol Pharmacol, 18*:737, 1977.
16. Bonner, H.W.; S.W. Leslie; A.B. Combs; and C.A. Tate: Effects of exercise training and exhaustion on ^{45}Ca uptake by rat skeletal muscle mitochondria and sarcoplasmic reticulum. *Res Commun Chem Pathol Pharmacol, 14*:767, 1976.
17. Bowers, W.D., Jr.; R.W. Hubbard; J.A. Smoake; R.C. Daum; and E. Nilson: Effects of exercise on the ultrastructure of skeletal muscle. *Am J Physiol, 227*:313, 1974.
18. Brooks, G.A.; K.J. Hittleman; J.A. Faulkner; and R.E. Beyer: Temperature, skeletal muscle mitochondrial functions, and oxygen debt. *Am J Physiol, 220*:1053, 1971.
19. Carafoli, E.: Mitochondria, Ca^{2+} transport and the regulation of heart contraction and metabolism. *J Mol Cell Cardiol, 7*:83, 1975.
20. Carafoli, E.: The interaction of Ca^{2+} with mitochondria, with special reference to the structural role of Ca^{2+} in mitochondrial and other membranes. *Mol Cell Biochem, 8*:133, 1975.
21. Carafoli, E.; R. Dabrowska; F. Crovetti; R. Tiozzo; and W. Drabikowski: An in vitro study of the interaction of heart mitochondria with troponin bound Ca^{2+}. *Biochem Biophys Res Commun, 62*:908, 1975.
22. Costill, D.L.; P.D. Gollnick; E.D. Jansson; B. Saltin; and E.M. Stein: Glycogen depletion pattern in human muscle fibers during distance running. *Acta Physiol Scand, 89*:374, 1973.
23. Cvorkov, N.; E.W. Banister; and K.S. Lisop: Effect of high-protein diet on rat heart mitochondria after exhaustive exercise. *Am J Physiol, 226*:996, 1974.
24. DeLeiris, J. and D. Feuvray: Ischaemia-induced damage in the working rat heart preparation: The effect of perfusate substrate composition upon subendocadial ultrastructure of the ischaemic left ventricular wall. *J Mol Cell Cardiol, 9*:365, 1977.
25. Dhalla, N.S.: Involvement of membrane systems in heart failure due to intracellular calcium overload and deficiency. *J Mol Cell Cardiol, 8*:661, 1976.
26. Dhalla, N.S.; P.V. Sulakhe; M. Fedelesova; and J.C. Yates: Molecular ab-

normalities in cardiomyopathy. *Comparative Pathology of the Heart Advances in Cardiology,* (Basel, Switzerland, Karger), *13*:282-300, 1974.
27. Dohm, G.L.; H. Barakat; T.P. Stephenson; S.N. Pennington; and E.B. Tapscott: Changes in muscle mitochondrial lipid composition resulting from training and exhaustive exercise. *Life Sci, 17*:1075, 1975.
28. Dohm, G.L.; R.L. Huston; E.W. Askew; and H.L. Fleshood: Effect of exercise, training, and diet on muscle citric acid cycle enzyme activity. *Can J Biochem, 51*:849, 1973.
29. Dohm, G.L.; R.L. Huston; E.W. Askew; and P.C. Weiser: Effects of exercise on activity of heart and muscle mitochondria. *Am J Physiol, 223*:783, 1972.
30. Ekelund, L.G.; A. Holmgren; and C.O. Ovenfors: Heart volume during prolonged exercise in the supine and sitting position. *Acta Physiol Scand, 70*:88, 1967.
31. Elbrink, J. and I. Bihler: Membrane transport: its relation to cellular metabolic rates. *Science, 188*:1177, 1975.
32. Ericson, S.: Determination of the isoelectric point of rat liver mitochondria by cross-partition. *Biochim Biophys Acta, 356*:100, 1974.
33. Ernster, L. and K. Nordenbrand: Skeletal muscle mitochondria. In *Methods in Enzymology, Vol. 10. Oxidation and Phosphorylation,* edited by R.W. Estabrook and M.E. Pullman. New York, Academic Press, 1967.
34. Fortes, P.H.: Glutaraldehyde as a probe of metabolism-linked changes in the mitochondrial proteins. In *Probes of Structure and Function of Macromolecules and Membranes,* edited by B. Chance, C. Lee, and J.K. Blaise. New York, Acad Pr, 1971
35. Franke, W.W.; S. Krien; and R.M. Brown, Jr.: Simultaneous glutaraldehyde-osmium tetroxide fixation with postosmication. *Histochemie, 19*:162, 1969.
36. Gale, J.B.: Differential effects of fixatives, buffers and ionic species on the ultrastructure of heart mitochondria from resting and exhausted rats. *J Electron Microsc (Tokoyo), 26*:185, 1977.
37. Gale, J.B.: Mitochondrial swelling associated with exercise and method of fixation. *Med Sci Sports, 6*:182, 1974.
38. Gale, J.B.: *Skeletal muscle mitochondria swelling with exhaustive exercise.* Presented to the Annual Meeting of American College of Sports Medicine, Philadelphia, May, 1972.
39. Gale, J.B. and F.J. Nagle: Skeletal muscle changes of ATP and creatine phosphate storage in rats trained at 900 and 7600 feet altitude. *Nature, 232*:342, 1971.
40. Gazzotti, P.: The effect of Ca^{2+} on the oxidation of exogenous NADH by rat liver mitochondria. *Biochem Biophys Res Commun, 67*:634, 1975.
41. Gobel, S.: Electron microscopical studies on the plasma membranes of cerebellar neurons and astrocytes. *J Ultrastruct Res, 15*:310, 1966.
42. Gollnick, P.D. and D.W. King: Effect of exercise and training on mitochondria of rat skeletal muscle. *Am J Physiol, 216*:1502, 1969.
43. Gonzalez-Serratos, H.; L.M. Borrero; and C. Franzini-Armstrong: Possible role of mitochondria in the development of fatigue. *J Gen Physiol,*

62:656, 1973.

44. Grinnell, F.; R.G.W. Anderson; and C.R. Hackenbrock: Glutaraldehyde induced alterations of membrane anionic sites. *Biochim Biophys Acta, 426*:772, 1976.

45. Hardonk, M.J.; T.J. Haarsma; F.W.J. Dijkhuis; M. Poel; and J. Koudstaal: Influence of fixation and buffer treatment on the release of enzymes from the pasma membrane. *Histochemistry, 54*:57, 1977.

46. Hashimoto, I.; W.L. Sembrowich; and P.D. Gollnick: Calcium uptake by isolated sarcoplasmic reticulum and homogenates in different fiber types following exhaustive exercise. Presented at the annual meeting of the Amer. College of Sports Med., Washington, D.C., May, 1978.

47. Hauser, H.; B.A. Levine; and R.J.P. Williams: Interactions of ions with membranes. *Trends in Biochem Sci, 1*:278, 1976.

48. Hayat, M.A.: *Principles and Techniques of Electron Microscopy; Biological Applications, Vol. 1.* New York, Van Nos Reinhold, 1970.

49. Hayat, M.A.: Speciman preparation. In *Electron Microscopy of Enzymes; Principles and Methods, Vol. 1.,* edited by M.A. Hayat. New York, Van Nos Reinhold, 1973.

50. Hearse, D.J.; S.M. Humphrey; D. Feuvray; and J. DeLeiris: A biochemical and ultrastructural study of the species variation in myocardial cell damage. *J Mol Cell Cardiol, 8*:759, 1976.

51. Hearse, D.J.; S.M. Humphrey; and W.G. Nayler: Cellular preservation or damage during myocardial anoxia: a biochemical and electron-microscopic investigation. *Biochem Soc Trans, 2*:1009, 1974.

52. Hicks, L. and H.D. Fahimi: Peroxisomes (microbodies) in the myocardium of rodents and primates. *Cell Tissue Res, 175*:467, 1977.

53. Holt, S.J. and R.M. Hicks: Studies on formalin fixation for electron microscopy and cytochemical staining purposes. *J Biophys Biochem Cytol, 11*:31, 1961.

54. Hulsmann, W.C.: Two types of mitochondria in heart muscle from euthyroid and hyperthyroid rats. *Biochem J, 116*:32 p. 1970.

55. Hultman, E. and J. Bergstrom: Local energy-supplying substrates as limiting factors in different types of leg muscle work in normal man. In *Limiting Factors of Physical Performance,* edited by J. Keul. Stuttgart, Georg Thieme Publishers, 1973.

56. Huston, R.L.; P.C. Weiser; and G.L. Dohm: Effects of training, exercise and diet on muscle glycolysis and liver gluconeogenesis. *Life Sci, 17*:369, 1975.

57. Jennings, R.B.; P.B. Herdson; and H.M. Sommers: Structural and functional abnormalities in mitochondria isolated from ischemic dog myocardium. *Lab Invest, 20*:548, 1969.

58. Jurkowitz, M.; K.M. Scott; R.A. Altschuld; A.J. Merola; and G.P. Brierley: Ion transport by heart mitochondria: Retention and loss of energy coupling in aged heart mitochondria. *Arch Biochem Biophys, 165*:98, 1974.

59. Kerpel-Fronius, S. and F. Hajos: Electron microscopic demonstration of energy production and coupled respiration of in situ mitochondria.

J Histochem Cytochem, 81:740, 1970.

60. King, D.W. and P.D. Gollnick: Ultrastructure of rat heart and liver after exhaustive exercise. *Am J Physiol, 218*:1150, 1970.

61. Korn, E.D.: A chromatographic and spectrophotometric study of the products of the reaction of osmium tetroxide with unsaturated lipids. *J Cell Biol, 34*:627, 1967.

62. Kretsinger, R.H.: Calcium-binding proteins. In *Annual Review of Biochemistry, Vol. 45*, edited by E.E. Snell, P.D. Boyer, A. Meister, and C.C. Richardson. Palo Alto, CA, Annual Reviews, 1976.

63. Laguens, R.P. and C.L.A. Gomez-Dumm: Fine structure of myocardial mitochondria in rats after exercise for one-half to two hours. *Circ Res, 21*:271, 1967.

64. Laguens, R.P.; B.B. Lozada; G. Gomez-Dumm; and A.R. Ruiz Beramendi: Effect of acute and exhaustive exercise upon the fine structure of heart mitochondria. *Experientia, 22*:244, 1966.

65. Leblanc, P. and H. Clausen: ADP and Mg^{2+} requirement for Ca^{2+} accumulation by hog heart mitochondria. Correlation with energy coupling. *Biochim Biophys Acta, 347*:87, 1974.

66. Lehninger, A.L.; A. Vercesi; and E.A. Bababunmi: Regulation of Ca^{2+} release from mitochondria by the oxidation-reduction state of pyridine nucleotide. *Proc Natl Acad Sci USA, 75*:1690, 1978.

67. Ling, G.N. and C.L. Walton: What retains water in living cells? *Science, 191*:293, 1976.

68. Luftig, R.B.; E. Wehrli; and P.N. McMillan: The unit membrane image: a re-evaluation. *Life Sci, 21*:285, 1977.

69. Maher, J.T.; A.L. Goodman; R. Francesconi; W.D. Bowers; L.H. Hartley; and E.T. Angelakos: Responses of rat myocardium to exhaustive exercise. *Am J Physiol, 222*:207, 1972.

70. Margoliash, E.; G.H. Barlow; and V. Byers: Differential binding properties of cytochrome c: possible relevance for mitochondrial ion transport. *Nature, 228*:723, 1970.

71. Maser, M.D.; T.E. Powell; and C.W. Philpott: Relationship among pH, osmolality, and concentration of fixative solutions. *Stain Tech, 42*:175, 1967.

72. Maunsbach, A.B.: The influence of different fixatives and fixation methods on the ultrastructure of rat kidney proximal tubule cells. *J Ultrastruct Res, 15*:283, 1966.

73. McMillan, P.N. and R.B. Luftig: Preservation of membrane ultrastructure with aldehyde or imidate fixatives. *J Ultrastruct Res, 52*:243, 1975.

74. Moore, D.H.; H. Ruska; and W.M. Copenhaver: Electron microscopic and histochemical observations of muscle degeneration after tourniquet. *J Biophys Biochem Cytol, 2*:755, 1956.

75. Munn, E.A.: *The Structure of Mitochondria*. London, Acad Pr, 1974.

76. Nayler, W.G.; J. Dunnett; and D. Berry: The calcium accumulating activity of subcellular fractions isolated from rat and guinea pig heart muscle. *J Mol Cell Cardiol, 7*:275, 1975.

77. Nayler, W.G.; J. Dunnett; and W. Burian: Further observations on species

determined differences in the calcium-accumulating activity of cardiac microsomal fractions. *J Mol Cell Cardiol, 7*:663, 1975.

78. Ohno, H.; H. Watanabe; C. Kishihara; N. Taniguchi; and E. Takakuwa: Effect of physical exercise on the activity of GOT isozyme in human plasma. *Tohoku J Exp Med, 126*:371, 1978.

79. Oram, J.F.; J.L. Bennetch; and J.R. Neely: Regulation of fatty acid utilization in isolated perfused rat hearts. *J Biol Chem, 248*:5299, 1973.

80. Packer, L.; M.P. Donovan; and J.M. Wrigglesworth: Probes of macromolecular and molecular structure in the membranes of mitochondria and submitochondrial vesicles. In *Probes of Structure and Function of Macromolecules and Membranes,* edited by B. Chance, C. Lee, and J.K. Blaise. New York, Acad Pr, 1971.

81. Packer, L. and G.D. Greville: Energy-linked oxidation of glutaraldehyde by rat liver mitochondria. *FEBS Lett, 3*:112, 1969.

82. Parr, D.R.; J.M. Wimhurst; and E.J. Harris: Calcium induced damage of rat heart mitochondria. *Cardiovas Res, 9*:366, 1975.

83. Poland, J.L. and D.A. Traunes: Adrenal influence on the supercompensation of cardiac glycogen following exercise. *Am J Physiol, 224*:540, 1973.

84. Poland, J.L. and D.A. Trauner: The effects of prior exercise on myocardial glycogenesis during a fast. *Proc Soc Exp Biol Med, 136*:1100, 1971.

85. Raczniak, T.J.; C.F. Chesney; and J.R. Allen: Oxidative phosphorylation and respiration by mitochondria from normal and failing rat hearts. *J Mol Cell Cardiol, 9*:215, 1977.

86. Sabatini, D.D.; K. Bensch; and R.J. Barrnett: The preservation of cellular ultrastructure and enzymatic activity by aldehyde fixation. *J Cell Biol, 17*:19, 1963.

87. Saito, H.: Species difference in experimentally induced heart failure from a viewpoint of mitochondrial respiration. *Res Commun Chem Pathol Pharmacol, 6*:1019, 1973.

88. Saltin, B.: Aerobic work capacity and circulation of exercise in man. *Acta Physiol Scand [Suppl], 62*:230, 1964.

89. Schmidt, H.; E. Gadermann; and K. Voigt: Zum Energiestoff welch sel von Leistungs—sportern unter Wettkampfeldingungen. *Med Welt Stg, 21*:1675, 1970. Cited by J. Keul, E. Doll, and D. Keppler: *Energy Metabolism of Human Muscle.* Baltimore, U Park Pr, 1972.

90. Schwartz, A.: Electron transport and mitochondria. *Cardiology, 56*:35, 1971/1972.

91. Schwartz, H.: Cell membrane Na^+, K^+-ATPase and sarcoplasmic reticulum: possible regulators of intracellular ion activity. *Fed Proc, 35*:1279, 1976.

92. Schwerzman, K.; P. Gazzotti; and E. Carafoli: Ruthenium red as a carrier of electrons between external NADH and cytochrome c in rat liver mitochondria. *Biochem Biophys Res Commun, 69*:812, 1976.

93. Seabra-Gomes, R.; C.E. Ganote; and W.G. Nayler: Species variation in anoxic-induced damage of heart muscle. *J Mol Cell Cardiol, 7*:929, 1975.

94. Sembrowich, W.L.; R.E. Shepherd; and P.D. Gollnick: The effects of exhaustive exercise on heart mitochondria from trained and sedentary

rats. *Med Sci Sports, 7*:69, 1975.

95. Senger, H.: Changes of the oxidative phosphorylation in mitochondria of rat skeletal muscle following strenuous exercise. *Acta Biol Med Ger, 34*:181, 1975.

96. Sjostrand, F.S.: The arrangement of mitochondrial membranes and a new structural feature of the inner mitochondrial membranes. *J Ultrastruct Res, 59*:292, 1977.

97. Sjostrand, F.S.: *Electron Microscopy of Cells and Tissues.* New York, Acad Pr, 1967.

98. Sjostrand, F.S.: The structure of mitochondrial membranes: A new concept. *J Ultrastruct Res, 64*:217, 1978.

99. Sjostram, M. and L. Thornell: Preparing sections of skeletal muscle for transmission electron analytical microscopy (TEAM) of diffusible elements. *J Miscros, 103*:101, 1975.

100. Sordahl, L.A.; G.K. Asimakis; R.T. Dowell; and H.L. Stone: Functions of selected biochemical systems from the exercised-trained dog heart. *J Appl Physiol, 42*:426, 1977.

101. Taylor, P.B.; D.R. Lamb; and B.C. Budd: Structure and function of cardiac mitochondria in exhausted guinea pigs. *Eur J Appl Physiol, 35*:111, 1976.

102. Terjung, R.L.; K.M. Baldwin; P.A. Molé; G.H. Klinkerfuss; and J.O. Holloszy: Effect of running to exhaustion on skeletal muscle mitochondria: a bio-chemical study. *Am J Physiol, 223*:549, 1972.

103. Terjung, R.L.; G.H. Klinkerfuss; K.M. Baldwin; W.W. Winder; and J.O. Holloszy: Effect of exhausting exercise on rat heart mitochondria. *Am J Physiol, 225*:300, 1979

104. Tomanek, R.J. and E.W. Banister: Myocardial ultrastructure after acute exercise stress with special reference to transverse tubules and intercalated discs. *Cardiovas Res, 6*:671, 1972.

105. Tooze, J.: Measurements of some cellular changes during the fixation of amphibian erythrocytes with osmium tetroxide solutions. *J Cell Biol, 22*:551, 1964.

106. Trump, B.F. and J.L.E. Ericsson: Ultrastructure of cells and tissues. A comparative analysis with particular attention to the proximal convoluted tubule of the rat kidney. *Lab Invest, 6*:507, 1965.

107. Utsumi, K. and L. Packer: Glutaraldehyde fixed mitochondria. I. Enzyme activity, ion translocation, and conformational changes. *Arch Biochem Biophys, 121*:633, 1967.

108. Vandenheuvel, F.A.: Structure of membranes and role of lipids therein. *Adv Lipid Res, 9*:161, 1972.

109. Vasington, F.D.; P. Gazzotti, R. Tiozzo; and E. Carafoli: The effect of ruthenium red on Ca^{2+} transport and respiration in rat liver mitochondria. *Biochim Biophys Acta, 256*:43, 1972.

110. Waite, M.; L.T.M. Van Deenan; T.R.C. Tuigrok; and P.F. Elbers: Relation of mitochondrial phospholipase A activity to mitochondrial swelling. *J Lipid Res, 10*:599, 1969.

111. Weibel, E.R.: Stereological principles for morphometry in electron micro-

scope cytology. *Int Rev Cytol, 26*:235, 1969.

112. Wilson, B.A. and W.N. Stainsby: Relation between oxygen uptake and developed tension in dog skeletal muscle. *J Appl Physiol, 45*:234, 1978.

113. Wollenberger, A.: Responses of the heart mitochondria to chronic cardiac overload and physical exercise. In *Myocardiology.* Baltimore, U Park Pr, 1972.

114. Wood, R.L. and J.H. Luft: The influence of buffer systems on fixation with osmium tetroxide. *J Ultrastruct Res, 12*:22, 1965.

115. Wrigglesworth, J.M. and L. Packer: pH-dependent confirmational changes in submitochondrial particles. *Arch Biochem Biophys, 133*:194, 1969.

116. Yarom, R.; P.D. Peters; M. Scripps; and S. Rogel: Effect of specimen preparation on intercellular myocardial calcium. *Histochemistry, 38*:143, 1974.

117. Yates, J.C. and N.S. Dhalla: Structural and functional changes associated with failure and recovery of hearts after perfusion with Ca^{2+}-free medium. *J Mol Cell Cardiol, 7*:91, 1975.

118. Zammit, V.A. and E.A. Newsholme: Effects of calcium ions and adenosine diphosphate on the activities of NAD^+-linked isocitrate dehydrogenase from the radular muscles of the whelk and flight muscles of insects. *Biochem J, 154*:677, 1976.

Chapter 8

SKELETAL MUSCLE ULTRASTRUCTURE AND FIBER TYPES IN PREPUBESCENT CHILDREN

J.D. MacDougall, R.D. Bell, and H. Howald

INTRODUCTION

THE ANABOLIC effects of sexual maturity upon skeletal muscle growth are well recognized, and it has been estimated that between the ages of 6 and 20 muscle mass increases by approximately fourfold (1). However, very little is known as to the effects of the growth process upon the chemical and structural characteristics of muscle. Increasing involvement of prepubescent children in highly organized and competitive sport has prompted a recent concern as to its possible effects on growth and development. In order to assess these effects, there is an obvious need for a greater understanding of the normal skeletal muscle characteristics of young children.

The purpose of this study was to determine whether prepubertal muscle differs from adult tissue with respect to (1) percent fiber type and (2) certain ultrastructural characteristics.

METHODS

Needle biopsies were taken from the vastus lateralis of 7 female and 6 male preschool children. The average age of the subjects was 6.4 years, and they were all considered to be healthy normoactive children. One portion of each biopsy was used for histochemical analysis and another for electron microscopy.

Following freeze-drying at −30° for a minimum of 4 days, the tissue for fiber typing analysis was subjected to a process of microdissection in an environmentally controlled atmosphere. Three small sections were cut from one end of each dissected fiber and adhered to appropriately labelled glass slides with distilled water. The sections were then stained for ATPase activity following preincubation at a pH of 10.6 and 4.3 (8) and NADH diaphorase (7). Fibers were then classified as slow twitch oxidative (ST), fast twitch glycolytic (FG), or fast twitch oxidative glycolytic (FOG) according to Peter et al. (10). One hundred single fibers were classified per biopsy.

Tissue for electron microscopy was fixed in 6.25% gluteraldehyde, separated into approximately 10 blocks and embedded in Epon®. According to the morphometric procedure developed by Weibel (13), 6 blocks were randomly selected, transversely sectioned, and mounted on 200 mesh grids. From each block, 8 micrographs were randomly taken under the Phillips EM200 to yield a final magnification of 75,000 (4). Stereological analysis was performed on each micrograph by means of a 168 point short line test system (14).

Maximal oxygen consumption was also directly determined for each child during progressive continuous treadmill running (5). In the instances where a plateauing effect was not evident, the highest value achieved was considered to represent $\dot{V}O_2$max.

RESULTS

Percent fiber type and $\dot{V}O_2$max for both males and females are shown in Table 8-I. Sex differences for the 3 muscle fiber types and for $\dot{V}O_2$max were all nonsignificant.

Similarly, at the ultrastructural level, the tissue from the 6 year old girls did not differ from that of the boys. Mean morphometric characteristics for the combined data are illusted in Figure 8-1. The volume density of the central mitochondria was 5.65 percent; that is, 5.56 percent of the total volume of the muscle fiber is composed of mitochondria. Similarly, 82.31 percent of the muscle was composed of myofibrils, 11.5 percent cytoplasm, and 0.45

TABLE 8-I
MUSCLE FIBER TYPES IN 6 YEAR OLD CHILDREN*

	ST (TYPE I)	FT, OX (IIA)	FT, GLYC (IIB)	
	FIBERS %	FIBERS %	FIBERS %	$\dot{V}O_2$max ml/kg/min
MALES (n = 6)	62.1 (±14.2)	17.3 (±10.3)	20.6 (±9.8)	47.2 (±3.0)
FEMALES (n = 7)	55.6 (± 8.5)	22.1 (± 8.8)	22.3 (±8.4)	43.1 (±5.8)
COMBINED (n = 13)	58.8 (±11.4)	19.7 (± 9.5)	21.5 (±9.1)	45.2 (±4.7)

*Mean (± SD) values for % fiber type in vastus lateralis and maximal oxygen uptake for 6 year old boys and girls.

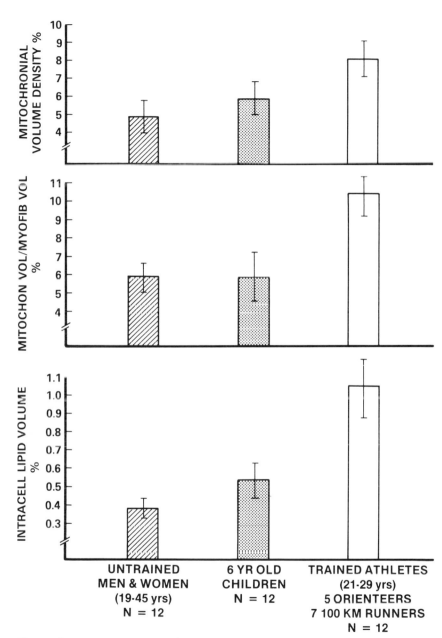

Figure 8-1. Mean (SD) morphometry results for 6 year olds compared with those of a group of sedentary adults and well-trained endurance athletes.

percent intracellular lipid. When these results were compared with those for a group of untrained men and women and a group of well-trained endurance athletes (4, 6), the values were found to lie between those for the other 2 groups (Fig. 8-1). There was a significant correlation ($r = 0.69$) between central mitochondrial volume density and the percent ST fibers for each subject as determined histochemically.

DISCUSSION

PERCENT FIBER TYPE. The mean value of 58.8 ($\pm$ 11.4) percent for ST fibers is similar to what one would expect in a normal group of adults (3, 11, 12). There is as yet very little data available as to the normally expected percent occurrence of the FT subtypes. The 32 percent occurrence for FOG fibers and 13 percent for FG fibers in a control sample of 70 physically active 16 year old boys reported by Saltin et al. (11) would appear to differ significantly from the 20 and 22 percent, respectively, occurrence of these subtypes in 6 year olds. However, these same authors acknowledge that one would expect a more equal proportion of these 2 fiber types in untrained subjects. The present data therefore suggest that percent fiber type is predetermined by 6 years of age or earlier and would appear to be altered very little by the maturation process.

MORPHOMETRY. Based on the ultrastructural parameters investigated, it is apparent that skeletal muscle of prepubescent children differs minimally from that of adults. In fact, based on the relative volume densities of mitochondria and intracellular lipid, the 6 year olds in the present study demonstrate an equivalent or slightly greater capacity for oxidative metabolism than do sedentary adults. The findings of similar mitochondrial to myofibrilar volume ratios in both prepubescent and adult tissue indicate that, with growth and maturation, the large increase in total contractile protein that occurs is paralleled by a similar increase in mitochondrial number and size. The correlation between percent ST fibers and mitochondrial volume density further supports findings of higher mitochondrial concentrations within these fibers (2, 9, 13).

In summary, the present study indicates that although there are large differences in total muscle size, histochemically and ultrastructurally skeletal muscle in 6 year old children does not differ from that of adults.

REFERENCES

1. Asmussen, E.: Growth in muscular strength and power. In *Physical Activity-Human Growth and Development,* edited by G.L. Rarick. New York, Acad Pr, 1973.
2. Cullen, M.J. and Weightman, D.: The ultrastructure of normal human muscle in relation to fiber type. *J Neurol Sci, 25*:43, 1975.
3. Gollnick, P.D.; Armstrong, R.B.; Saubert, C.W.; Piehl, K.; and Saltin, B.: Enzyme activity and fiber composition in skeletal muscle of untrained and trained man. *J Appl Physiol, 33*:312, 1972.
4. Hoeppler, H.; Luthi, P.; Claassen, H.; Weibel, E.R.; and Howald, H.: The ultra-structure of the normal human muscle. A morphometric analysis of untrained men, women and well-trained orienteers. *Pflügers Arch, 244*:217, 1973.
5. Howald, Hans.: Eine Ergospirometrie-Anlage mit on-line Datenverarbeitung durch Mikrocomputer. *Acta Mediocotech, 21*:115, 1973.
6. Howald, Hans.: Ultrastructure and biochemical function of skeletal muscle in twins. *Ann Hum Biol, 3*:455, 1976.
7. Novokoff, A.B.; Shin, W.; and Druker, J.: Mitochondrial localization of oxidative enzymes: Staining results with two tetrazolium salts. *J Biophys Biochem Cytol, 9*:47, 1961.
8. Padykula, H.A. and Herman, E.: The specificity of the histochemical method of adenosine triphosphatase. *J Histochem Cytochem, 3*:170, 1955.
9. Payne, C.M.; Stern, L.Z.; Curless, R.C.; and Hannapel, L.K.: Ultrastructure fiber typing in normal and diseased human muscle. *J Neurol Sci, 25*:99, 1975.
10. Peter, J.B.; Barnard, R.J.; Edgerton, V.R.; Gillespie, C.A.; and Stempel, K.E.: Metabolic profiles of three fiber types of skeletal muscle in guinea pigs and rabbits. *Biochemistry, 11*:2627-2634, 1972.
11. Saltin, B.; Henriksson, J.; Hygaard, E.; Anderson, P.; and Jansson, E.: Fibre types and metabolic potentials of skeletal muscles in sedentary men and endurance runners. *Ann NY Acad Sci, 301*:3, 1977.
12. Taylor, A.W.; Lavoie, J.; Lemieux, G.; Durfresne, D.; Skinner, J.S.; and Vallee, J.: The effects of endurance training on the number, area and enzyme activity of skeletal muscle fibers on French Canadian women. *Med Sci Sports, 8*:54, 1976.
13. Tomanek, R.J.; Asmundson, C.R.; Cooper, R.R.; and Barnard, R.J.: Fine structure of fast-twitch and slow-twitch guinea pig muscle fibers. *J Morphol, 139*:47, 1973.
14. Weibel, E.R.: Stereological techniques for electron microscopic morphometry. In *Principles and Techniques of Electron Microscopy,* edited by M.A. Hayatt. Vol. 3 New York, Van Nos Reinhold, pg. 237, 1973.

Chapter 9

THE DEVELOPMENT OF FATIGUE DURING HIGH INTENSITY AND ENDURANCE EXERCISE

R.H. FITTS, D.H. KIM, AND F.A. WITZMANN

ALTHOUGH MANY studies on the etiology of muscle fatigue have been conducted and alterations in muscle function reported, little is known about the mechanisms responsible for muscle fatigue. The problem is complex as muscle fatigue is dependent on work intensity, environmental factors, the percent of fast (type II) fibers, and the percent of slow (type I) fibers, as well as the individual's degree of fitness. For example, fatigue experienced in high intensity short duration exercise (e.g. one-mile race) is dependent on different factors than those precipitating fatigue in endurance events (e.g. marathon run). Muscle fatigue produced during these 2 general types of activity will be discussed, with the authors' results as well as selected work of others being presented. Due to the limitations inherent in a symposium, no attempt is made to present a complete review.

HIGH INTENSITY EXERCISE

Exercise of this nature involves an energy demand that exceeds one's maximal aerobic capacity, and thus requires a high level of anaerobic metabolism. As a consequence, a build-up in muscle lactate occurs, cell pH falls, and high energy phosphagen stores [phosphocreatine (PC) and ATP] decrease. All of these changes have been suggested as possible fatigue-inducing agents (54). The concentration here will be on the relationship between muscle lactate and the contractile properties of muscle during the development of fatigue and recovery. The effect of lactic acid production on cell pH and the potential role of an elevated H^+ ion in fatigue will be discussed.

LACTIC ACID PRODUCTION: High intensity work is characterized by a high component of anaerobic metabolism and, con-

118

sequently, results in high muscle lactate. As early as 1907 lactic acid was implicated as a possible fatigue agent (23). This hypothesis linking muscle lactic acid build-up to fatigue gained popularity following the work of Hill and Kupalov in the late 1920s (31, 33). Following a void of 20 years, Asmussen and co-workers (2) revived the concept of muscle lactate as a causative agent in fatigue. However, the real renewal of interest in lactate and other muscle substrates occurred following the development of the needle biopsy technique (6). Karlsson and Saltin (39) used the biopsy technique to evaluate substrate changes following exercise to exhaustion at 3 different work loads. At the highest and medium loads (performed for 2 and 6 minutes), muscle lactate at exhaustion was 16.1 $mmole \cdot kg^{-1}$ wet muscle, while ATP and PC were depleted to the same amount after 2 minutes of work at all loads. These results not only linked muscle lactate accumulation to exhaustion but suggested that high energy phosphagen depletion was not limiting under their experimental conditions.

As a result of the indication that lactate may be a causative agent in muscle fatigue, Fitts and Holloszy (21) evaluated the relationship between muscle lactate and force during the development of and recovery from fatigue in frog sartorius muscle. Muscle fatigue was produced by *in vitro* electrical stimulation in an anaerobic frog Ringers environment. After 2, 6, 10, or 15 minutes of stimulation, the muscles were quick-frozen in isopentane precooled in liquid N_2. In the recovery studies, muscles were permitted to recover in oxygenated solution for selected periods of time or until complete recovery had occurred. Figure 9-1 presents a summary of the results. The most important finding was the extremely high negative correlation between the decrease in twitch tension and the increase in muscle lactate ($r = -0.99$, $p < 0.000001$), further supporting a role for lactate in the development of muscle fatigue. Muscle PC concentrations decreased approximately 85 percent. However, the decrease followed a different time course from the decrease in muscle twitch tension (Fig. 9-1). ATP was the only substrate other than lactate to show a statistically significant correlation with twitch tension during the development of fatigue ($r = 0.82$, $p < 0.05$).

The muscles recovered from fatigue in 2 phases. A rapid increase representing 27 percent of the total recovery occurred in the first 10 seconds, followed by no change for about 10 minutes,

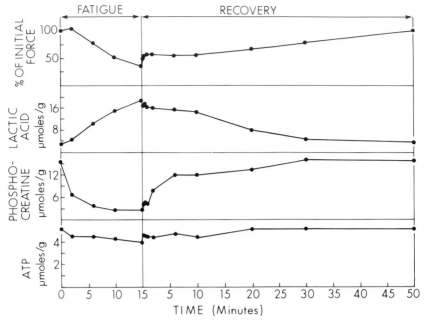

Figure 9-1. Changes in contractile force and in lactic acid, ATP, and PC concentrations during the development of fatigue in isolated frog sartorius muscles stimulated at 30 shocks/min for 15 minutes under anaerobic conditions and during subsequent recovery in oxygenated solution. [Data from Fitts and Holloszy (20).]

after which twitch tension increased linearly until prefatigue levels were reached (Fig. 9-1). Although a significant inverse correlation between muscle lactate and twitch tension ($r = -0.92$, $p < 0.00001$) was also observed during the recovery period, no change in lactate occurred during the early rapid phase of recovery. This suggests that some factor other than lactate must have contributed to the development of fatigue. One cannot dismiss the possibility that a limited availability of ATP at the cross bridges played a role in fatigue development. ATP did not decrease extensively during contractile activity (3.9 μMol/g after 15 min of stimulation); however, a close relationship was observed between an increase in ATP (3.9 to 4.6 μMol/g) and twitch tension during the first 15 seconds of recovery.

In subsequent experiments evaluating soleus muscle *in situ* (19), one of the earliest signs of fatigue was a decrease in the rate of tension development (dp/dt). Thus, the rapid early phase of twitch

TABLE 9-I

MUSCLE CONTRACTION TIME (C.T.), ONE-HALF RELAXATION TIME (½R.T.), TWITCH TENSION (P_t), PEAK RATE OF TWITCH TENSION DEVELOPMENT (P_t, dP/dt), AND MAXIMAL ISOMETRIC TENSION (P_o), DURING DEVELOPMENT OF AND RECOVERY FROM FATIGUE

Group*	C.T. (msec)†	½R.T. (msec)†	P_t (g/cm²)†	P_t, dP/dt (g/msec/cm²)†	P_o (g/cm²)†
Control (20)	42 ± 1	45 ± 1	863 ± 43	31.9 ± 1.5	2673 ± 52
Fatigue development (under anaerobic conditions)					
2 min Stimulation (8)	54 ± 2‡	61 ± 3‡	886 ± 46	30.4 ± 1.2	2339 ± 74‡
6 min Stimulation (14)	60 ± 2	80 + 4	734 ± 39§	23.8 ± 1.3‡	2041 ± 34
10 min Stimulation (13)	61 ± 2	85 ± 4	531 ± 28	16.5 ± 1.1	1729 ± 71
15 min Stimulation (19)	59 ± 2	82 ± 3	353 ± 18	10.5 ± 0.8	1272 ± 47
Recovery (under aerobic conditions)					
0.25 min Recovery (6)	53 ± 3	69 ± 6	590 ± 65∥	17.1 ± 1.3∥	1407 ± 48
2 min Recovery (8)	51 ± 3	62 ± 5	646 ± 57	19.5 ± 1.6	1823 ± 63∥
6 min Recovery (8)	49 ± 2	57 + 4	688 ± 55	21.5 ± 1.5	1837 ± 58
10 min Recovery (10)	46 ± 2	55 ± 3	705 ± 60	22.5 ± 1.7	2004 ± 83
20 min Recovery (6)	39 ± 2	45 ± 2	724 ± 91	26.9 ± 2.3	2235 ± 118
30 min Recovery (6)	38 ± 2	44 ± 2	812 + 96	29.9 + 3.0	2486 + 124

*Number of muscles per group is given in parentheses.
†Values are means ± SE.
‡Significantly different from control, $p < 0.01$.
§Significantly different from control, $p < 0.05$.
∥Significantly different from 15 minute stimulation value, $p < 0.01$.
Data from Fitts et al. (20).

tension recovery observed in frog sartorius following cessation of contractile activity may have been due to an increase in twitch dp/dt rather than to a change in the number of active cross bridges. This possibility was evaluated by repeating the earlier frog studies using a combined force and displacement transducer capable of completely characterizing the contractile properties (20). The results of this study are shown in Table 9-I. As in the earlier study (21), twitch tension (P_t) recovered in 2 phases following cessation of contractile activity. In the early (0–15 sec) phase of recovery, P_t increased from 41 to 68 percent of control and was paralleled by a similar increase in twitch dp/dt from 33 to 54 percent of control. Notably, the peak tetanic tension (P_o), an indicator of the number of active cross bridges, did not change significantly during this period. This suggests that the early phase of P_t recovery is due to a rapid recovery in dp/dt rather than to any change in ATP. The correlation between ATP and P_t (21) thus appears to be coincidental rather than cause and effect, since any increase in ATP from a limiting level would effect P_o as well as P_t.

These results illustrate the danger of utilizing P_t to assess the force-generating capacity of muscle during fatigue studies (9, 14, 18, 20, 21, 41, 42). It is clear that even at a constant temperature P_t can be influenced by dp/dt as well as the duration of the twitch. To obtain a reliable indicator of the force-generating capacity of muscle, P_o should be measured (20).

MECHANISMS OF LACTIC ACID EFFECT—AN ALTERATION IN CELL PH: When the P_o and P_t values obtained in the second frog study (20) were correlated to the earlier muscle lactate data (21), P_o showed an even higher inverse correlation than P_t with lactate (20). It is apparent that lactate somehow interferes with the force-generating capacity of muscle. The mechanism of this deleterious effect is unknown but probably involves a change in cell pH (an increase in free H^+ ion) rather than a direct effect of the lactate molecule (29, 49). A highly significant negative correlation was found between intracellular lactate and cell pH during recovery from exhaustive exercise (49). Resting skeletal muscle pH determined by a variety of techniques (Table 9-II) is approximately 7.00 (1, 29, 48, 49) and with maximal continuous exercise to exhaustion decreases to values below 6.5 (Table 9-II). A free H^+ ion concentration of this magnitude could interfere with muscle function by (1) inhibiting ATP formation from glycolysis by suppressing the rate-limiting enzyme phosphofructokinase (55), (2) affecting the activation of or the force-generating capacity of individual cross bridges (7, 15, 24), and (3) altering the ability of the sarcoplasmic reticulum (SR) to load and release Ca^{++} (15, 44).

At least 2 observations lend support to the concept that an elevated H^+ ion inhibits glycolysis. Hill (32) found lactate formation during muscle stimulation to stop when the intracellular pH dropped to 6.3, and Hermansen and Osnes (29) observed no change in pH during the 60 second measurement period for the most acidic homogenates of fatigued muscle. In contrast, the pH values of the homogenates from resting muscle showed a marked fall. Sahlin et al. (49) suggest that this inhibition of glycolysis by the

TABLE 9-II

SKELETAL MUSCLE pH

Method	Rest Value*	Fatigue Value*	Reference
Muscle Homogenate	6.92 ± 0.03	6.41 ± 0.04	Hermansen and Osnes (29)
Calculated from	7.04 ± 0.05	6.37 ± 0.11	Sahlin et al. (49)
HCO_3^- and PCO_2			
Micro-electrode	7.07 ± 0.007		Aickin and Thomas (1)
DMO Method	7.06 ± 0.02		Roos (48)

*Values are means ± SE except for Sahlin et al., where means ± SD are listed.

H^+ ion may be the limiting factor for performance of intense exercise. Although possible, frog studies (20, 21) and the human studies of Karlsson and Saltin (39) give indirect evidence that ATP does not fall enough to limit the force-generating capacity of muscle.

Although acidosis has long been known to cause a negative inotropic effect on cardiac muscle (7, 15, 25, 40, 45), the effect on skeletal muscle is less pronounced. In fact, Pannier et al. (46) observed acidosis (pH 6.86) caused by increasing PCO_2 to potentiate soleus P_t and P_o tension. Recently, however, studies on skinned fibers (7, 15) have definitively shown acidosis to depress the force output of skeletal as well as cardiac muscle. Decreasing pH from 7.4 to 6.2 not only reduced the maximal tension generated in the presence of optimal free Ca^{++}, but also increased the threshold of free Ca^{++} required for contraction, and shifted the force-pCa curve to the right such that higher free Ca^{++} was required to reach a given tension (15). Fast twitch fibers were found to be more sensitive to the acidotic depression of maximal tension that slow soleus muscle fibers (7). These effects may be mediated by a H^+ ion interference with Ca^{++} binding to troponin (24). However, the results of Bolitho-Donaldson and Hermansen (7) and Fabiato and Fabiato (15) indicate that the effect is not due to a simple competitive inhibition of Ca^{++} binding to troponin. The observed depression of maximal tension was completely reversible on returning to neutral pH but could not be overcome by increasing free Ca^{++} (15). Fabiato and Fabiato (15) suggest that the H^+ ion effect may be acting at some step after Ca^{++} interaction with troponin, perhaps affecting the troponin or tropomyosin molecule directly. The fact that maximum rigor tension is reduced by 33 percent when pH is changed from 7.00 to 6.20 (with a pCa 9.50) suggests that the H^+ ion may directly alter the actin myosin interaction independent of any Ca^{++} regulatory effect (15).

The third possibility is that an elevated H^+ ion deleteriously affects the functional capacity of the sarcoplasmic reticulum (SR). Nakamaru and Schwartz (44) found a decrease in pH to increase the Ca^{++} binding capacity of isolated SR membranes and suggested that a drop in pH might reduce the amount of Ca^{++} released from SR during excitation. Fabiato and Fabiato (15) observed that the pH optimal for Ca^{++} loading of SR is dependent on free Ca^{++}. With a low free Ca^{++} (pCa 7.75), maximal loading—as determined by the amplitude of caffeine-induced contractions of skinned fibers—occurred with a pH optimal between 7.00 and 7.40, while at high free Ca^{++} (pCa 6.00) the optimal pH was 6.60 to 6.20. The physiological significance of these findings depends upon the actual *in vivo* cell free Ca^{++} concentration. If the free Ca^{++} concentration is pCa 7.00, the pH optimal for Ca^{++} loading by the SR would be between 7.00 and 6.60. Since the resting muscle cell pH is approximately 7.0 (1, 29, 48, 49), one would not expect a drop in cell pH between 7.0 and 6.60 to adversely affect the SR. In fact, a small acidosis may potentiate Ca^{++} loading by the SR and as a result increase both the amount of tension generated on excitation and the rate of relaxation. This effect could explain Pannier et al. (46) observation of an acidotic potentiation of soleus twitch tension. A cell pH fall below 6.60 would adversely affect SR function and thus contribute to a depression in muscle force (15).

ENDURANCE EXERCISE

Numerous factors have been linked to fatigue resulting from prolonged endurance activity. These include depletion of muscle (30, 52), and liver (3, 27) glycogen, decreases in blood glucose levels (11, 47), dehydration (50), and increases in body temperatures (8, 26, 27, 51). Undoubtedly each of these factors contributes to fatigue to a varying degree, their relative importance depending on the environmental conditions and the nature of the activity. This section will (1) review some of these potential fatigue factors, particularly body carbohydrate depletion and (2) present evidence linking an alteration in the contractile properties and sarcoplasmic reticulum function of muscle to the development of fatigue during prolonged exercise.

GLYCOGEN DEPLETION: In 1896, Chauveau suggested that the rate of carbohydrate utilization was dependent on the intensity of work (10). This belief was based on the observation that the respiratory exchange ratio (RQ) increased from 0.75 during rest to 0.95 during exercise (10). With the development of the muscle biopsy technique (6), these early theories based on RQ were proven correct by direct measurements of glycogen utilization at different work intensities (30, 52). Glycogen utilization was found to increase from 0.3 to 3.4 glucose units $\times$ Kg^{-1} $\times$ min^{-1} as the relative work load increased from 25 to 100 percent of the maximal oxygen uptake ($\dot{V}O_2max$) (52). Muscle glycogen depletion coincided with exhaustion during prolonged work bouts requiring approximately 75 percent of $\dot{V}O_2max$. With work loads below 50 or above 90 percent of $\dot{V}O_2max$, ample muscle glycogen remained at exhaustion (52). The rate of body carbohydrate usage is dependent not only on the intensity of the work but also on the individual's state of fitness (30, 52, 53). Trained individuals have a lower RQ (12, 30, 52) and deplete glycogen at a slower rate (30, 52, 53) than untrained men. The lower RQ, increased rate of CO_2 production from fatty acids (37), and the slower rate of glycogen utilization are all indicative of a shift toward a higher fat oxidation (34).

Baldwin et al. (3) found the glycogen sparing effect of exercise training to exist in all 3 fiber types and liver (Table 9-III). Following a 45 minute treadmill running test, swimming-trained rats had significantly higher glycogen levels in all 3 fiber types than untrained animals (Table 9-III). The liver glycogen levels were supercompensated at rest in the trained rats (75% greater than controls) and the rate of utilization during exercise was significantly lower than for the untrained controls (Table 9-III).

Exercise training has been shown to induce an increase in the size and number of mitochondria (27) as well as a change in the mitochondrial composition in all 3 fiber types (34). The activities of a number of mitochondrial enzymes involved in fat and carbohydrate metabolism and the capacity to oxidize these substrates increases up to twofold in hindlimb muscle of rats subjected to a regular program of exercise training (34, 35). It has been suggested that these changes in skeletal muscle mitochondria are responsible for the slower utilization of carbohydrate by trained compared to untrained during submaximal exercise (34, 36). As a consequence, the trained individual is protected from fatigue that would result from depletion of body carbohydrate stores.

In an attempt to further characterize the relationship between

TABLE 9-III

RESPONSE OF LIVER AND MUSCLE GLYCOGEN CONCENTRATIONS TO A 3-STAGE TREADMILL
EXERCISE TEST IN EXERCISE-TRAINED AND UNTRAINED RATS

Tissue	Group	Glycogen concentration, mg/g wet weight*			
		Resting	15 min	30 min	45 min
Liver	Trained	72.1 ± 5.0‡	70.9 ± 5.5‡	61.5 ± 4.8§	52.6 ± 7.5§
	Untrained	42.3 ± 6.6	36.7 ± 2.8	21.7 ± 5.0	5.3 ± 2.1
Gastrocnemius	Trained	10.51 ± 0.40†	9.10 ± 0.90†	7.16 ± 0.18	6.04 ± 0.46‡
	Untrained	9.20 ± 0.30	7.00 ± 0.17	6.64 ± 0.32	3.01 ± 0.74
Red vastus	Trained	8.18 ± 0.38	6.60 ± 0.42	5.20 ± 0.37†	5.14 ± 0.25§
	Untrained	8.05 ± 0.68	5.62 ± 0.41	3.88 ± 0.48	2.29 ± 0.31
White vastus	Trained	10.10 ± 0.10	8.48 ± 0.43	7.10 ± 0.40	5.57 ± 0.38§
	Untrained	9.80 ± 0.20	8.58 ± 0.19	6.87 ± 0.55	2.82 ± 0.59
Soleus	Trained	5.08 ± 0.29	3.33 ± 0.42	2.76 ± 0.23	2.76 ± 0.20§
	Untrained	4.66 ± 0.29	3.07 ± 0.26	2.36 ± 0.12	1.72 ± 0.10

*Each value is the mean ± SE for 6 animals.
†Trained vs untrained, $p < 0.05$.
‡Trained vs untrained, $p < 0.01$.
§Trained vs untrained, $p < 0.001$.
Data from Baldwin et al. (3).

TABLE 9-IV

EFFECTS OF 10, 30, 60, AND 120 MINUTES OF DAILY RUNNING
ON RAT GASTROCNEMIUS MUSCLE MITOCHONDRIAL
CONTENT AND ENDURANCE*

Groups	Oxygen Uptake (μl/g·min)	Citrate Synthase μmole/g·min	Cytochrome C (nmole/g)	Run Time to Exhaustion (min)
Sedentary	36.6 ± 0.8	20.0 ± 0.7	10.0 ± 0.5	
Runners ·				
(min/day)				
10	39.6 ± 1.3	22.9 ± 1.0	11.6 ± 0.7	$22 \pm\ \ 2$
30	44.5 ± 3.2	31.4 ± 2.7	13.1 ± 1.1	41 ± 11
60	57.1 ± 2.0	37.3 ± 2.4	13.8 ± 0.7	50 ± 12
120	75.6 ± 2.3	45.5 ± 2.3	19.2 ± 0.6	111 ± 16

*O_2 consumption of whole muscle homogenates was measured during uncontrolled respiration with pyruvate plus malate as substrate. Citrate synthase and cytochome c were used as additional markers for evaluating mitochondrial content. For the endurance exercise test, the animals ran at 1.2 mph (0.5 m/sec) up a 15% grade for the first 10 minutes, and then at 1.5 mph (0.7 m/sec) up a 15% grade until they became exhausted. Values are means + SE Data from Fitts et al. (17).

muscle mitochondrial content, body carbohydrate usage, and endurance, rats were trained on a treadmill for 10, 30, 60, or 120 minutes per day (16, 17). As can be seen in Table 9-IV, the mitochondrial content of the gastrocnemius muscle, as reflected in a number of mitochondrial markers, increased in proportion to the duration of the daily running and varied over a wide range. The endurance capacity, as measured by a run time to exhaustion, was directly related to the duration of daily training and highly correlated ($p < 0.001$) with gastrocnemius cytochrome c concentration (correlation coefficient of 0.79) and oxygen uptake capacity (correlation coefficient of 0.69). When total body carbohydrate was estimated following a 30 minute exercise test, a high correlation ($p < 0.001$) between glycogen remaining and gastrocnemius muscle respiratory capacity was observed (Fig. 9-2) with a correlation coefficient of 0.90. Although these results do not prove a causative relationship, they do support the concept that the exercise-induced increase in the muscle mitochondria content improves endurance by sparing glycogen and postponing the fatigue associated with body carbohydrate depletion (11, 30, 47, 52, 53).

CONTRACTILE PROPERTIES: While body carbohydrate depletion is undoubtably one causative factor in fatigue associated with prolonged exercise, it is unlikely to be the exclusive factor. As a first step in an attempt to elucidate other causative agents in fatigue, Fitts and Holloszy (19) studied the contractile properties

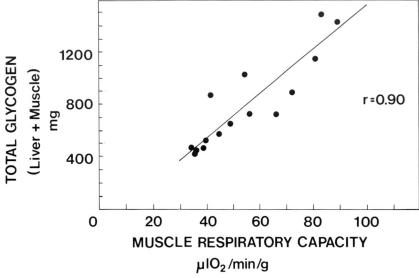

Figure 9-2. Correlation between gastrocnemius muscle respiratory capacity and total glycogen remaining in the liver and muscles of rats after a 30 minute exercise test. [Data from Fitts et al. (17).]

of trained and control rat soleus muscle *in situ* during and after 30 minutes of electrical stimulation. Following the training period (2 hour/day of treadmill running for 18 weeks), the animals were anesthetized and the soleus dissected free of surrounding tissues with its blood supply intact. The muscles were attached to a combined tension and displacement transducer and stimulated indirectly via the nerve with 250 ms trains at a rate of 110/minute. Train tension (P_{tr}) and rate of train tension development (P_{tr}, dp/dt) were monitored continually, while peak tetanic tension (P_o) and peak tetanic rate (P_o, dp/dt) were determined after 0, 6, 12, 24, and 30 minutes of stimulation. The force-velocity relations were measured and the maximal velocity of shortening (Vmax) calculated before and after the 30 minutes of stimulation. The muscles from the exercise-trained animals showed only an 8 percent decrease in P_o during the 30 minutes of electrical stimulation compared to a 32 percent decrease in the untrained muscles. The P_{tr} decreased with a similar pattern as P_o with the trained muscles relatively resistant to fatigue. In contrast, [P_o, dp/dt] changed significantly in both groups with a 48 and 40 percent decrease in the soleus muscles of the untrained and exercise-trained animals respectively during the 30 minutes of electrical stimulation. Similar to the frog studies described earlier (20), the fall in dp/dt was rapid with more than 50 percent of the decrease occurring in the first 6 minutes of contractile activity. It is apparent that a fall in dp/dt is one of the first signs of fatigue under a variety of experimental conditions (19, 20). The decrease in dp/dt during contractile activity is not simply due to a decrease in the number of active actin-myosin cross bridges, as $[P_o, dp/dt]$ falls more rapidly and to a greater extent than P_o (19). The fall in dp/dt is thus suggestive of a decrease in the rate of activation of the actin-myosin interactions. At present, the limiting step in this process is unknown (38). If Ca^{++} availability is limiting, the decreased dp/dt might reflect a reduced rate and/or extent of Ca^{++} release from the sarcoplasmic reticulum. Alternatively, the rate constant for cross bridge attachment may be rate-limiting in tension development (38); consequently, the depressed dp/dt during the development of fatigue might be indicative of a direct change in one of the contractile proteins.

With contractile activity in both anaerobic (20) and aerobic (19) conditions, Vmax appears relatively resistant to fatigue. Table 9-V shows a comparison of Vmax and P_o at rest and following electrical stimulation for frog sartorius (anaerobic conditions, 22°C) and rat soleus (aerobic conditions, 37.5°C) muscles (19, 20). In the case of frog sartorius, Vmax was not significantly altered following 15 minutes of contractile activity despite a greater than 50 percent fall in P_o. The Vmax of rat soleus muscle showed a similar resistance to change. These results imply that the activity of ac-

TABLE 9-V

EFFECT OF FATIGUE ON MAXIMUM SHORTENING VELOCITY AND
P_o OF FROG SARTORIUS AND RAT SOLEUS MUSCLE

Muscle	Vmax*		P_o
	cm/sec	Lo/sec	g/cm²
Frog Sartorius (22°C)			
Rest	17.3 ± 0.3	5.2 ± 0.1	2673 ± 52
Fatigued	15.9 ± 0.3	4.8 ± 0.2	1272 ± 47†
Percent decrease	8	8	52
Rat Soleus (37.5°C)			
Rest	6.99 ± 0.28	2.90 ± 0.13	2185 ± 68
Fatigued	6.04 ± 0.36	2.56 ± 0.18‡	1465 ± 118†
Percent decrease	14	12	33

*Values are means ± SEM.
†Fatigue versus rest, $p < 0.01$.
‡Fatigue versus rest, $p < 0.05$.

tomyosin ATPase, the enzyme thought to be rate limiting in muscle shortening (5), is relatively resistant to alteration during prolonged contractile activity.

The altered contractile properties in response to electrical stimulation (19, 20) suggest that muscle fatigue during prolonged activity is due to a complex interaction of factors. In an attempt to characterize some of these fatigue factors, the authors recently studied the effects of a prolonged swim on muscle function (22, 56). Female rats were fasted overnight and then swam to exhaustion (7 hours) with 2 percent body weight tied to their tails. This exercise protocol has been shown to deplete muscle glycogen in all 3 fiber types (13). At exhaustion, the rats were killed by decapitation and exsanguination and the myofibrils (MF) and sarcoplasmic reticulum (SR) isolated by differential centrifugation (58) from the slow, type I soleus (SOL), the fast, type IIA deep vastus lateralis (DVL) (4), the fast, type IIB, superficial vastus lateralis (SVL) (4), and the mixed fast, type IIA and IIB, extensor digitorum longus (EDL). In addition, the contractile properties of the SOL, SVL, and the EDL were determined *in vitro* (21°C).

The prolonged swim produced significant alterations in the contractile properties of the slow soleus (type I) and fast EDL (type IIA and IIB) but not the fast SVL (type IIB). As can be seen in Table 9-VI, 7 hours of swimming significantly depressed both twitch tension (P_t) and P_o in the SOL and EDL muscles, while the SVL was unaltered. The EDL isometric contraction and one-half relaxation (½RT) times were significantly shortened to 77 and 66 percent of control values respectively. In contrast, the slow soleus

TABLE 9-VI

EFFECT OF A PROLONGED SWIM TO EXHAUSTION ON THE
TWITCH (P_t) AND TETANIC TENSION (P_o)

Muscle	P_t g/cm²*	P_o g/cm²*
Soleus		
Control	374 ± 36	2466 ± 76
Post Swim	243 ± 36†	1651 ± 228†
EDL		
Control	636 ± 36	2397 ± 171
Post Swim	205 ± 67†	633 ± 190†
SVL		
Control	780 ± 54	1757 ± 88
Post Swim	751 ± 34	1713 ± 86

*Values are means ± SEM.
†Post swim significantly different from control, $p < 0.05$.

had a slightly prolonged ½RT at exhaustion compared to control muscles. The maximal rates of tension development (positive dp/dt) and decline (negative dp/dt) were also significantly depressed in the fatigued EDL and soleus muscles. The greatest decrease occurred in the EDL where the positive dp/dt of both twitch and tetanic contractions were only 43 percent of the control values. In agreement with the earlier fatigue studies (19, 20), the Vmax of both the fast and slow muscles studied was found to be relatively resistant to fatigue compared to the changes observed in P_o.

Following partial purification (58) the ATPase activity of the MF and SR, as well as the Ca^{++} uptake of the SR, were measured in fatigued and control samples. The MF Ca^{++} stimulated ATPase activity (μMoles P_i/mg/min) of the fast muscles was unaltered (range 0.250 to 0.300); however, the activity of the slow soleus MF 0.074 ± 0.011 was significantly depressed compared to the control activity of 0.099 ± 0.009. The prolonged swim had no effect on the SR yield from any of the fast muscles (1.5 to 2.0 mg/g) but produced a significant decrease in the amount of SR isolated from the soleus muscle (0.57 ± 0.17 mg/g for fatigued versus 0.81 ± 0.17 mg/g for control). None of the muscles studied exhibited any changes in the SR Ca^{++} stimulated ATPase activity. Ca^{++} uptake by the SR vesicles (μMoles Ca^{++}/mg SR) measured by the millipore filtration procedure (43, 57) was depressed in all muscles studied. The greatest decrease occurred in the slow soleus (0.955 ± 0.064 control versus 0.630 ± 0.120 fatigued) and fast red DVL (2.607 ± 0.157 control versus 1.537 ± 0.170 fatigued).

It is apparent from these results that muscle fatigue is related primarily to the degree of usage during prolonged endurance exercise and not directly to the amount of glycogen depletion. Although muscle glycogen was low in all 3 fiber types at exhaustion, the alterations in contractile properties and SR function were confined to muscles with a high percentage of type I and/or type IIA fibers. The SVL, a 100 percent type IIB muscle, was essentially unaltered. Type IIB fibers were recruited less frequently during the endurance activity (3, 35), but due to their glycolytic nature the amount of glycogen used was similar to the oxidative type I and IIA fibers.

The observation that MF ATPase was unaltered in fast muscle and decreased only slightly in the slow soleus at exhaustion supports the physiological findings of a small decline in Vmax (56). Together with the electrical stimulation studies (19, 20), these results illustrate the fatigue resistant nature of the MF ATPase. In contrast to the MF, the SR appears quite susceptible to alteration during prolonged contractile activity (22, 28). The reduced functional capacity of the SR may in part explain the decrease in positive and negative dp/dt observed in fast and slow muscles as well as the prolonged ½RT of the slow soleus.

In conclusion, the experimental studies described in this chapter illustrate the complex nature of muscle fatigue. The discussion of this topic has been simplified by considering the potential causative agents of fatigue in 2 general types of work. In short duration, high intensity exercise, there is a high degree of anaerobic metabolism and muscle lactate production. A high negative correlation has been established between muscle lactate and the force generating capacity of muscle. The fatigue associated with the build-up in muscle lactate is thought to be a direct result of an elevated free H^+ concentration. Potential mechanisms of the deleterious effect of the H^+ ion are described.

In prolonged endurance activity, the depletion of body carbohydrate stores frequently occurs at exhaustion. Undoubtably other factors are involved as type I and IIA fibers fatigued, but type IIB fibers, despite low glycogen concentration, were unaltered by a 7 hour swim. Myofibrils and the maximal velocity of shortening were found to be resistant to fatigue. Other muscle organelles (see Chapter 7) probably are involved in the fatigue progress. The sarcoplasmic reticulum, a membrane system involved in the regulation of cell Ca^{++}, is altered by prolonged exercise; the decreased capacity of this system may contribute to the observed physiological changes in muscle with exhaustion.

REFERENCES

1. Aickin, C.C. and Thomas, R.C.: Micro-electrode measurement of the intracellular pH and buffering power of mouse soleus muscle fibres. *J Physiol (Lond)*, 267:791, 1977.
2. Asmussen, E.; von Döbeln, W.; and Nielsen, M.: Blood lactate and oxygen debt after exhaustive work at different oxygen tensions. *Acta Physiol Scand*, 15:57, 1948.
3. Baldwin, K.M.; Fitts, R.H.; Booth, F.W.; Winder, W.W.; and Holloszy, J.O.: Depletion of muscle and liver glycogen during exercise: Protective effect of training. *Pflügers Arch*, 354:203, 1975.

4. Baldwin, K.M.; Klinkerfuss, G.H.; Terjung, R.L.; Molé, P.A.; and Holloszy, J.O.: Respiratory capacity of white, red, and intermediate muscle: adaptative responses to exercise. *Am J Physiol, 222*:373, 1972.
5. Barany, M.: ATPase activity of myosin correlated with speed of muscle shortening. *J Gen Physiol, 50*:197, 1967.
6. Bergström, J.: Muscle electrolytes in man. *Scand J Clin Lab Invest [Suppl], 68*, 1962.
7. Bolitho-Donaldson, S.K. and Hermansen, L.: Differential, direct effects of H^+ on Ca^{++}-activated force of skinned fibers from the soleus, cardiac and adductor magnus muscles of rabbits. *Pflügers Arch, 376*:55, 1978.
8. Brooks, G.A.; Hittelman, K.J.; Faulkner, J.A.; and Beyer, R.E.: Temperature, skeletal muscle mitochondrial functions, and oxygen debt. *Am J Physiol, 220*:1053, 1971.
9. Brust, M.: Changes in contractility of frog muscle due to fatigue and inhibitors. *Am J Physiol, 206*:1043, 1964.
10. Chauveau, A.: Source et nature du potential directement utilisé dans le trovail musculaire, d'oprés les échanges respiratoires, chez l'homme en d'abstinence. *CR Acad Sci (Paris), 122*:1163, 1896.
11. Christensen, E.H. and Hansen, O.: Hypoglykamie, arbeitsfähigkeit and ermüdung. *Scand Arch Physiol, 81*:172, 1939.
12. Christensen, E.H. and Hansen, O.: Respiratorischen quotient und O_2-Augnahme. *Scand Arch Physiol, 81*:180, 1939.
13. Conlee, R.K.; Rennie, M.J.; and Winder, W.W.: Skeletal muscle glycogen content: diurnal variation and effects of fasting. *Am J Physiol, 231*:614, 1976.
14. Eberstein, A. and Sandow, A.: Fatigue in phasic and tonic fibers of frog muscle. *Science, 134*:383, 1961.
15. Fabiato, A. and Fabiato, F.: Effects of pH on the myofilaments and the sarcoplasmic reticulum of skinned cells from cardiac and skeletal muscles. *J Physiol (Lond), 276*:233, 1978.
16. Fitts, R.H.: The effects of exercise-training on the development of fatigue. *Ann NY Acad Sci, 301*:424, 1977.
17. Fitts, R.H.; Booth, F.W.; Winder, W.W.; and Holloszy, J.O.: Skeletal muscle respiratory capacity, endurance, and glycogen utilization. *Am J Physiol, 228*:1029, 1975.
18. Fitts, R.H.; Campion, D.R.; Nagle, F.J.; and Cassens, R.G.: Contractile properties of skeletal muscle from trained miniature pig. *Pflügers Arch, 343*:133, 1973.
19. Fitts, R.H. and Holloszy, J.O.: Contractile properties of rat soleus muscle: effects of training and fatigue. *Am J Physiol, 2*:C86, 1977.
20. Fitts, R.H. and Holloszy, J.O.: Effects of fatigue and recovery on contractile properties of frog muscle. *J Appl Physiol, 45*:899, 1978.
21. Fitts, R.H. and Holloszy, J.O.: Lactate and contractile force in frog muscle during development of fatigue and recovery. *Am J Physiol, 231*:430, 1976.
22. Fitts, R.H.; Kim, D.H.; and Witzmann, F.A.: The effect of prolonged activity on the sarcoplasmic reticulum and myofibrils of fast and slow skeletal

muscle. *Physiologist, 22*:38, 1979.

23. Fletcher, W.W. and Hopkins, F.G.: Lactic acid in mammalian muscle. *J Physiol (Lond), 35*:247, 1907.

24. Fuchs, F.; Reddy, V.; and Briggs, F.N.: The interaction of cations with the calcium-binding site of troponin. *Biochim Biophys Acta, 221*:407, 1970.

25. Gaskell, W.H.: On the tonicity of the heart and blood vessels. *J Physiol (Lond), 3*:48, 1880.

26. Gollnick, P.D. and Ianuzzo, C.D.: Colonic temperature response of rats during exercise. *J Appl Physiol, 24*:747, 1968.

27. Gollnick, P.D. and King, D.W.: Effect of exercise and training on mitochondria of rat skeletal muscle. *Am J Physiol, 216*:1502, 1969.

28. Hashimoto, I.; Sembrowich, W.L.; and Gollnick, P.D.: Calcium uptake by isolated sarcoplasmic reticulum and homogenates in different fiber types following exhaustive exercise. *Med Sci Sports, 10*:42, 1978.

29. Hermansen, L. and Bjorn-Osnes, J.: Blood and muscle pH after maximal exercise in man. *J Appl Physiol, 32*:304, 1972.

30. Hermansen, L.; Hultman, E.; and Saltin, B.: Muscle glycogen during prolonged severe exercise. *Acta Physiol Scand, 71*:129, 1967.

31. Hill, A.V.: The absolute value of the isometric heat coefficient Tl/H in a muscle twitch, and the effect of stimulation and fatigue. *Proc R Soc, Lond [Biol], 103*:163, 1928.

32. Hill, A.V.: The influence of the external medium on the internal pH of muscle. *Proc R Soc Lond [Biol], 144*:1, 1955-56.

33. Hill, A.V. and Kupalov, P.: Anaerobic and aerobic activity in isolated muscles. *Proc R Soc Lond [Biol], 105*:313, 1929.

34. Holloszy, J.O.: Biochemical adaptations to exercise: aerobic metabolism. In *Exercise and Sport Sciences Reviews,* edited by J.H. Wilmore. New York, Acad Pr, Vol. 1, pp. 45, 1973.

35. Holloszy, J.O. and Booth, F.W.: Biochemical adaptations to endurance exercise in muscle. *Ann Rev Physiol, 38*:273, 1976.

36. Holloszy, J.O.; Molé, P.A.; Baldwin, K.M.; and Terjung, R.L.: Exercise induced enzymatic adaptations in muscle. In *Limiting Factors of Physical Performance,* edited by K. Keul. Stuttgart, Georg Thieme, pp. 65, 1973.

37. Issekutz, B.; Miller, H.I.; and Rodahl, K.: Lipid and carbohydrate metabolism during exercise. *Fed Proc, 25*:1415, 1966.

38. Julian, F.J. and Moss, R.L.: The concept of active state in striated muscle. *Circ Res, 38*:53, 1976.

39. Karlsson, J. and Saltin, B.: Lactate, ATP, and CP in working muscles during exhaustive exercise in man. *J Appl Physiol, 29*:598, 1970.

40. Lorkovic, H.: Influences of changes in pH on the mechanical activity of cardiac muscle. *Circ Res, 19*:711, 1966.

41. Mainwood, G.W. and Lucier, G.E.: Fatigue and recovery in isolated frog sartorius muscle: the effects of bicarbonate concentration and associated potassium loss. *Can J Physiol Pharmacol, 50*:132, 1972.

42. Mainwood, G.W. and Worsley-Brown, P.: The effects of extracellular pH and buffer concentration on the efflux of lactate from sartorius muscle. *J Physiol (Lond), 250*:1, 1975.

43. Martonosi, A. and Feretos, F.: Sarcoplasmic reticulum. 1. The uptake of Ca^{++} by sarcoplasmic reticulum fragments. *J Biol Chem, 239*:648, 1964.

44. Nakamura, Y. and Schwartz, A.: The influence of hydrogen ion concentration on calcium binding and release by skeletal muscle sarcoplasmic reticulum. *J Gen Physiol, 59*:22, 1972.

45. Pannier, J.L. and Levsen, I.: Contraction characteristics of papillary muscle during changes in acid-base composition of the bathing fluid. *Arch Int Physiol Biochim, 76*:624, 1968.

46. Pannier, J.L.; Weyne, J.; and Levsen, I.: Effects of PCO_2, bicarbonate and lactate on the isometric contractions of isolated soleus muscle of the rat. *Pflügers Arch, 320*:120, 1970.

47. Pruett, E.D.R.: Glucose and insulin during prolonged work stress in men living on different diets. *J Appl Physiol, 28*:199, 1970.

48. Roos, A.: Intracellular pH and distribution of weak acids across cell membranes: A study of *D*- and *L*-lactate and of DMO in rat diaphragm. *J Physiol, 249*:1, 1975.

49. Sahlin, K.; Alvestrand, A.; Brandt, R.; and Hultman, E.: Intracellular pH and bicarbonate concentration in human muscle during recovery from exercise. *J Appl Physiol, 45*:474, 1978.

50. Saltin, B.: Aerobic work capacity and circulation during exercise in man. *Acta Physiol Scand [Suppl], 230*:5, 1964.

51. Saltin, F.; Gagge, A.P.; Bergh, U.; and Stolwijk, J.A.J.: Body temperature and sweating during exhaustive exercise. *J Appl Physiol, 32*:635, 1972.

52. Saltin, B. and Karlsson, J.: In *Muscle Metabolism During Exercise,* edited by B. Pernow and B. Saltin. New York, Plenum Pr, pp. 289, 1971.

53. Saltin, B. and Karlsson, J.: In *Muscle Metabolism During Exercise,* edited by B. Pernow and B. Saltin. New York, Plenum Pr, pp. 395, 1971.

54. Simonson, E.: Accumulation of metabolites. In *Physiology of Work Capacity and Fatigue,* edited by E. Simonson. Springfield, Thomas, pp. 9, 1971.

55. Trivedi, B. and Danforth, W.H.: Effect of pH on the kinetics of frog muscle phosphofructokinase. *J Biol Chem, 241*:4110, 1966.

56. Witzmann, F.A.; Kim, D.H.; and Fitts, R.H.: The effect of prolonged activity on the contractile properties of fast and slow skeletal muscle. *Physiologist, 22*:135, 1979.

57. Worsfold, M. and Peter, J.B.: Kinetics of calcium transport by fragmented sarcoplasmic reticulum. *J Biol Chem, 245*:5545, 1970.

58. Zak, R.; Etlinger, J.; and Feshman, D.A.: Studies on the fractionation of skeletal and heart muscle. In *Research in Muscle Development and the Muscle Spindle,* edited by F. Przybyeski, J. Van der Meullen, M. Victor, and B. Barker. New York, Elsevier, pp. 163, 1971.

Chapter 10

HISTOCHEMICAL CHARACTERISTICS OF SELECTED LOCOMOTOR AND RESPIRATORY MUSCLES OF THE RAT

H.J. GREEN AND K. GREENE

Introduction

SKELETAL MUSCLE is the biological machine for generating force (5), a requirement that is necessary for a wide variety of load transmitting functions necessary for survival. Since animals are characterized by their ability to perform diverse motor functions, ranging from the most delicate tasks requiring the coordination of a number of muscle groups to locomotor activities that either must be sustained over prolonged periods or that require the generation of large torque outputs, it might be expected that proficiency of movement would best be accomplished by having some degree of specialization both in terms of the character of the muscle cell and the selective manner in which individual muscle cells are recruited (8).

It has long been realized that skeletal muscle cells are not uniform but are composed of different fiber types with specific ultra-structural, metabolic, and physiologic characteristics (8). There has been a continuing quest to interrelate these properties so that a system can be developed for identification of fundamental "fiber types" (2). To date, however, no universal scheme has proved applicable to all species and all muscles.

At present, the only generally acceptable procedure for subdivision of mammalian muscle fibers is based upon a histochemical stain for myofibrillar ATPase after alkaline preincubation (15). This enables the fiber to be classified into 2 distinct categories (Type I and Type II). More recently, such a classification has been proven to correlate with the contractile characteristics in both human and nonhuman muscle (2, 3, 6).

136

The relationship of the metabolic differentation of the muscle tissue of these 2 "fundamental" fiber types remains obscure (17). At the extremes, Type I (Slow Twitch or ST) and Type II (Fast Twitch or FT) represent widely contrasting forms of specialization that can be characterized by marked differences in their enzyme activity patterns of energy metabolism (17). In selective skeletal muscles of a number of species, an inverse relationship exists in the ST fibers between the levels of glycolytic enzymes and the enzymes representative of aerobic substrate metabolism. It has consistently been found that ST fibers are high in oxidative potential and low in glycolytic potential (15). Such a finding is consistent with the proposed function of the ST fibers that have been classified as fatigue resistant and that appear to be selectively recruited in low intensity activity (8, 20). The FT fibers, although characterized by relatively high activities of glycolytic enzymes, appear to be heterogenous in the enzyme activities of oxidative metabolism. This has led Peter et al. (15) to propose a subclassification system for the FT fibers labelled fast twitch glycolytic (FG) and fast twitch oxidative-glycolytic (FOG). Although a number of species have been used in the development of the Peter et al. (15) classification schema, observations have been restricted to locomotor muscles. This chapter reports on some initial findings regarding the appropriateness of the Peter et al. (15) fiber type classification system to selected respiratory muscles (internal and external intercostals, diaphragm). In addition, a number of supporting properties (aerobic potential, size, capillarization) were compared for each fiber type between both respiratory and locomotor muscles. This seemed particularly relevant in view of the different patterns of utilization between these two different muscle groups. While most limb skeletal muscles contract at irregular intervals, between which occur long periods of rest, the respiratory muscles and particularly the diaphragm are required to sustain regular rhythmic contractions throughout the entire life span (21).

Methods

Samples of selected muscles (soleus, red and white gastrocnemius) and respiratory muscles (diaphragm, internal and external intercostals) were obtained from adult male Wistar rats (200–250 gm) following cervical dislocation. The respiratory muscles were removed initially, mounted, and quickly frozen in isopentane cooled to liquid nitrogen temperatures. Histochemistry was accomplished on a midportion of the anterior left hemodiaphragm while intercostal muscles were excised from the fourth intercostal space. Following removal of these muscles, the hind leg muscles on the right side were obtained and frozen in similar fashion.

Muscle cross sections (10 μm) were cut in a cryostat at $-20°C$ and stained for myofibrillar adenosine triphosphatase (ATPase) according to the procedures of Padykula and Herman (14), for NADH tetrazoleum reductase (NADH-TR) according to Novikoff et al. (13), and for alpha glycerophosphate dehydrogenase according to Wattenburg and Leong (19). Approximately 600 fibers were randomly sampled from 8 to 10 fasicules distributed throughout the cross sectional area of the sample. Fiber areas were determined from the NADH-TR stained sections by projecting the slides at a known magnification and tracing the fiber borders with a Numonics digitizer (7).

Capillary supply was determined for each muscle fiber according to the amylase-PAS method reported by Anderson (1). Where possible, at least 20 fibers were sampled from each category used in the classification. Capillarization was expressed in terms of the total number of capillaries per muscle fiber and on a ratio of capillaries to the cross-sectional area of the fiber.

This chapter summarizes the preliminary data on a single animal. For each histochemical stain, individual sections from all muscles for a given animal were placed in the same Columbia jars and treated identically. This precaution was taken to eliminate any variability that might occur between staining sessions.

Results

Table 10-I summarizes the distribution of fiber types within FT and ST categories according to the intensity of the NADH-TR stain. Four stain intensities were used to differentiate the oxidative potential of each muscle cell. In the ST muscle fibers, moderate to dark activity predominates for all 6 muscle tissues examined. However, different oxidative potentials appear to exist between muscle fibers within this range. The diaphragm muscle, for example, contains only 27 percent dark-staining fibers as contrasted to external and internal intercostals, which contain 69 and 100 percent dark-staining fibers respectively. For this animal, the gastroc-white

TABLE 10-I

HISTOCHEMICAL CHARACTERISTICS OF SELECTED LOCOMOTOR AND
RESPIRATORY MUSCLES OF THE RAT (PERCENT DISTRIBUTION)

	FT NADH-DIAPHORASE*				ST NADH-DIAPHORASE			
	1	2	3	4	1	2	3	4
DIAPHRAGM	1	41	24	34	—	12	61	27
EXTERNAL INTERCOSTAL	55	22	13	10	—	—	31	69
INTERNAL INTERCOSTAL	39	35	7	19	—	—	—	100
SOLEUS	—	—	70	30	1	7	89	3
GASTROC-RED	22	20	53	5	—	—	88	12
GASTROC-WHITE	32	68	—	—	—	—	—	—

*Staining intensity is indicated by 4 (dark), 3 (moderate), 1 (light), and 0 (no activity).

contained no ST fibers. The distribution of oxidative potential is more heterogenous in the FT cells. The gastroc-white, as an example, contained no fibers that stained moderate to dark for NADH-TR, whereas the soleus contained only cells with an oxidative potential in this range. Differences were also evident in the respiratory muscles examined. For both the external and internal intercostal muscles, in excess of 70 percent of the cells contained very little oxidative activity. The diaphragm appears the most heterogenous as large percentages of fibers are represented as having either dark, moderate, or light activity.

Table 10-II examines the areas of a sample of fibers from each of the categories examined. In general, fibers classified as FT have the largest areas; however, there are considerable differences

TABLE 10-II

MUSCLE FIBER AREAS OF SELECTED LOCOMOTOR AND
RESPIRATORY MUSCLES OF THE RAT

	FT NADH-DIAPHORASE				ST NADH-DIAPHORASE			
	1	2	3	4	1	2	3	4
DIAPHRAGM	5118*	4109	1636	1123	—	1672	1381	1017
EXTERNAL INTERCOSTAL	4415	3172	1307	1057	—	—	1029	849
INTERNAL INTERCOSTAL	5144	4316	2300	1794	—	—	—	1519
SOLEUS	—	—	2502	2188	4004	3554	2476	1917
GASTROC-RED	3141	2607	1469	1310	—	—	1788	1161
GASTROC-WHITE	4789	3841	—	—	—	—	—	—

*$\bar{X}$ in $(\mu m)^2$

within each subclassification. For both the ST and FT groups, a relationship is evident between the oxidative potential and fiber size. For all muscles, size is inversely related to the aerobic potential of the cell. For the FT cells, a clear demarcation in size exists between fibers staining light to moderate in NADH-TR. Approximately a twofold difference in size is evident between these subclassifications. Within each classification of oxidative potential, the type of fiber (FT or ST) does not appear to influence the size.

The capillary distribution as determined by the number of capillaries surrounding each fiber is presented in Table 10-III. No trend appears evident for either FT or ST groups between capillary number and oxidative potential. In general, capillary numbers ranged between 3.8 and 7.0 per muscle fiber. A comparison between muscles revealed that the external intercostal and gastroc-white contained fewer capillaries within each subclassification examined.

TABLE 10-III
CAPILLARIES PER MUSCLE FIBER OF SELECTED LOCOMOTOR AND
RESPIRATORY MUSCLES OF THE RAT

	FT NADH-DIAPHORASE				ST NADH-DIAPHORASE			
	1	2	3	4	1	2	3	4
DIAPHRAGM	6.7	6.3	5.2	5.5	—	5.6	5.6	5.6
EXTERNAL INTERCOSTAL	4.0	4.7	4.7	4.8	—	—	4.0	3.8
INTERNAL INTERCOSTAL	5.8	5.6	5.7	5.4	—	—	—	4.8
SOLEUS	—	—	5.5	5.7	7.0	5.5	5.6	5.7
GASTROC-RED	5.9	6.4	6.1	6.2	—	—	5.9	6.0
GASTROC-WHITE	3.8	3.9	—	—	—	—	—	—

When the number of capillaries were divided by the area of each muscle cell to obtain a ratio of the number of capillaries per unit area, a direct relationship was observed between oxidative potential and capillarization (Table 10-IV). This was evident for both FT and ST fibers in all muscle sections. It is of interest that the capillary density of the soleus muscle is less than the other muscles examined. The diaphragm and gastroc-red muscles, on the other hand, appear to rank highest on this measure of capillary density.

TABLE 10-IV

CAPILLARY TO FIBER AREAS OF SELECTED LOCOMOTOR AND
RESPIRATORY MUSCLES OF THE RAT

	FT NADH-DIAPHORASE				ST NADH-DIAPHORASE			
	1	2	3	4	1	2	3	4
DIAPHRAGM	1.3*	1.5	3.2	4.9	—	3.3	4.0	5.5
EXTERNAL INTERCOSTAL	0.9	1.5	3.6	4.5	—	—	3.9	4.5
INTERNAL INTERCOSTAL	1.1	1.3	2.5	3.0	—	—	—	4.8
SOLEUS	—	—	2.2	2.6	1.8	1.5	2.2	3.0
GASTROC-RED	1.9	2.4	4.2	4.7	—	—	3.3	5.2
GASTROC-WHITE	0.8	1.0	—	—	—	—	—	—

*10^{-3} $(\mu m)^2$

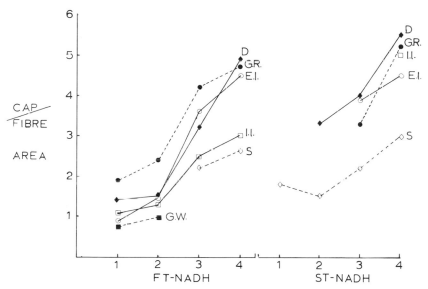

Figure 10-1. Comparison of fiber type and capillary to fiber ratios in selected locomotor and respiratory muscles. S = soleus; G.W. = gastroe-white; G.R. = gastroe-red; D = diaphragm; E.I. = external intercostal; I.I. = internal intercostal.

The distribution of fiber types according to the classification of Peter et al. (15) for each muscle section appears in Table 10-V. In contrast to Peter et al. (15), two categories of ST fibers have been recognized, one low in oxidative activity (SO$_1$) and one moderate to high in oxidative activity (SO$_2$). Fast glycolytic (FG) and fast oxidative-glycolytic (FOG) types have been established by combin-

TABLE 10-V
MUSCLE FIBER TYPE DISTRIBUTIONS OF SELECTED LOCOMOTOR AND
RESPIRATORY MUSCLES OF THE RAT*

	FG	FOG	SO_1	SO_2
DIAPHRAGM	30	42	3	25
EXTERNAL INTERCOSTAL	72	22	—	6
INTERNAL INTERCOSTAL	63	22	—	15
SOLEUS	—	20	6	74
GASTROC-RED	32	45	—	23
GASTRO-WHITE	100	—	—	—

*Classified according to Peter et al. (15).

ing the subclassifications for the two lowest and two highest staining intensities on NADH-TR respectively. Based on this schema,
the soleus muscle is basically a slow twitch muscle, whereas the
gastrocnemius is basically fast twitch. The gastroc-white, however,
contains 100 percent FG fibers, while the gastroc-red contains a
relatively high percentage of both FG and FOG fibers. While fiber
distribution of the diaphragm is much like the gastroc-red, both
the internal and external intercostal muscles are relatively
homogenous in fast twitch fiber distribution with a preponderance of the fast fibers classified as FG.

Table 10-VI provides a summary of the histochemical characteristics examined and averaged over all muscles. For both ST and
FT fiber classifications, oxidative potential is inversely proportional to size and directly proportional to capillary to fiber size
ratios. No relationship is evident between oxidative potential and
capillary number.

TABLE 10-VI
SUMMARY OF SELECTED HISTOCHEMICAL FEATURES
AVERAGED OVER ALL MUSCLES

	FT NADH-DIAPHORASE				ST NADH-DIAPHORASE			
	1	2	3	4	1	2	3	4
FIBER SIZE $(\mu m)^2$	4521	3609	1843	1494	4004	2613	1669	1293
CAPILLARIES/FIBRE (N)	5.2	5.4	5.4	5.5	7.0	5.6	5.3	5.2
CAPILLARY TO FIBER RATIOS $(10^{-3} \mu m^2)$	1.2	1.5	3.1	3.9	1.8	2.4	3.4	4.6

Discussion

Identification of the muscle fiber types according to the Peter et al. (15) schema indicates that the soleus muscle is basically composed of SO fibers, while the gastroc-red and the gastroc-white, both high in FT fibers, have a preponderance of FOG and FG fibers respectively. This finding is consistent with previous work (3, 13, 15) and, in fact, represents the reason for selection of these particular limb muscles for comparison with the respiratory muscles. Both the diaphragm and gastroc-red muscles appear similar in the distribution of these 3 fiber types. The intercostals are basically FT fibers, and in particular, both contain a high percentage of FG fibers, similar to the gastroc-white muscle. Keens et al. (10) using the same classification system have found an approximately similar distribution for the 3 respiratory muscles examined.

However, closer comparison of the oxidative potential of the FT and ST fibers between the respiratory and locomotor muscles reveals some differences. When 4 levels of oxidative potential are used, as determined by the NADH-TR stain intensity, the diaphragm contains a relatively high percentage of dark-staining FT fibers as compared to the gastroc-red fibers. The intercostals, on the other hand, have a large percentage of FT fibers that appear to have minimal oxidative activity. In contrast, the ST intercostal muscle fibers are distinguished by having a greater percentage of dark-staining cells than the limb muscles, which are to a great extent moderate staining.

Although histochemical techniques are, at best, semiquantitative, these results suggest that the utilization of 4 categories of NADH-TR activity can lead to considerably more information regarding muscle fiber differentiation than the high and low oxidative activity categories proposed by Peter et al. (15). This speculation is further supported by the relationship of the oxidative potential to fiber size. Using 4 subclassifications of NADH-TR, a clear relationship exists between the size of the fiber and aerobic potential. This association exists regardless of the muscle examined and whether the cells are slow or fast twitch. For both ST and FT cells, there is an approximate threefold difference in fiber size between the extreme staining intensities. Neither size nor oxidative potential appear to relate to the number of capillaries surrounding each fiber type. This conclusion applies to both the respiratory and the limb muscles examined. This finding is at odds with a number of investigators (1, 13, 18) who have found that the number of capillaries surrounding each individual muscle fiber was directly proportional to the activity of the oxidative enzymes in the fibers. Myrhage (12) has also reported a positive relation between the number of capillaries and average diameter of muscle cells in a number of cat hind limb muscles. It is possible that part of this discrepancy may be explained by the procedures used to determine capillary density. In this study, individual fiber types were identified and the size and capillary number determined. Capillaries shared between fibers were included as belonging to the fiber being measured.

The functional significance of the 3 basic fiber types (SO, FOG, FG) remains uncertain. Henneman and Olsen (8) have proposed that during low intensity activity smaller alpha motoneurons and consequently small muscle fibers are recruited preferentially to develop the necessary tension. For these muscles to be fatigue resistant, it is necessary that their mode of energy metabolism be primarily aerobic while relying essentially on exogenous substrates derived from the blood for maintaining fuel homeostasis (9). The findings of this study would tend to confirm the aerobic nature of both the small ST and the FT fibers in all of the muscles studied. In addition, the high capillary density found in these fibers may be essential in minimizing the fatigue that occurs with sustained function (16). The large fibers that are recruited normally only under conditions of intense contraction rely mainly on anaerobic glycolysis for ATP regeneration (9). The low oxidative capacity and capillary density observed in these fibers is consistent with this proposed function.

The respiratory muscles investigated contain a mixture of all 3 fiber types; however, there is a decided preponderance of FG and FOG fibers. The diaphragm, which is required to contract during each inspiratory maneuver, is composed of an excess of 65 percent of moderate to high oxidative fibers of both fast and slow twitch. The size and capillary density of these fibers is very similar to the gastrocnemius red muscle in the limb, a muscle known for its ability to resist fatigue (16). Recently, it has been postulated that diaphragmatic fatigue occurs when the rate of energy consumption by the muscle is greater than the rate of energy supplied to the muscle by the blood. An energy deficit develops that leads to ultimate failure of the diaphragm as a force generator (4). It is possible that the ability of the diaphragm to maintain function during chronic overload is closely related to its oxidative fiber composition (11). On the basis of the histochemical evidence presented and the known fatigue-resistant properties of other muscles of comparable characteristics, this appears to be a reasonable hypothesis.

REFERENCES

1. Anderson, P.: Capillary density in skeletal muscle of man. *Acta Physiol Scand, 95*:203, 1975.
2. Barnard, R.J.; R. Edgerton; T. Furukawa; and J.B. Peter: Histochemical, biochemical and contractile properties of red, white and intermediate fibres. *Am J Physiol, 220*:410, 1971.
3. Burke, R.E. and V.R. Edgerton: Motor unit properties and selective involvement in movement. *Exerc Sport Sci Rev, 3*:31, 1975.
4. Derenne, J.P.H.; P.T. Macklem; and C.H. Roussos: The respiratory muscles: mechanics, control and pathophysiology. *Am Rev Respir Dis, 118*:581, 1978.
5. Edwards, R.H.T.: Physiological and metabolic studies of the contractile machinery of human muscle in health and disease. *Phys Med Biol, 24*:237, 1979.
6. Essén, B.; F. Jansson; J. Henriksson; A.W. Taylor; and B. Saltin: Metabolic characteristics of fibre types in human skeletal muscles. *Acta Physiol Scand, 95*:153, 1975.
7. Green, H.; J.A. Thomson; W.D. Daub; M.E. Houston; and D.A. Ranney: Fibre composition, fiber size and enzyme activities in vastus lateralis of elite athletes involved in high intensity exercise. *Eur J Appl Physiol, 41*:109, 1979.
8. Henneman, E. and C.B. Olsen: Relations between structure and function in the design of skeletal muscles. *J Neurol, 28*:581, 1965.
9. Hooker, A.M. and K. Baldwin: Substrate oxidation specificity in different types of mammalian muscle. *Am J Physiol, 236(1)*:C66, 1979.
10. Keens, T.G.; V. Chen; P. Patel; P. O'Brien; H. Kevison; and C.D. Ianuzzo: Cellular adaptation of the ventilatory muscles to a chronic increased respiratory load. *J Appl Physiol, 44(6)*:905, 1978.
11. Lieberman, D.A.; J.A. Faulkner; A.B. Craig, Jr.; and L.C. Maxwell: Performance and histochemical composition of guinea pig and human diaphragm. *J Appl Physiol, 34*:233, 1973.
12. Myrhage, R.: Capillary supply of the muscle fibre population in hind limb muscles of the cat. *Acta Physiol Scand, 103*:19, 1978.
13. Novikoff, A.B.; W. Shin; and J. Drucker: Mitochondrial localization of oxidative enzymes: Staining results with two tetrazolium salts. *J Biophy Biochem Cytol, 9*:47, 1961.

14. Padykula, H.A. and E. Herman: The specificity of the histochemical method of adenosine triphosphatase. *J Histochem Cyto Chem, 3*:170, 1955.
15. Peter, J.B.; R.J. Barnard; V.R. Edgerton; C.A. Gillespie; and K.E. Stempel: Metabolic profiles of three fiber types of skeletal muscle in guinea pigs and rabbits. *Biochemistry II*:2627-2634, 1972.
16. Petrofsky, J.S. and A.R. Lind: Isometric endurance in fast and slow muscles of the cat. *Am J Physiol, 236(5)*:C185-C191, 1979.
17. Pette, D. and C. Spamer: Metabolic subpopulations of muscle fibers: A quantitative study. *Diabetes 28*: Suppl. 1, 25, 1979.
18. Romanul, F.C.A.: Capillary supply and metabolism of muscle fibers. *Arch Neurol, 12*:497, 1965.
19. Wattenburg, L.W. and J. Leong: Effects of co-enzymes Q_{10} and menadione on saccinate dehydrogenase activity as measured by tetrazoleum salt reduction. *J Histochem Cyto Chem, 8*:296-3, 1961.
20. Wuerker, R.B.; A.M. McPhredran; and E. Henneman: Properties of motor units in heterogenous pale muscle (M. gastrocnemius) of the cat. *J Physiol (Lond), 28*:85, 1965.
21. Yellin, H.: Differences in histochemical attributes between diaphragm and hind leg muscles of the rat. *Anat Rec, 173*:333, 1972.

Chapter 11

OXYGEN CONSUMPTION DURING EXERCISE AND RECOVERY

J.M. HAGBERG

SINCE THE first metabolic rate determinations during exercise were made in the 1880s, the measurement of oxygen consumption ($\dot{V}O_2$) during maximal and submaximal exercise has proven to be the most useful method for determining energy expenditure (2). The $\dot{V}O_2$ methodology used then, and that still used today, involves the collection of the expired air of the subject in Douglas bags or spirometers. While this technique is excellent for steady state $\dot{V}O_2$ determinations, it is very difficult to accurately describe the time course of the change in $\dot{V}O_2$ from the onset of exercise or recovery because of the difficulty in collecting very frequent, accurately timed samples. In spite of this inherent difficulty, Hill and Lupton (14) in 1922 first presented data concerning the approach of $\dot{V}O_2$ towards steady state at the onset of exercise. It is interesting, from a historical standpoint, that they thought the lag in the rise of $\dot{V}O_2$ was the result of the gradual increase in tissue lactate, which in turn caused the progressive rise in muscle respiration (14). They also were the first to study the time course of the repayment of the oxygen debt (14). In fact, much of the interest since the early days of exercise physiology has centered on the oxygen debt, the excess metabolism during recovery from exercise, as well as on the changes that occur at the onset of exercise.

In recent years, with the advent of rapidly responding respiratory gas analyzers, interest in the transient phases of $\dot{V}O_2$ during exercise and recovery has been revived. In 1972, Whipp and Wasserman first began using a computer-based system with a rapidly responding mass spectrometer to analyze gas fractions and a pneumotachometer to measure expired flow; this system calculated all respiratory gas exchange values ($\dot{V}O_2$, $\dot{V}_E$, $\dot{V}CO_2$, RQ,

$P_{ET}O_2$, $P_{ET}CO_2$) on a breath-by-breath basis (1). Similar systems were later designed and used at the University of Wisconsin (9, 10, 11) and Washington University in St. Louis (8, 13). The major advantage of these breath-by-breath systems for describing the time course of the changes in $\dot{V}O_2$ is the large number of points (10–40/min) on the $\dot{V}O_2$ versus time curve generated during an exercise or recovery transient, as opposed to the limited number (2–4/min) generated with the Douglas bag system.

TIME COURSE OF THE INCREASE IN $\dot{V}O_2$ AT THE ONSET OF EXERCISE

It was commonly believed, before the development of computer-based breath-by-breath $\dot{V}O_2$ systems, that the half time ($t_{1/2}$) of the exponential rise in $\dot{V}O_2$ at the onset of exercise was 30 seconds, regardless of work intensity or the training status of the subject (4, 6). In the first study using the breath-by-breath methodology, however, Whipp and Wasserman (21) demonstrated that the $t_{1/2}$ of the $\dot{V}O_2$ response was clearly related to exercise intensity. They also stated that the $t_{1/2}$ of the response was related to the cardiovascular fitness of the subject; however, they compared only 2 subjects.

In order to more clearly assess the role of fitness in the relationship of the $t_{1/2}$ of the $\dot{V}O_2$ response to leg cycling, the responses, at the same absolute and relative work rates, of 2 groups of subjects of similar age—one untrained with an average $\dot{V}O_2$ max of 49.7 ml/kg/min and the second a group of highly trained cross-country runners with an average $\dot{V}O_2$ max of 70.2 ml/kg/min—were compared (11). The $t_{1/2}$ of the response for the trained subjects was significantly shorter at the same absolute work rates, indicating a more rapid adaptation to the exercise stress (Fig. 11-1). The same trend was evident when the groups were compared at equal relative work rates, but the differences were not significant (Fig. 11-2).

Two more recent reports have investigated the oxygen uptake kinetics of the same subject before and after a program of intensive training (8, 13). They have both shown that the response of trained subjects was more rapid even at the same relative work rates following training. The magnitude of the change in the $t_{1/2}$ of the $\dot{V}O_2$ response at the onset of exercise with training was such that the oxygen deficit was significantly reduced at the same absolute work rate following training, while it was unchanged at the

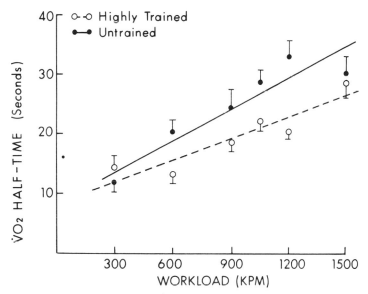

Figure 11-1. The half-time of the $\dot{V}O_2$ response at the onset of exercise versus the absolute work rate. Values are means ± SEM. (From Hagberg et al.: *J Appl Physiol, 44*:90, 1978, with permission of The American Physiological Society).

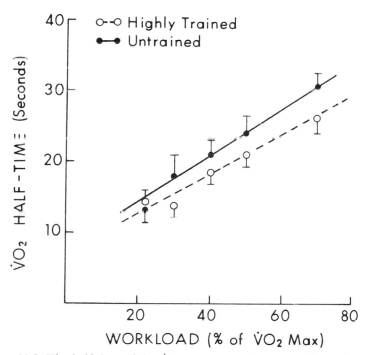

Figure 11-2. The half-time of the $\dot{V}O_2$ response at the onset of exercise versus the relative work rate. Values are means ± SEM. (From Hagberg et al.: *J Appl Physiol, 44*:90, 1978, with permission of The American Physiological Society).

same relative work rate following training despite the 24 percent higher absolute work rate (Table 11-I). The second of these 2 studies also showed that the time courses of the increase in $\dot{V}CO_2$, $\dot{V}_E$, and heart rate at the onset of exercise were more rapid at both the same absolute and the same relative work rates following training (8).

TABLE 11-I
EFFECTS OF TRAINING ON MAGNITUDE OF THE O_2 DEFICIT

	Before Training*	After Training* Same Absolute Work Rate	Same Relative Work Rate
50% of $\dot{V}O_2$max			
O_2 Deficit (liters)	0.66 ± 0.04	0.48 ± 0.07†	0.69 ± 0.06
Work Rate (kpm/min)	675 ± 31	675 ± 31	875 ± 28†
70% of $\dot{V}O_2$max			
O_2 Deficit (liters)	1.18 ± 0.11	0.93 ± 0.14†	1.29 ± 0.07
Work Rate (kpm/min)	994 ± 50	994 ± 50	1275 ± 44†

*Values are means ± SE of 8 subjects.
†Before versus after training, $p < 0.05$.

The decrease in oxygen deficit that results from the more rapid adaptation of $\dot{V}O_2$ in trained subjects agrees with the data of Hultman et al. (16) and Karlsson et al. (17), who found that trained subjects deplete their creatine phosphate (CP) and ATP stores less and produce less lactate in the first minutes of exercise.

TIME COURSE OF THE $\dot{V}O_2$ CHANGES AFTER THE INITIAL MINUTES OF EXERCISE

At work rates above approximately 65–70 percent of $\dot{V}O_2$max, a second component of the rise in $\dot{V}O_2$ during exercise is present. This is shown in Figure 11-3 as the slow rise in $\dot{V}O_2$ that occurs after the rapid increase during the first 2–3 minutes of exercise. The second component can be seen more clearly in the semilogarithmic plot of the $\dot{V}O_2$ change in Figure 11-4. The second component is clearly related to relative work intensity. In a group of untrained subjects, the second component was evident at 70 percent of $\dot{V}O_2$max but not at 50 percent of $\dot{V}O_2$max. Following training, which elicited a 24 percent increase in $\dot{V}O_2$max, the second component was not present at the absolute work rate equal to 50 percent of their pretraining $\dot{V}O_2$max, at 50 percent of their new $\dot{V}O_2$max, or at the absolute work rate equal to 70 percent of their pretraining $\dot{V}O_2$max (now equal to 58% of their $\dot{V}O_2$max).

The second component was still present at 70 percent of their new $\dot{V}O_2$max and the slope of the second component was the same as before training. However, steady state ($\leq 1\%$ $\dot{V}O_2$ change for 2+ minutes) was attained earlier because of the more rapid and larger first component of the $\dot{V}O_2$ response.

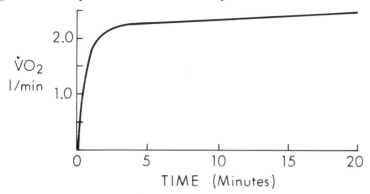

Figure 11-3. Schematic of the $\dot{V}O_2$ changes during exercise showing the slow rise in $\dot{V}O_2$ that occurs after the initial minutes of exercise at higher work intensities.

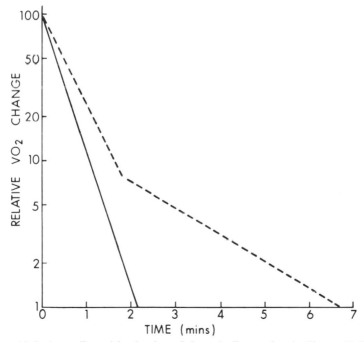

Figure 11-4. A semilogarithmic plot of data similar to that in Figure 11-3. The solid line shows a one-component exponential rise towards steady state while the dashed line shows a two-component $\dot{V}O_2$ response.

The second component of the $\dot{V}O_2$ response during exercise has been attributed to a "lactacid" mechanism (20); however there is no theoretical or experimental support for such a mechanism. The causes of the increase in $\dot{V}O_2$ between minutes 5 and 20 of exercise at 65 and 80 percent of $\dot{V}O_2$max were investigated (10). Most of this increase (i.e. the second component) can be attributed to the direct and indirect effects of temperature (Fig. 11-5). The Q_{10} effect, the increase in metabolic rate that results from the action of temperature on enzyme kinetics, could account for 30 percent of the rise in $\dot{V}O_2$ between minutes 5 and 10 of exercise at both work intensities (Fig. 11-5). The rise in ventilation across this

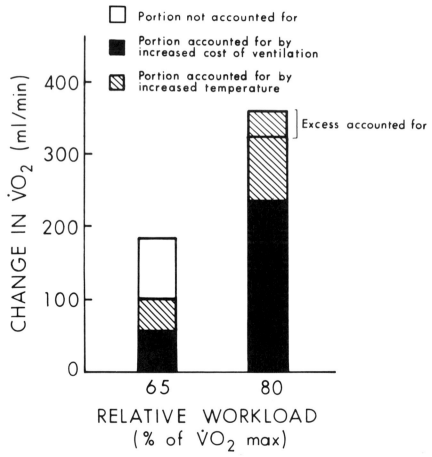

Figure 11-5. Causes of the rise in $\dot{V}O_2$ observed between minutes 5 and 20 of exercise at 65 and 80% of $\dot{V}O_2$max (From Hagberg et al.: *J Appl Physiol, 45*:381, 1978, with permission of The American Physiological Society).

same time period was significantly correlated with the rise in temperature; this suggests that this slow rise in ventilation may be due to the slowly increasing temperatures (7). The estimated cost of the increase in ventilation could account for another 30 percent of the rise in $\dot{V}O_2$ at 65 percent of $\dot{V}O_2$max and for slightly over 75 percent of the rise at 80 percent of $\dot{V}O_2$max (Fig. 11-5).

These data, along with those of Hubbard (15), imply that the second component of the $\dot{V}O_2$ response is due to the direct and indirect effects of increasing body temperature, not to a "lactacid" phenomenon.

TIME COURSE OF THE DECLINE IN $\dot{V}O_2$ AT THE ONSET OF RECOVERY

The excess $\dot{V}O_2$ following the cessation of exercise has received considerable attention since it was first observed in 1845 by Vierordt (2). It was commonly believed, until only recently, that the $t_{1/2}$ of the exponential decline of $\dot{V}O_2$ towards the resting level was 30 seconds, regardless of work intensity or the training state of the individual (4, 6). However, as with the time course of the response to exercise, the $t_{1/2}$ of the decrease in $\dot{V}O_2$ has, with the use of breath-by-breath $\dot{V}O_2$ systems, been shown to also be proportional to the relative work intensity and to be influenced by the subject's level of training (8). Following a program of endurance exercise training, the decline of $\dot{V}O_2$ occurred more rapidly at both the same absolute and the same relative work rates. As a result of the more rapid recovery of $\dot{V}O_2$, oxygen debt is lower at the same absolute work rate and unchanged at the same relative work rate following training. This was true despite the fact that $\dot{V}O_2$ was 24 percent higher at the same relative work rate following training (Table 11-II). The heart rate, $\dot{V}CO_2$, and $\dot{V}_E$ also decreased towards

TABLE 11-II
EFFECTS OF TRAINING ON MAGNITUDE OF THE O_2 DEBT

	Before Training*	After Training*	
		Same Absolute Work Rate	Same Relative Work Rate
50% of $\dot{V}O_2$max			
O_2 Debt (liters)	0.70 ± 0.07	0.49 ± 0.04†	0.76 ± 0.06
Work Rate (kpm/min)	675 ± 31	675 ± 31	875 ± 28†
70% of $\dot{V}O_2$max			
O_2 Debt (liters)	1.41 ± 0.15	1.04 ± 0.07†	1.47 ± 0.12
Work Rate (kpm/min)	994 ± 50	994 ± 50	1275 ± 44†

*Values are means ± SE of 8 subjects.
†Before versus after training, $p < 0.05$.

baseline more rapidly at both the same absolute and the same relative work rates following training. The $t_{1/2}$ of the course of each of the variables during exercise and recovery were closely correlated; in fact, the $t_{1/2}$ of $\dot{V}O_2$, $\dot{V}CO_2$, and $\dot{V}_E$ courses were essentially the same in exercise and recovery while the recovery heart rate $t_{1/2}$ was significantly longer than the exercise $t_{1/2}$.

The time course of $\dot{V}O_2$ during recovery also follows a 2 component exponential curve at higher work intensities. No evidence (8) was found of a second component following work requiring 50 percent of $\dot{V}O_2$max before or after training; following training, recovery after work equal to 70 percent of the pretraining $\dot{V}O_2$max (now equal to 58% of $\dot{V}O_2$max) also exhibited a single exponential curve. A second component was clearly evident at 70 percent of $\dot{V}O_2$max before training. It is questionable if a second component existed at 70 percent of the subject's new $\dot{V}O_2$ following training; if one was present, it accounted for only 2 percent of the total change in $\dot{V}O_2$.

The oxygen debt associated with the first component of the decline in $\dot{V}O_2$ during recovery is usually termed the "alactacid" debt and is attributed to the repletion of creatine phosphate, ATP, venous oxygen, and myoglobin oxygen stores. The cause of the slower second component, previously termed the "lactacid" phase, is widely debated (9).

In an attempt to ascertain the cause of the slower second phase of $\dot{V}O_2$ during recovery, the 2 components of oxygen debt following 5 and 20 minutes of exercise at 3 work intensities (50, 65, and 80% of $\dot{V}O_2$max) were compared (9). The magnitude of the "alactacid" debt was proportional to exercise intensity and was not affected by work duration. This is very much in line with the concept that CP-ATP repletion is the cause for this component, since it has been shown that phosphagens are decreased early in exercise and are not further depleted during long-term submaximal exercise (16). The magnitude of the slow component of the oxygen debt was not altered by exercise duration at 50 and 65 percent of $\dot{V}O_2$max; however at 80 percent of $\dot{V}O_2$max the slow debt was 5 times higher following the longer exercise. It has been hypothesized that the excess $\dot{V}O_2$ of the second component is used in the metabolism of lactate; however, the biochemical basis for such a mechanism is not clear. Theoretical and experimental data can be best summarized as offering little or no support for a lactacid mechanism except for reports supporting muscle gluconeogenesis from lactate (12, 18). Blood lactate levels were higher following the longer exercise at 80 percent of $\dot{V}O_2$max, but only by 20 mg% (9). Making numerous assumptions, it is possible to attribute only 30 percent of the excess slow debt following 20 minutes of exercise at 80 percent of $\dot{V}O_2$max to the metabolism of lactate. Thus, it appears that lactate can account for only a small part of the second component of oxygen debt.

As in the second component of the increase in $\dot{V}O_2$ during exercise, an increase in temperature appears to play a large role in the second component of the O_2 debt. The Q_{10} effect of temperature, assuming the increase in skeletal muscle temperature to be twice the observed increase in rectal temperature (5), completely accounted for that portion of the slow component of the oxygen debt not attributable to lactate metabolism following the longer exercise at 80 percent of $\dot{V}O_2$max (9). In addition, the increase in temperature observed between the 5 and 20 minute exercise bouts at 50 and 65 percent of $\dot{V}O_2$max could completely account for the average difference in the slow component of the oxygen debt between these 2 work durations. This finding is supported by a number of other investigators who attribute the majority of the second component of recovery $\dot{V}O_2$ to the effect of temperature rather than to the metabolism of lactate (3, 5, 19)

SUMMARY

The time course of the rise in $\dot{V}O_2$ following the onset of exercise and of the decline in $\dot{V}O_2$ following the cessation of exercise have been shown to be proportional to the relative exercise intensity. However, the state of training also plays an independent role in determining the time course of the response; that is, the trained subject will approach steady state or baseline $\dot{V}O_2$ more rapidly than an untrained subject, even at the same relative work intensity. The second component of $\dot{V}O_2$ in exercise can best be attributed to the effects of temperature on metabolism and ventilation. The second component in recovery may be caused by a combination of the temperature effect and the energetic costs of muscle gluconeogenesis from lactate.

REFERENCES

1. Beaver, W.L.; K. Wasserman; and B.J. Whipp: On-line computer analysis and breath-by-breath graphical display of exercise function tests. *J Appl Physiol, 34*:128, 1973.

2. Benedict, F.G. and E.P. Cathcart. *Muscular Work,* Pub. #187. Washington, D.C., Carnegie Inst, 1913.
3. Brooks, G.A.; H.J. Kittelman; J.A. Faulkner; and R.E. Beyer: Temperature, skeletal muscle mitochondria function, and oxygen debt. *Am J Physiol, 220*:1053, 1971.
4. Cerretelli, P.; R. Sikand; and C.E. Farhi: Readjustments in cardiac output and gas exchange during onset of exercise and recovery. *J Appl Physiol, 21*:1345, 1966.
5. Claremont, A.D.; F.J. Nagle; W.D. Reddan; and G.A. Brooks: Comparison of metabolic, temperature, heart rate, and ventilatory responses to exercise at extreme ambient temperatures. *Med Sci Sports,* 7:150, 1975.
6. Davies, C.T.M.; P.E. DiPrampero; and P. Cerretelli: Kinetics of cardiac output and respiratory exchange during exercise and recovery. *J Appl Physiol, 32*:618, 1972.
7. Dempsey, J.A. and W.D. Reddan: Hyperventilation during prolonged work: cause and effect. *Med Sci Sports,* 8:62, 1976.
8. Hagberg, J.H.; R.C. Hickson; A.A. Ehsani; and J.O. Holloszy: Faster adjustment to and recovery from submaximal exercise in the trained state. *J Appl Physiol, 48*:218, 1980.
9. Hagberg, J.M.; J.P. Mullin; and F.J. Nagle: Effect of work intensity and duration on recovery $\dot{V}O_2$. *J Appl Physiol, 48*:540, 1980.
10. Hagberg, J.M.; J.P. Mullin; and F.J. Nagle: Oxygen consumption during constant load exercise. *J Appl Physiol, 45*:381, 1978.
11. Hagberg, J.M.; F.J. Nagle, and J.L. Carlson: Transient O_2 uptake response at the onset of exercise. *J Appl Physiol, 44*:90, 1978.
12. Hermansen, L. and O. Vaage: Lactate disappearance and glycogen synthesis in human muscle after maximal exercise. *Am J Physiol, 233*:E422, 1977.
13. Hickson, R.C.; H.A. Bomze; and J.O. Holloszy: Faster adjustment of O_2 uptake to the energy requirement of exercise in the trained state. *J Appl Physiol, 44*:877, 1978.
14. Hill, A.V. and H. Lupton: Muscular exercise, lactic acid, and the supply and utilization of oxygen. *Q J Med, 16*:135, 1922.
15. Hubbard, J.L.: The effect of exercise on lactate metabolism. *J Physiol (Lond), 231*:1, 1973.
16. Hultman, E.; J. Bergstrom; and N. McLennan Anderson: Breakdown and resynthesis of phosphorylcreatine and adenosine triphosphate in connection with muscular work in man. *Scand J Clin Lab Invest, 19*:56, 1967.
17. Karlsson, J.; L.O. Nordesjo; L. Jorfeldt; and B. Saltin: Muscle lactate, ATP, and CP levels during exercise after physical training in man. *J Appl Physiol, 33*:199, 1972.
18. McLane, J.A. and J.O. Holloszy: Glycogen synthesis from lactate in three types of skeletal muscle. *J Biol Chem, 254*:6548, 1979.
19. Varene, P.; C. Jacquemin; J. Durand; and J. Raynaud: Energy balance during moderate exercise at altitude. *J Appl Physiol, 34*:633, 1973.
20. Volkov, N.I.; V.N. Cheremisinov; and E.N. Razumovskii: Oxygen exchange in man during muscular activity. In *The Oxygen Regime of the Organism and*

Its Regulation, edited by N.V. Lauer and A.Z. Kolchinskaya. NASA Technical Translation, 1969.

21. Whipp, B.J. and K. Wasserman: Oxygen uptake kinetics for various intensities of constant load work. *J Appl Physiol, 33*:351, 1972.

Chapter 12

ARM AND LEG MAXIMAL AND SUBMAXIMAL $\dot{V}O_2$ AMONG ARM- AND LEG-TRAINED ATHLETES

J. DANIELS AND J. BALES

INTRODUCTION

NUMEROUS studies have focused on comparing the aerobic demands of arm and leg work and on differences that might exist in heart rate and ventilatory responses to work performed by the arms alone, legs alone, and arms and legs combined. (1–3, 12, 13). There has been general agreement that more work can be performed by the legs, relative to the arms (2, 12, 13); that the arms demand a higher $\dot{V}O_2$ for a given work load than do the legs (13); and that heart rate maximum (HRmax) and maximum ventilation ($\dot{V}_E$max) are lower during arm work than during leg work (1–3, 13, 15). Some studies have included arm-trained athletes among their subjects to shed light on the limits of upper-extremity aerobic capacity and efficiency (6, 11, 12, 14, 15). The results of some of these experiments suggest that the arms may be capable of reaching $\dot{V}O_2$max values greater than those related to maximal leg work among the same athletes (12, 14). Often it is suggested that the assessment of various physiological responses of athletes to exercise is best accomplished while the subjects are performing their specific sport, using the same muscles in the same way they would in training or in competition. From a strictly practical point of view, the attainment of, or improvement of, work capacity during an athlete's specific performance may be the only real point of concern.

Athletes and coaches who are involved with endurance sports where work is done by the arms often perform a great deal of off-season training where the legs do most or all of the work. The idea is to condition the cardiovascular system in "general," or to improve the "central" factors that may limit performance. If cardiac output is limiting, then this general conditioning would seem appropriate; however, if peripheral circulation or mass of the exercising muscles limit the amount of work possible, then it would appear far better to concentrate on performing specifically during all training sessions.

The present study was conducted to investigate further the aerobic responses of arm-trained endurance athletes to arm and leg work in performing their specific sport. A secondary purpose was to compare the aerobic responses of arm-trained athletes to those of athletes who perform both arm and leg endurance activities, and to some nontrained individuals.

METHODS

Subjects included 8 highly proficient male competitive paddlers (*arm athletes*) from Ottawa, Ontario, Canada; 8 male pentathletes, members of the United States Modern Pentathlon training center in San Antonio, Texas (*arm and leg athletes* who compete in horseback riding, fencing, pistol shooting, 300 meter swimming, and 4000 meter running events), and 8 male college students who were enrolled in a beginning physical education class at the University of Texas, Austin, Texas. The latter group was considered representative of individuals who are not arm trained but are involved in occasional physical activity. The paddlers were in the middle of their competitive season and the pentathletes were considered in good condition and performed all 5 events on a daily basis.

All subjects performed a running $\dot{V}O_2$max test on a treadmill, with speed and grade increments added to produce exhaustion in 5–8 minutes. All subjects also performed a 5–8 minute increasing-load (beginning at 300 kpm) arm-cranking $\dot{V}O_2$max test on a Monarch mechanically breaked bicycle ergometer. In addition, submaximal data were collected on the athletes at 300, 450, and 600 kpm while arm cranking at 50 rpm and at 600 kpm peddling 50 rpm on the bicycle. Finally, data were collected on the paddlers during on-the-water submaximal and maximum effort paddling, over a smooth, calm course 1500 meters long. In all tests, the apparatus described by Daniels (9) was used. In $\dot{V}O_2$max tests in the laboratory, consecutive 30 to 60 second collections began after 4 minutes of work; the highest $\dot{V}O_2$ reached was considered $\dot{V}O_2$max. In all submaximal laboratory collections, a single 60 second sample was taken from 5 to 6 minutes after the exercise began.

In paddling tests 2 man racing canoes were used with a special rig employed, which allowed the back paddler to open and close a collection valve attached to the boat. (see Fig. 12-1). The exact time of collection (after at least 4 minutes in each case) was determined by the investigators who ran beside the paddling canal and called out 50 meter splits and timed the bag collections. Expired gas samples were collected for approximately 90 seconds in submaximal tests and 60 seconds in maximal paddling tests. Pace was kept steady by maintaining predetermined 50 meter splits. In the maximal paddling tests (2 runs were made by each subject and the greatest value taken as maximal) a preset near maximal speed was held for 3 to 4 minutes, after which time the paddlers worked all-out for a final 2 minutes. The maximal collection was made during the final 60 seconds of each maximal run. A Parkinson-Cowan flow meter and Lloyd Gallenkamp gas analyzer were used in measuring and analyzing all gas samples. Heart rates were measured by palpation for 10 seconds during the first 15 seconds after completion of each test. Heart rates were not taken in the paddling tests. Data were analyzed with an analysis of variance and post-hoc techniques.

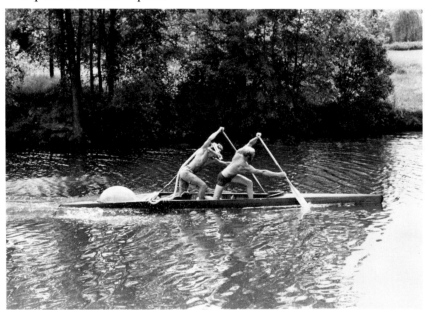

Figure 12-1. Paddling test, showing the equipment used in collecting expired gas samples.

RESULTS

Table 12-I shows the anthropometric and maximum work data on the athletes and nonathletes. The only difference among the subjects in anthropometric characteristics was that the nonathletes had a greater 6 site skinfold sum than either group of athletes, not an unexpected finding. During the running maximal test, the nonathletes had a greater HRmax than either group of athletes and a lower $\dot{V}O_2$max than the pentathletes, who also had a greater $\dot{V}O_2$max than did the paddlers. The pentathletes also had a higher HRmax and higher $\dot{V}_E$max than the paddlers, who looked surprisingly similar to the nonathletes in $\dot{V}O_2$ and $\dot{V}_E$. During the arm maximal tests, the nonathletes attained a significantly lower $\dot{V}O_2$max and a higher HR than either group of athletes. The paddlers and pentathletes did not differ in any of the parameters recorded. The percentages of running $\dot{V}O_2$max reached during arm work were 79, 67, and 58 for the paddlers, pentathletes, and nonathletes respectively. All values are significantly different ($p <$ .05).

Table 12-II gives the submaximal values recorded for the pentathletes and paddlers during work on the bicycle ergometer. Since no significant differences existed between the 2 groups on any of the measured responses to submaximal arm work, the data (Fig. 12-2) were pooled and various regression equations were generated relating the variables. These relationships can be used, for example, to compare the heart rate values of arm and leg work at any constant $\dot{V}O_2$, since the same load produces a different heart rate for the 2 modes of work (1, 4, 13).

Maximal and submaximal data, collected during actual paddling, are presented in Table 12-III and Figure 12-3, respectively. The two items of significance ($p <$ .05) in Table 12-III are (1) the low $\dot{V}_E$ recorded in paddling relative to running (Table 12-I) and (2) the significantly greater $\dot{V}O_2$max reached paddling compared with arm cranking. In fact, even though canoe paddling uses primarily upper body muscles, 5 of the 8 subjects reached between 96 percent and 100 percent of their running $\dot{V}O_2$max. Interestingly, the two lowest relative $\dot{V}O_2$max values reached during paddling (79% and 87%) were by the two subjects considered to be in the poorest condition by their coach. Figure 12-3 shows the relationship between paddling speed and $\dot{V}O_2$ to be quite linear, at

TABLE 12-I

ANTHROPOMETRIC AND ARM WORK AND RUNNING $\dot{V}O_2$max DATA*

	Paddlers		Pentathletes		Nonathletes	
Age yr	19.1	(17-24)	22.0	(20-24)	19.8	(18-21)
Ht cm	178.4	(175-183)	180.3	(168-193)	182.0	(179-193)
Wt kg	73.1	(65.4-75.8)	71.6	(65.8-85.7)	73.3	(63.3-88.5)
6-site skinfold† mm	48.4‡	(38.8-61.3)	43.0‡	(38.3-56.5)	73.1	(50.0-99.8)
RUN MAX						
$\dot{V}O_2$ l/min	4.07§	(3.38-4.72)	4.88‡§	(4.58-5.09)	4.07	(3.55-4.89)
$\dot{V}O_2$ ml/kg × min^{-1}	55.6§	(45.1-63.1)	68.2‡§	(57.8-77.2)	55.5	(47.7-58.6)
HR B/min	183.0‡§	(168-192)	191.0§	(184-200)	198.0	(184-204)
$\dot{V}_E$ l/min	152.1§	(123-184)	182.0‡§	(168-191)	162.9	(143-191)
R	1.25	(1.08-1.49)	1.17	(1.09-1.26)	1.22	(1.13-1.26)
ARM MAX						
$\dot{V}O_2$ l/min	3.23‡	(2.88-3.60)	3.25‡	(2.56-3.49)	2.37	(2.17-2.58)
$\dot{V}O_2$ ml/kg × min^{-1}	44.2‡	(38.3-48.1)	45.4‡	(35.1-53.0)	32.3	(29.1-37.9)
HR B/min	172.1‡	(164-180)	177.2‡	(160-192)	184.3	(142-204)
$\dot{V}_E$ l/min	114.0	(71-138)	124.0	(84-161)	117.2	(98-138)
R	1.24‡	(1.04-1.43)	1.21‡	(1.07-1.35)	1.37	(1.23-1.46)

*Data are presented as means and ranges.

†Sum for tricep, subscapular, suprailiac, umbilical, pectoral, anterior thigh.

‡Significantly different from nonathletes ($p < .05$).

§Significantly different from other group of athletes ($p < .05$).

TABLE 12-II

BICYCLE ERGOMETER SUBMAX DATA*

	300 KPM—Arms	450 KPM—ARMS	600 KPM—Arms	600 KPM—Legs
Paddlers				
$\dot{V}O_2$ l/min	1.13 (.98-1.27)	1.52 (1.34-1.71)	1.87 (1.73-2.13)	1.48 (1.15-1.85)
HR B/min	91.1 (78-108)	107.4 (92-120)	124.2 (108-156)	107.0 (94-128)
$\dot{V}_E$ l/min	34.2 (22.9-46.9)	45.4 (33.0-61.8)	56.7 (42.2-81.7)	37.9† (31.1-50.1)
Pentathletes				
$\dot{V}O_2$ l/min	1.17 (1.03-1.26)	1.53 (1.36-1.69)	1.88 (1.72-2.05)	1.57 (1.41-1.79)
HR B/min	89.2 (67-104)	107.0 (73-116)	119.1 (86-152)	111.3 (80-124)
$\dot{V}_E$ l/min	27.4 (18.5-36.8)	30.9 (31.7-46.8)	49.5 (40.2-62.7)	31.5† (23.8-38.5)

*Data are presented as means and ranges.

†Significantly different at the .05 level, paddlers compared to pentathletes.

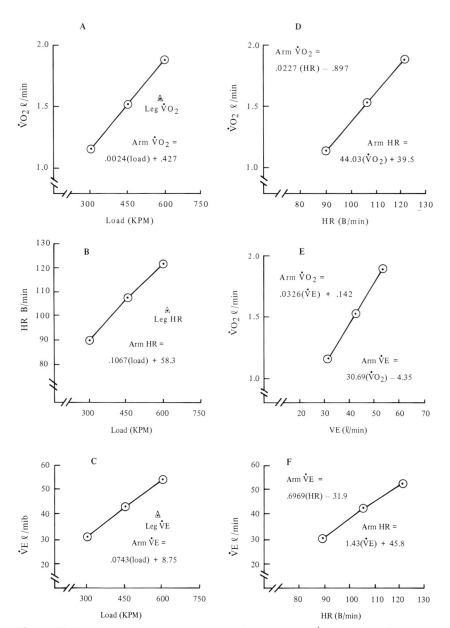

Figure 12-2. Regression curves constructed from mean $\dot{V}O_2$ submax data during arm cranking. Leg $\dot{V}O_2$ at 600 kpm is also shown.

least over the range of speeds tested. The relatively tight grouping of the individual values around the regression curve would appear to speak well for the subject's ability to hold an even pace and to perform their gas-sampling duties effectively.

TABLE 12-III
DATA FROM ON-THE-WATER MAX PADDLING TESTS*

$\dot{V}O_2$max ml/kg × min^{-1}	51.7	(44.3-61.1)
$\dot{V}O_2$max l/min	3.78	(3.32-4.44)
% of running $\dot{V}O_2$max	93.3	(79-100)
% of arm VO_2max	117.2	(105-130)
$\dot{V}_E$max l/min	127.4	(99-149)
R at $\dot{V}O_2$max	1.10	(1.01-1.27)

*Data are presented as means and ranges.

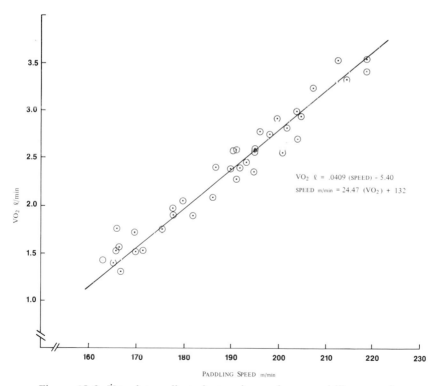

$$VO_2 \; \ell = .0409 \; (\text{SPEED}) - 5.40$$
$$\text{SPEED} \; \text{m/min} = 24.47 \; (VO_2) + 132$$

Figure 12-3. V̇O₂ data collected at various submax paddling speeds.

DISCUSSION

During the running $\dot{V}O_2$max tests (Table 12-I) all groups of subjects appear to have performed maximally, as evidenced by the consistently high R values. The higher $\dot{V}O_2$max found among the pentathletes would be expected since endurance running is one of their disciplines. Two of the pentathlon subjects have consistently been among the best runners in World and Olympic competition, and their $\dot{V}O_2$max values of 68.5 and 75.7 ml/kg/min compare favorably with world-class middle-distance runners (8). That the nonathletes had a $\dot{V}O_2$max equal to the paddlers is probably more a function of the nonathletes being moderately active college students and a little fitter than average young adults than it is the paddlers being of a poor aerobic fitness. The paddlers in the present study had a running $\dot{V}O_2$max equal to that reported earlier on Belgium and Canadian paddlers (11, 15) but lower than reported by Tesch et al. (14) for elite Swedish paddlers. Running HRmax was lower in the paddlers than among nonathletes, presumably a result of the conditioning of the heart through strenuous paddling training. The higher HRmax reached by the pentathletes can only be construed to be a function of their familiarity to performing hard running. However, even with their higher HRmax, the pentathletes had a higher O_2 pulse (25.6 ml/beat) than either the paddlers (22.2 ml/beat) or nonathletes (20.6 ml/beat). $\dot{V}_E$ at $\dot{V}O_2$max running was also highest among the pentathletes, but it was not higher than would be expected to support their higher $\dot{V}O_2$max and certainly in line with values reported for runners (8).

In the arm-cranking maximal tests (Table 12-I), the two groups of athletes showed nearly identical results in all measured parameters. Both groups of athletes reached a much greater $\dot{V}O_2$max than did the nonathletes, obviously a function of the regular arm training demanded by their sports. The fraction of run $\dot{V}O_2$max reached during maximum arm work was greatest for the paddlers (.79) because of their combination of a good arm $\dot{V}O_2$max and a not-so-high run $\dot{V}O_2$max. Vrijens et al. (15) found an arm/leg $\dot{V}O_2$max fraction of .89 among paddlers and .81 among conditioned controls, but their leg $\dot{V}O_2$max was determined during a cycling test and not running on a grade as in the present study. The paddlers tested by Tesch et al. (14) had a .85 arm/running $\dot{V}O_2$max similar to the results we found. The pentathletes had a lower arm/run $\dot{V}O_2$max fraction (.67) even though they reached a good $\dot{V}O_2$max with their arms, because of their higher running maximum. It might be expected that pentathletes, who train both arms and legs for endurance work, would show an arm/run $\dot{V}O_2$max ratio similar to individuals who are not trained specifically for either arm or leg work. In fact, an arm/leg $\dot{V}O_2$max fraction of about .70 has been reported by several investigators (2, 3, 13). These nonathletes, however, had an arm/run $\dot{V}O_2$max fraction of .58, a little lower than referred to above; the fact that the subjects did their leg maximal test on a treadmill and were relatively more active with their legs could easily account for this discrepancy.

Maximal heart rates recorded during the arm-cranking tests showed a similar pattern to those reached in running, i.e. the paddlers were significantly lower than the nonathletes ($p < .05$), who in turn had the highest values of all groups. In support of findings of other investigators (1–3, 13), the heart rate reached in maximal arm cranking was lower for all groups ($p < .05$) compared with their running tests. The arm/run HR fraction was either .93 or .94 for each group of subjects, indicating that the lower HRmax with the arms did not seem to be greatly influenced by the fitness of the subjects' arms. If arm fitness were a factor, then the arm $\dot{V}O_2$max values should have shown similar differences from those reached in running as was the case with heart rates. The O_2/pulse values (ml/beat) during maximal arm work were 18.8, 18.4, and 12.9 for the paddlers, pentathletes, and nonathletes, respectively. These are very similar to those reported by Zwiren and Bar-or (16) for active (17.9) and sedentary (10.0) subjects. Previous investigators (1, 13) have shown that heart rate is higher with the arms, compared with leg work at any particular submaximal work load. Some (5, 11) have found no difference between arm and leg heart rate, however, when compared with the same $\dot{V}O_2$ rather than the same work load. The authors' results support this finding, as can be seen in Table 12-II and Figure 12-2. If the average $\dot{V}O_2$max of the athletes (3.241, from Table 12-I) is used to predict the related arm heart rate from Figure 12-2D, a value of 182 beats per minute is obtained. This is higher than the maximum recorded for these subjects and offers further evidence that the factor limiting heart rate is not metabolic in nature. It is more likely that the limit is hemodynamic, possibly a result of an increase in intrathoracic pressure during strenuous arm cranking.

Maximum ventilation reached in the arm tests were significantly lower ($p < .05$) for all groups of subjects, which supports the findings of Secher et al. (12), who also reported no difference in the $\dot{V}_E/\dot{V}O_2$ fraction when comparing arm and leg work. The data collected on the athletes in the authors' study agree with this ventilatory equivalent finding, but the same did not hold true for the nonathletes. This latter group had a $\dot{V}_E/\dot{V}O_2$ ratio of 49.5 during maximal arm work (compared with 40.0 in maximal leg work), which, along with their significantly higher R at arm maximum, indicates that these subjects were hyperventilating in their arm maximal tests, even though their $\dot{V}_E$max was only 72 percent of that reached in running. The paddlers and pentathletes showed a similar difference in $\dot{V}_E$max during arm work (75% and 68% of leg max, respectively), but in their case $\dot{V}_E/\dot{V}O_2$ did not differ from that reached during running (37.4 running, 36.8 arms).

The submaximal arm and leg peddling data presented in Table 12-II and Figure 12-2 support the findings of others, that at a submaximal work load arm $\dot{V}O_2$, HR, and $\dot{V}_E$ are higher than recorded for leg work at the same load (1, 13) and that, at a given submax $\dot{V}O_2$ (for our subjects at 450kpm arms and 600kpm legs), heart rate does not differ between arm and leg work (5, 11).

The high $\dot{V}O_2$max reached during paddling (Table 12-III) supports the idea of specific-task tests (7, 11, 12) when assessing the response of athletes to physical performance. The trunk muscles undoubtedly come more into play in paddling than in arm cranking, and the additional active muscle mass undoubtedly contributed to a paddling $\dot{V}O_2$max in excess of that reached during arm cranking ($p < .05$). That none of the subjects exceeded his running $\dot{V}O_2$max while paddling (5 of the 8 had nearly identical values, however) suggests that running during the nonpaddling season can adequately stimulate cardiac output and the ventilatory system to keep pace with in-season paddling needs. However, it would seem far better, off-season, to choose a demanding arm endurance sport, such as swimming, or an arm and leg sport, such as cross-country skiing, if active paddling is not possible.

Maximum ventilation was significantly less during paddling than in running ($p < .05$) and a little greater than during arm cranking; however, there was no evidence that $\dot{V}_E$ limited the $\dot{V}O_2$ reached in paddling. The regression equation relating $\dot{V}_E$ to $\dot{V}O_2$ paddling is $\dot{V}_E = .032 \times \dot{V}O_2 - 10.6$. From this, the paddling $\dot{V}O_2$ of 3.78 liters, which was reached, would demand a $\dot{V}_E$ of 110.4 liters. The subjects reached a $\dot{V}_E$ of 127.4 liters (see Table 12-III), which should handle the demand quite easily.

The apparent linearity of the paddling speed/$\dot{V}O_2$ relationship (Fig. 12-3) is probably due to the narrow range of speeds over which such a test is reasonable. It would be expected that in water the increasing energy demands of increasing speed of movement would not be linear. This certainly speaks well for the design of the racing canoes used in competition today. The data in Figure 12-3 should prove useful in preparing on-the-water paddling workouts when $\dot{V}O_2$max, or some percentage thereof, is to be demanded of the athletes.

CONCLUSION

Within the limits of this study the following conclusions seem appropriate.

1. Any difference reached between arm and leg $\dot{V}O_2$max is dependent upon the state of training of the particular muscle groups involved and the specific work task employed.

2. Maximum $\dot{V}_E$ is lower during arm work than in running, but does not in itself limit arm $\dot{V}O_2$max.

3. Arm HRmax, although it appears in absolute terms to be related to running HRmax, is lower during arm cranking; the decrement appears not to be related to the fitness level of the arms or legs.

4. During submaximal arm cranking, HR, $\dot{V}_E$, and $\dot{V}O_2$ are higher than during leg work at the same submaximal work load; at the same submaximal $\dot{V}O_2$, however, arm and leg HR do not differ.

5. O_2/pulse and $\dot{V}_E/\dot{V}O_2$ differences between arm and leg work are dependent upon the fitness of the muscle groups tested.

6. $\dot{V}O_2$max during canoe paddling can reach values equal to those reached during running; $\dot{V}_E$max paddling does not equal that of running.

7. The relationship between speed of canoe paddling and $\dot{V}O_2$ is linear in the range 160–220 m/min. $\dot{V}O_2 \, 1 = .0409 \times$ speed $-$ 5.40.

REFERENCES

1. Asmussen, E. and I. Hemmingsen: Determination of maximum working capacity at different ages in work with the legs or with the arms. *Scand J Clin Lab Invest, 10*:67, 1958.
2. Astrand, P-O. and B. Saltin: Maximal oxygen uptake and heart rate in various types of muscular activity. *J Appl Physiol, 16*:977, 1979.
3. Astrand, P-O.; B. Ekblom; R. Messin; B. Saltin; and J. Stenberg: Intraarterial blood pressure during exercise with different muscle groups. *J Appl Physiol, 20*:235, 1965.
4. Bevegard, S.; U. Freyhuss; and T. Standell: Circulatory adaptation to arm and leg exercise in supine and sitting position. *J Appl Physiol, 21*:37, 1966.
5. Bobbert, A.C.: Physiological comparison of three types of ergometers. *J Appl Physiol, 15*:1007, 1960.
6. Cermak, J.; I. Kuta; and J. Parizkova: Some predispositions for top performance in speed canoeing and their changes during the whole year training program. *J Sports Med Phys Fitness, 15*:243, 1975.
7. Cunningham, D.A.; P.B. Goode; and J.B. Critz: Cardiorespiratory response to exercise on a rowing and bicycle ergometer. *Med Sci Sports, 7*:37, 1975.
8. Daniels, J. and N. Oldridge: The effects of alternate exposure to altitude and sea level on world-class middle-distance runners. *Med Sci Sports, 2*:107, 1970.
9. Daniels, J.D.: Portable respiratory gas-collection equipment. *J Appl Physiol, 31*:164, 1971.
10. Gleser, M.A.; D.H. Horstman; and R.B. Mello: The effect on $\dot{V}O_2$max of adding arm work to leg work. *Med Sci Sports, 6*:104, 1974.
11. Pyke, F.S.; J.A. Baker; R.J. Hoyle; and E.W. Scrutton: Metabolic and circulatory responses of canoeists to work on a canoeing and bicycle ergometer. *Aust J Sports Med, 5*:22, 1973.
12. Secher, N.H.; N. Ruberg-Larsen; R.A. Binkhorst; and F. Bonde-Petersen: Maximal oxygen uptake during arm cranking and combined arm plus leg exercise. *J Appl Physiol, 36*:515, 1974.
13. Stenberg, J.; P-O. Astrand; B. Ekblom; J. Royce; and B. Saltin: Hemodynamic response to work with different muscle groups, sitting and supine. *J Appl Physiol, 22*:61, 1967.
14. Tesch, P.; K. Piehl; G. Wilson; and J. Karlsson: Physiological investigations of Swedish elite canoe competitors. *Med Sci Sports, 8*:214, 1976.
15. Vrijens, J.; P. Hoekstra; J. Bonckaert; and P. Van Uytvanck: Effects of training on maximal working capacity and hemodynamic response during arm and leg-exercise in a group of paddlers. *Eur J Appl Physiol, 34*:113, 1975.
16. Zwiren, L.D. and O. Bar-or: Response to exercise of paraplegics who differ in conditioning level. *Med Sci Sports, 7*:94, 1975.

Chapter 13

THE EXCRETION OF CATECHOLAMINES AS AN INDEX OF EXERCISE STRESS

E.T. HOWLEY

IN A 1969 report (6) on the sympathoadrenal response to exercise, von Euler indicated that while the parameters of oxygen uptake, pulmonary ventilation, and heart rate were quantitatively related to the work rate, these data gave no direct information on the degree of effort or stress experienced by the subject. He indicated the need for a quantitative "effort index" that could relate the degree of effort to a given work rate and suggested, on the basis of his earlier work (3) that the measurement of the urinary excretion of catecholamines might be useful in that regard. Three studies that attempted to examine this proposition will be summarized.

The purpose of the first study, conducted at Pennsylvania State University (11), was to determine if catecholamine (CA) excretion could be used as an "effort index" to permit comparisons between subjects differing in work capacity. Four males, whose maximal aerobic power ($\dot{V}O_2$max) ranged from 48 to 68 ml(kg·min)$^{-1}$, were used as subjects. The protocol selected was based on data showing that circulatory adjustments are similar among individuals when a work task is set at a percentage of $\dot{V}O_2$max, even though intraindividual differences in $\dot{V}O_2$max exist. The subjects worked at 60, 70, and 80 percent $\dot{V}O_2$max for 30 minutes and at 90 percent $\dot{V}O_2$max until exhaustion (duration ranged from 20–25 min). Only 1 test was conducted per week. The following procedures were used for each test day:

1. Subject reported to lab, voided.
2. Subject drank 200 ml water and sat for 1 hour.
3. Subject voided again (preexercise sample).
4. Subject ran on treadmill at appropriate %$\dot{V}O_2$max (30 min).
5. Subject sat for 1 hour and voided (exercise sample).

The total free catecholamines (epinephrine and norepine-phrine) were measured in duplicate according to the method of Viktora, Baukal, and Wolff (19), with the only modification being the use of 8 ml of 4% boric acid to elute the catecholamines from the resin. The values for the CA excretion during exercise were calculated by subtracting the output during the nonwork period (60 min) following exercise from the total (work + non-work) excretion (90 min). The remainder was divided by 30 min and expressed in ng/min. The preexercise CA excretion was used as the value for the CA excretion in the nonwork period. The values reported here have been corrected to 100 percent recovery based on data collected in subsequent studies.

The preexercise (rest) value for CA excretion was 46 ± 3 ng/min ($\bar{X}$ ± SE). The CA response for the 4 subjects to the different exercise intensities is shown in Figure 13-1. While the average response, indicated by the wide line, shows a smooth increase in the rate of CA excretion as the work load is increased, it is quite obvious that there was considerable individual variation in the response. One subject showed little change until 90 percent $\dot{V}O_2$max, while another had the same rate of CA excretion across work loads. Because of this variability (both between and within subjects) it was concluded that it would be very difficult to precisely express the "effort" experienced by any one subject using CA excretion alone.

In the second study, at The University of Tennessee (2), an assay was used to separate epinephrine (E) from norepinephrine (NE) in urine samples. The proposition of von Euler was tested again by having subjects work at two different work loads. The 9 subjects in this study followed a protocol similar to the previous study:

1. Subject reported to the lab, voided.
2. Subject sat for 1 hour, voided (preexercise sample).
3. Subject worked for 15 minutes at either 78 or 95 percent $\dot{V}O_2$max.
4. Subject sat for 1 hour, voided (exercise sample).

The adsorption and elution of the CA was performed as previously described (19). An internal standard, to measure recovery, was run with each urine sample and both samples and recoveries were analyzed in duplicate. The NE was differentiated from E by oxidizing the eluate at pH 6.0 to determine total CA and at pH 3.5

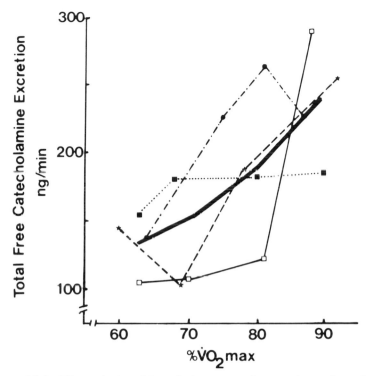

Figure 13-1. The relationship of the rate of excretion of total free catecholamines (epinephrine plus norepinephrine) to the relative work load (percent of maximal aerobic power—%$\dot{V}O_2$max). The wide line represents the average response of the four subjects.

to determine E. The NE was calculated according to von Euler and Floding (4). The CA excretion for the exercise period was calculated as described above. Briefly, the expected CA output for the 1 hour nonwork period of the exercise sample was subtracted from the total output. The excess was assumed due to the exercise. This value was divided by 15 minutes and expressed in ng/min. An average preexercise (resting) value for CA excretion was used as an estimate of the value for the nonwork period. All values were corrected to 100 percent recovery.

Table 13-I shows the results of the experiments. While the E excretion remained unchanged in spite of the large change in work load, the NE excretion was significantly elevated ($p < .05$). In a manner similar to the first study, the change in the average rate of NE excretion suggests its use as index of stress or effort. However, the individual variability in response was quite large.

TABLE 13-I

THE RATE OF EXCRETION OF EPINEPHRINE (E) AND
NOREPINEPHRINE (NE) TO TWO DIFFERENT WORK TASKS*

Work Load %$\dot{V}O_2$max	E Excretion ng/min	NE Excretion ng/min
95 ± 1	49 ± 10	262 ± 35
78 ± 2	52 ± 10	207 ± 43

*Values are $\bar{X}$ ± SE; N = 9.

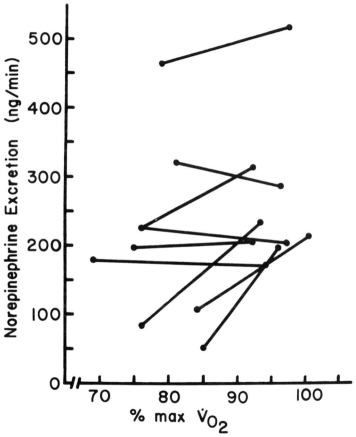

Figure 13-2. The norepinephrine response of 9 subjects to 2 work loads expressed as a percent of maximal aerobic power (%$\dot{V}O_2$max).

Figure 13-2 shows that only 6 of the 9 subjects had an increase in the rate of NE excretion with the increase in work load. The intersubject variability should be noted.

An interesting observation was made when the NE values (Table 13-I) were compared with the value for NE excretion for the 88 percent $\dot{V}O_2$max load used in the training portion of the study (2). The NE value for the 88 percent $\dot{V}O_2$max load was 263 ± 35 ng/min, or the same as the value for the 95 percent $\dot{V}O_2$max load. This plateau in NE excretion occurred at a work load (%$\dot{V}O_2$max) where the plasma NE concentration has been shown to increase logarithmically. In Figure 13-3, data from Howley (12) and Cronan and Howley (2) are used to show NE excretion values from 50

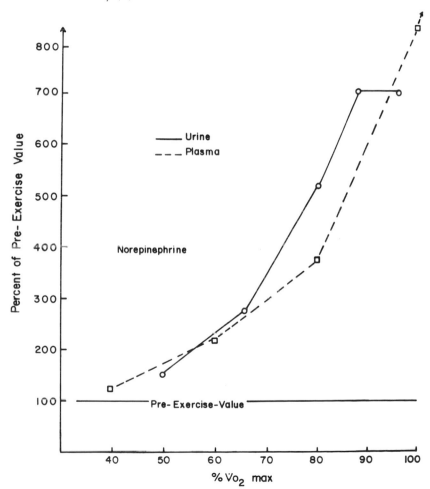

Figure 13-3. Comparison of the rate of norepinephrine excretion and the plasma concentration of norepinephrine to various work loads expressed as a percent of maximal aerobic power (%$\dot{V}O_2$max).

to 95 percent $\dot{V}O_2$max along with plasma NE values averaged from Haggendal, Hartley, and Saltin (10), Galbo, Holst, and Christensen (7), and Painter, Howley, and Liles (16). A restriction in blood flow to the kidney (9) and liver (17) at very high work loads may explain this anomaly in response. At heavy work rates, changes in kidney and liver blood flow would tend to cause the steep increase in the plasma NE concentration (due to the decreased rate of removal) and, simultaneously, a levelling off or possibly a decrease in the rate of excretion of NE. This could explain some of the observed responses in Figure 13-2. These data suggest that the reductions in renal function at high metabolic requirements might limit the use of urinary CA measurements as an index of stress or effort. However, as shown in Figure 13-3, changes in the concentration of plasma NE seem to be similar to the changes in the rate of excretion of NE up to about 80 percent $\dot{V}O_2$max.

The variation in the urinary CA response to work that was observed in the previous two studies could have been due to several factors. These include—

1. Inadequate or inconsistent hydration of the subject before the experiment.
2. Inadequate control of the subject's activity pattern immediately before the experiment.
3. Day-to-day variability of the subject.
4. Day-to-day variability in analytical procedure.
5. The intensity of work load being too high to permit adequate excretion of CA via the kidneys.

In the third study, these factors were controlled and E and NE excretion at various work rates again examined. The assay (with a Turner 430 spectrofluorometer) had previously been refined in terms of sensitivity, specificity of separating E from NE, and the recovery of standards added to each sample (in excess of 75% for both E and NE, with little variation from sample to sample). In addition, many experiments were conducted to determine the time course of the E and NE excretion pattern following exercise. The data indicated that within 30 minutes following exercise both E and NE had returned close to the preexercise values.

Based on these findings and the factors mentioned above, the following experiments were conducted. Six male subjects worked for 15 minutes at 50, 65, and 80 percent $\dot{V}O_2$max. On the day before the tests, the subject was instructed to drink water before retiring to assure adequate hydration. In addition, water was given as requested during all phases of the test. The following protocol was used:

1. Reported to laboratory, sat quietly for 20–30 minutes, then voided. This controlled for the previous physical activity of the subject.
2. Sat quietly again for 30 minutes, then voided (preexercise sample).
3. Exercised for 15 minutes, sat quietly for 30 minutes, then voided.
4. Exercised for 15 minutes, sat quietly for 30 minutes, then voided.
5. Exercised for 15 minutes, sat quietly for 30 minutes, then voided.
6. Sat quietly for 30 minutes, then voided (postexercise sample).

Doing all the work tests within 1 day controlled for the day-to-day variability of the subject. In addition, the work test order (6 possible combinations) was randomly assigned to the subject. Each subject had a different work test order and the subject was naive to the test order.

A timed volume of each urine sample (a volume equivalent to 3 minutes excretion) was analyzed for E and NE in duplicate, with a duplicate recovery made for each sample. All values were corrected to 100 percent recovery based on the added internal standards. The average recovery based on 63 urine samples was 77 ± 1 percent ($\bar{X} \pm SE$). All 5 urine samples of each subject were analyzed on the same day to control for the day-to-day variability of the assay. The excretion of E and NE for the exercise period was calculated as described above.

Table 13-II and Figure 13-4 show the results of the experiments. The NE excretion increased as the work load was increased and each subject showed a similar pattern of response. The NE value at 65 percent $\dot{V}O_2max$ was significantly higher ($p < .05$) than that at 49 percent $\dot{V}O_2max$ and the NE value at 82 percent $\dot{V}O_2max$ was significantly higher than that at 65 percent $\dot{V}O_2max$ ($p < .05$). The NE returned to the preexercise value during the 30–60 minute interval after work. The E response was less consistent among subjects, and there was no significant difference in response across work loads. The postexercise value was significantly higher than

TABLE 13-II*
THE EXCRETION OF EPINEPHRINE, NOREPINEPHRINE, AND
URINE AT REST BEFORE EXERCISE, FOR THREE WORK LOADS,
AND IN RECOVERY FROM EXERCISE

Workload %$\dot{V}O_2$max	Norepinephrine Excretion ng/min	Epinephrine Excretion ng/min	Urine Excretion ml/min
Pre-exercise rest	32 ± 4	10 ± 1	9.1 ± 1.4
49 ± 1	50 ± 12	21 ± 5	9.5 ± 0.7
65 ± 1	90 ± 17	18 ± 3	7.8 ± 0.6
82 ± 1	146 ± 12	20 ± 3	4.6 ± 0.4
Post-exercise rest	30 ± 7	14 ± 1	9.9 ± 1.4

*Values are $\overline{X}$ ± SE. N = 6. From *Medicine and Science in Sports*, Vol. 8, No. 4, pp. 219-222, 1976. Copyright 1976, The American College of Sports Medicine. Reprinted by Permission.

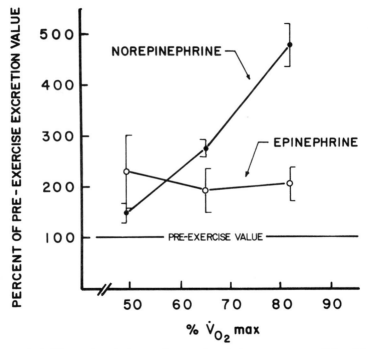

Figure 13-4. The epinephrine and norepinephrine responses of 6 subjects to 3 work loads expressed as a percent of maximal aerobic power (%$\dot{V}O_2$max). Values are $\overline{X}$ ± SE.

the preexercise value ($p < .05$). The individual responses of the subjects are shown in Figures 13-5 and 13-6. The NE response was consistent for each subject while the E response was extremely variable.

The use of the randomly assigned test order and subject's lack of knowledge of the test order did not appear to alter the NE response to exercise. The relationship observed between the work load and the average rate of NE excretion was consistent with earlier reports and did not appear to be affected by the changing rate of urine excretion (see Table 13-II). The small but significant rise in NE excretion at the 49 percent $\dot{V}O_2$max work load was followed by a fivefold increase (times rest) at the 82 percent

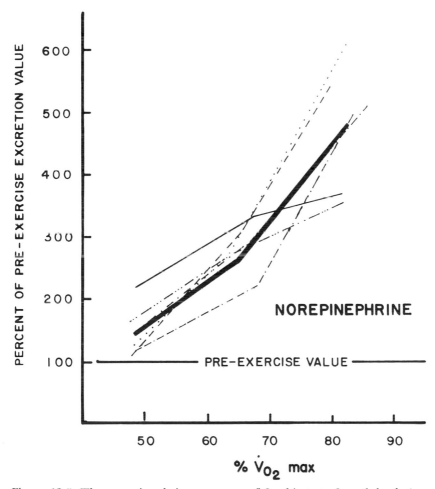

Figure 13-5. The norepinephrine response of 6 subjects to 3 work loads (expressed as %$\dot{V}O_2$max). The average response is indicated by the wide line. From *Medicine and Science in Sports,* Vol. 8, No. 4, pp. 219-222, 1976. Copyright 1976, The American College of Sports Medicine. Reprinted by Permission.

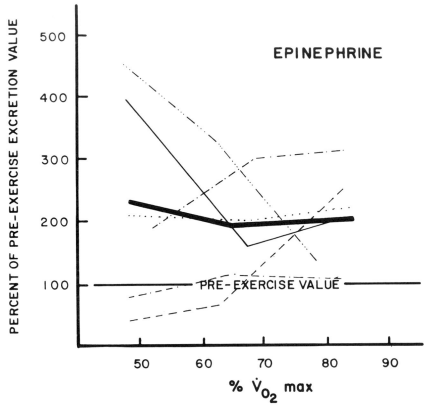

Figure 13-6. The epinephrine response of 6 subjects to 3 work loads (expressed as %$\dot{V}O_2$max). The average response is indicated by the wide line. From *Medicine and Science in Sports*, Vol. 8, No. 4, pp. 219-222, 1976. Copyright 1976, The American College of Sports Medicine. Reprinted by Permission.

$\dot{V}O_2$max work load. This relative increase in the rate of excretion of NE at the 82 percent $\dot{V}O_2$max work load was similar to that found by Haggendal et al. (10) and Galbo et al. (7) for plasma NE.

In contrast to this consistent NE response among subjects and among various studies, Figure 13-6 shows the excretion of E to be variable across work loads. In fact, 1 subject showed essentially no change in E excretion above the preexercise value, while 2 subjects showed the greatest rate of excretion at the lightest work load. The fact that the 5 samples of each subject were analyzed side by side, in duplicate, suggests that reasons other than the analytical procedure be sought to explain these results. Reports of such variability in the E response to exercise are not new (8, 10) but are in contrast to reports by Banister and Griffiths (1) and Galbo et al. (7) who found changes in Plasma E to parallel changes in plasma NE. In one of these studies (7), the subjects were tested on 1 day with a protocol in which the intensity was increased with each successive test. The test order was not specified in the other study. While it is not possible to conclude that test order or knowledge of the test order are critical factors for determining the E or NE response to exercise, it is known that anticipation of a potentially stressful situation can influence the E and NE responses (14, 15). In the above study (12), the 2 most inexperienced subjects showed the greatest rate of E excretion (4–4.5 times the resting value) compared to the other subjects and showed this response at the lightest (50 percent $\dot{V}O_2$max) work load.

DISCUSSION

These studies were conducted to test the proposition of von Euler that CA excretion might be useful as an "effort index" in evaluating the perception of the subject to a work task. On the basis of the studies reported above, NE excretion might be considered for such a role. The NE response increased as the intensity of exercise was increased up to about 80 percent of the subject's maximal aerobic power. Beyond this load, the alterations in splanchnic blood flow could complicate the use of NE excretion as an indicator of exercise intensity.

The implication throughout this chapter is that the CA response to exercise is a function of exercise intensity and not duration. The use of a constant duration in these urinary CA studies did not permit an examination of the influence of this variable. It must be noted, however, that the plasma concentrations of E (7) and NE (13) have been shown to increase over time at a constant work load.

Another point that needs to be mentioned is the casual versus causal nature of the relationship of the CA response to the subjective perception of effort. The observation that both increase with exercise intensity might lead the reader to assume that one is the cause of the other. This might be an erroneous assumption. The normal cardiovascular response to exercise includes an increase in the force and rate of contraction of the heart and an increase in the constriction of the vasculature in the splanchnic area (18). These changes are brought about by an increase in activity in the sympathetic nervous system, especially in the sympathetic nerves innervating the above structures. While a portion of the NE, the neurotransmitter mediating these responses, is taken back up into the neuron, some NE overflows into the vascular compartment (10). Consequently, the change in plasma or urine NE with increasing intensities of work may simply reflect the level of sympathetic activity needed to maintain homeostasis in the cardiovascular system and may not be causally related to the perception of effort of the subject.

REFERENCES

1. Banister, E.W. and Griffiths, J.: Blood levels of adrenergic amines during exercise. *J Appl Physiol, 33*:674, 1972.
2. Cronan, T.L., III and Howley, E.T.: The effect of training on epinephrine and norepinephrine excretion. *Med Sci Sports, 6*:122, 1974.
3. Euler, U.S. von and Hellner, S.: Excretion of noradrenaline and adrenaline in muscular work. *Acta Physiol Scand, 26*:183, 1952.
4. Euler, U.S. von and Floding, I.: A fluorimetric micromethod for differential estimation of adrenaline and noradrenaline. *Acta Physiol Scand (Suppl 118), 33*:45, 1955.
5. Euler, U.S. von: Quantitation of stress by catecholamine analysis. *Ciba Pharmacal Therap, 5*:398, 1965.
6. Euler, U.S. von: Sympatho-adrenal activity and physical exercise. In *Biochemistry of Exercise Medicine and Sport,* edited by J.R. Poortmans. Vol. 3. New York, Karger, 1969.
7. Galbo, H.; Holst, J.J.; and Christensen, N.J.: Glucagon and plasma catecholamine responses to graded and prolonged exercise in man. *J Appl Physiol, 38*:70, 1975.
8. Gray, I. and Beetham, W.P.: Changes in plasma concentration of epinephrine and norepinephrine with muscular work. *Proc Soc Exp Biol Med, 96*:636, 1957.
9. Grimby, G.: Renal clearances during prolonged supine exercise at different loads. *J Appl Physiol, 20*:1294, 1965.
10. Haggendal, J.; Hartley, L.H.; and Saltin, B.: Arterial noradrenaline concentration during exercise in relation to the relative work levels. *Scand J Clin Lab Invest, 26*:337, 1970.
11. Howley, E.T.; Skinner, J.S.; Mendez, J.; and Buskirk, E.R.: Effect of different intensities of exercise on catecholamine excretion. *Med Sci Sports, 2*:193, 1970.
12. Howley, E.T.: The effect of different intensities of exercise on the excretion of epinephrine and norepinephrine. *Med Sci Sports, 8*:219, 1976.
13. Howley, E.T.; Cox, R.; Welch, H.; and Adams, R.P.: Effect of hyperoxia on selected metabolic responses to prolonged work. *Abstract, Med and Sci in Sports and Ex 12*:107, 1980.

14. Mason, J.W.: A review of psychoendocrine research on the sympathetic-adrenal medullary system. *Psychosom Med, 30*:631, 1968.
15. Mason, J.W.; Hartley, L.H.; Kotchen, T.A.; Mougey, E.H.; Ricketts, P.T.; and Jones, L.R.G.: Plasma cortisol and norepinephrine responses in anticipation of muscular exercise. *Psychosom Med, 35*:406, 1973.
16. Painter, P.C.; Howley, E.T.; and Liles, J.: Changes in plasma epinephrine, norepinephrine and cyclic AMP with progressive work in man. Abstract. *Med Sci Sports, 8*:70, 1976.
17. Rowell, L.B.; Blackmon, J.R.; and Bruce, R.A.: Indocyanine green clearance and estimated hepatic blood flow during mild to maximal exercise in upright man. *J Clin Invest, 43*:1677, 1964.
18. Rowell, L.B.: Human cardiovascular adjustments to exercise and thermal stress. *Physiol Rev, 54*:75, 1974.
19. Viktora, J.K.; Baukal, A.; and Wolff, F.: New automated fluorometric methods for estimations of small amounts of adrenaline and noradrenaline. *Anal Biochem, 23*:513, 1968.

Chapter 14

THE 1979 CANADIAN SKI MARATHON:
A NATURAL EXPERIMENT
IN HYPOTHERMIA

J.A. FAULKNER, T.P. WHITE, AND J.M. MARKLEY, JR.

THE CANADIAN Ski Marathon is a 2 day event covering a 160 km wilderness cross-country trail parallel to the Ottawa River in the province of Quebec, Canada. The trail is divided into 10 sections varying in length from 12 to 24 km. Checkpoints with out-of-doors dispersal of soup, warm honey water, and cookies are located at the end of each section. On the first day, skiing occurs on the 5 sections between Lachute and Montebello, and on the second day on the sections between Montebello and Quinnville (Fig. 14-1).

The Marathon includes 3 classes of participants: touring, touring-team competition, and racing. Within each class there are several categories. The touring class has categories for open tourers of any age who may ski from 1 to 8 sections, as well as 3 coureur de bois categories. All coureur de bois must ski 80 km (five sections) each of 2 consecutive days. Bronze coureurs de bois are not required to carry a pack, but silver must carry a minimum 5 kg pack, and gold must carry a minimum 5 kg pack and be self-sufficient for overnight camping on the trail. The touring team class is for teams of 4 skiers classified by age and sex. These teams are credited with the total number of sections skied by their members. In the racing class, single racers ski the first 4 sections each day, for a 2 day total of 128 km. Racing teams consist of 2

The data on minute ventilation and oxygen uptake of JF during cross country skiing were collected by G.J.F. Heigenhauser. We thank Steve Cushing, Executive Director, of the Canadian Ski Marathon for permission to use data from the Official Results of the 1978 and 1979 marathons and R.G. Lawford, Chief, Scientific Services Divisions, Atmospheric Environment Service, Ontario Region, for the weather data. Supported in part by a grant from Michigan Heart Association.

184

skiers of which, each day, one skier completes the first 2 sections and the second skier completes the second 2.

In 1978 and 1979, the authors took part in the Canadian Ski Marathon. The first year, ideal weather and snow conditions prevailed, but the 1979 event was held during one of the coldest periods in recent history. The purpose of this chapter is to report the conditioning program that prepared skiers to complete the bronze coureur de bois in 1978 and a comparison of performances in all classes in the 1978 and 1979 Marathons.

Methods

Three asymptomatic males (Table 14-I) were in long-term stabilized physical activity programs for several years prior to preparation for competition in the bronze coureur de bois category of the Marathon. In the coureur de bois class, one starts at 6 AM and must finish the first 4 sections of the trail by 3 PM to prevent disqualification. The fifth section of the day is skied without further time requirements. This required an average skiing velocity of 7.1 km/hr for 9 hours. However, with 4 checkpoint stops of approximately 10 minutes and the possibility of lost time for waxing or repairs, a skier must maintain an 8 to 10 km/hr velocity over the first 4 sections to meet the minimum requirement. To condition for the competition, each of the 3 ran 4 to 6 times per week over distances from 6 to 16 kms, at a pace of from 11 to 13 km/hr during the 6 months prior to the Marathon. From mid-December 1978 and mid-January 1979 until the Marathon in mid-February, the 3 men cross-country skied 3 to 5 times a week, for 1 to 2 hours, at speeds of 10 to 14 km/hr. On weekends, 25 to 35 km were first skied at a 10 to 11 km/hr pace, and later, 30 to 40 km per day were covered at a 9 to 10 km/hr speed over more difficult terrain. During the week prior to the Marathon 2 light workouts were held.

TABLE 14-I

PHYSICAL CHARACTERISTICS OF THE THREE MARATHON SKIERS

	Age (years)	Height (cm)	Weight (kg)	Fat Free Body wt. (kg)	$\dot{V}O_2$max ml·kg^{-1}·min^{-1}
JF	55	180	71	63	53.1
JM	38	186	71	64	58.7
TW	29	190	89	76	56.2

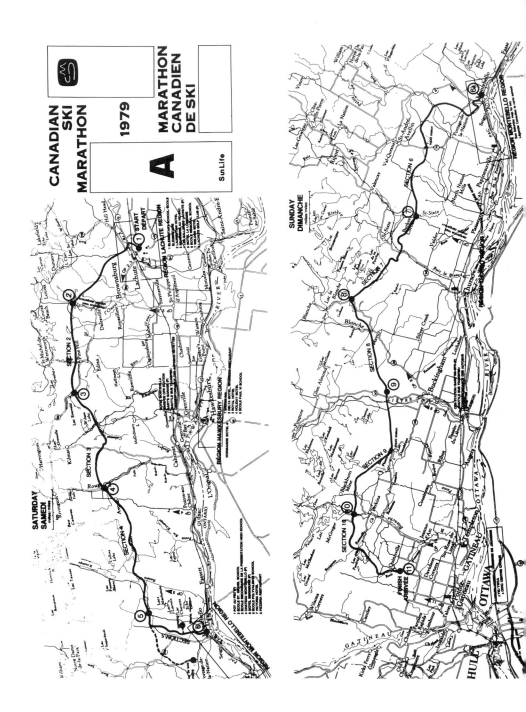

Figure 14-1*A*. Map of 160 km Canadian Ski Marathon. The upper portion indicates the five sections skied on the first day, the bottom portion contains the five sections skied on the second day. Reprinted with permission of the Canadian Ski Marathon.

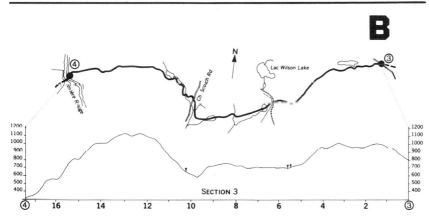

Figure 14-1*B*. Expanded map of Section 3, a typical section showing horizontal (upper portion) and vertical (lower portion) profiles. Elevation is expressed in meters. Reprinted with permission of the Canadian Ski Marathon.

In 1979, a maximum oxygen uptake ($\dot{V}O_2$max) test (11) was administered to each of the 3 men 2 weeks after the Marathon. The subjects ran on a treadmill at 11.3 km/hr for 2 minutes at grades of 0, 2.5, 5.5 percent and additional percentage grades until voluntary exhaustion was reached. Heart rate was monitored continuously, and expired gas was collected in bags during the last minute of each exercise intensity. Expired volume was measured by pumping the gas collected through a dry gas meter. Oxygen content of the expired gas was determined by a paramagnetic oxygen analyzer and carbon dioxide content by an infrared gas analyzer. The analyzers were calibrated with gases of known composition.

Oxygen uptake was measured for 1 subject while skiing on level terrain at 4, 10.5, and 12 km/hr. During the last minute of each 5 minute period of cross-country skiing, expired gas was collected in a bag carried on the skier's back. Analyses were made by the same procedures as for the treadmill run.

The data on minute ventilation and $\dot{V}O_2$ collected during cross-country skiing on JF (74 kg) and BL (83 kg) published by

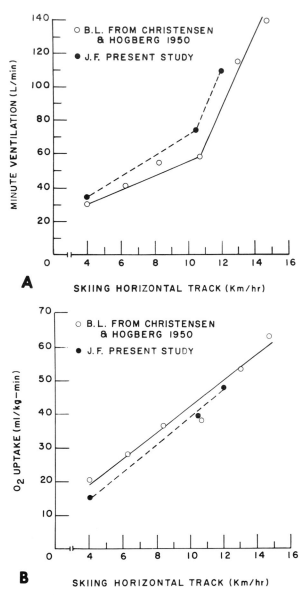

Figure 14-2. *(A)* Minute ventilation (STPD) and *(B)* oxygen uptake (STPD) expressed as a function of skiing velocity.

Christensen and Hogberg (2) are plotted as a function of skiing velocity (Fig. 14-2). The intercept and the slope of the $\dot{V}O_2$:skiing velocity relation is similar for the 2 skiers. Since the velocity of skiing during the Marathon is within the range observed and no significant differences between trained skiers were apparent, the energy expenditure of cross-country skiers during the Marathon was estimated from their skiing speed. Similar procedures have been effective in estimating the energy expenditure during marathon running (9). An estimate from skiing on level terrain, however, likely underestimates the actual energy expenditure skiing on the rugged terrain of the wilderness trail (Fig. 14-1B).

Results and Discussion

Under normal circumstances, ski racers wear lightweight racing boots, knee length socks, lightweight racing suits, minimal underclothing to absorb sweat, lightweight gloves, and head gear. Tourers, on the other hand, dress appropriate to their expected metabolic expenditure. Fast to slow tourers wear progressively heavier underwear, boots, trousers, jackets, and touques. In Figure 14-3, a gold coureur de bois is shown competing in the 1978 Marathon. In 1979, in deference to the exceptionally cold conditions, some skiers wore gaiters or socks over their ski boots; long underwear; an extra layer of underclothing; leather mittens with wool liners; a ballaclava to shield ears, forehead, cheeks, chin, and neck; and a heavy layer of petroleum jelly over all exposed areas of the face. Those who did not take such precautions, and even some of those who did, suffered minor to severe frostbite.

During the Canadian Ski Marathon, caloric and fluid replacement is provided for along the trail and at the four checkpoints, in addition to that carried by a skier. Fluid replacement may vary from 1 to 2 liters a day, depending on weather conditions, the type of clothing worn, and the sweat loss. Weight loss after the 2 days varied from 2 to 5% but the weight loss was reversed within 48 hours.

The physical characteristics of the skiers are presented in Table 14-I and the respiratory and metabolic results of the running and skiing tests in Table 14-II. The three men had $\dot{V}O_2$max between 53 and 59 ml/kg/min, equivalent to 15–17 METS. These values for $\dot{V}O_2$max are slightly higher than the values reported by Grimby et al. (7) for active middle-aged athletes but less than those reported by Hanson (8) for the United States Nordic Team.

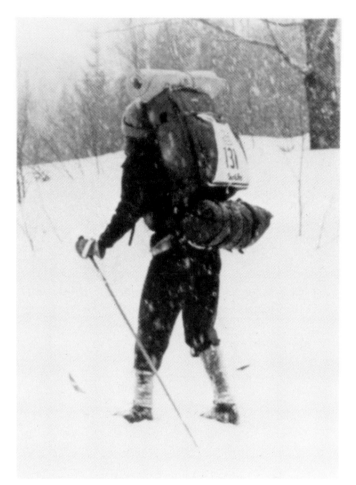

Figure 14-3. A gold coureur de bois competing in 1978 Marathon.

The estimates of the energy cost of the different classes of racers and fast and slow tourers (Table 14-III) indicate that the skiers in each of these classes maintained approximately 75 percent of their $\dot{V}O_2$max for 5 to 10 hours on 2 days in succession. The total energy costs, of the racers skiing 128 km and those of the slow and fast tourers skiing 160 km, in 2 days ranged from 11,000 to 13,000 kcal (Table 14-III). This is comparable to the 8,000 to 10,000 kcal expended by swimmers during a 12 to 14 hour crossing of the English Channel (10).

The total heat loss to respired air has never been measured at the ambient air temperatures and alveolar ventilations reported

TABLE 14-II

RESPIRATORY AND METABOLIC VARIABLES OF THE THREE MARATHON SKIERS DURING TREADMILL RUNNING AND FOR JF* DURING CROSS-COUNTRY SKIING

	Speed (km)	Grade (%)	HR (beats·min⁻¹)	$\dot{V}_E$ STPD (L·min⁻¹)	$\dot{V}O_2$ (L·min⁻¹)	R
			Submaximal Exercise			
JF*	10	0	130	74.00	2.92	0.96
JF	11.3	0	126	54.94	2.59	0.97
JM	11.3	0	144	60.35	2.90	1.00
TW	11.3	0	144	56.97	2.96	0.92
			Maximal Exercise			
JF*	12	0	156	110.00	3.56	1.09
JF	11.3	9.0	169	105.39	3.77	1.18
JM	11.3	10.0	176	116.85	4.16	1.24
TW	11.3	12.0	180	150.74	5.00	1.07

TABLE 14-III

ESTIMATED $\dot{V}_E$, $\dot{V}O_2$, AND TOTAL CALORIC EXPENDITURE FOR A 70 KG MAN SKIING THE MARATHON AT DIFFERENT VELOCITIES

	Velocity (km·hr⁻¹)	Distance (km)	$\dot{V}_E$ (liters·min⁻¹)	$\dot{V}O_2$ (ml·kg⁻¹·min⁻¹)	Total Energy Expenditure (Kcal)
Racers	13	128	120	55	11,100
Fast Tourers	10	160	60	40	13,100
Slow Tourers	8	160	50	30	12,300

here. During the Marathon, the racers and fast tourers skied at metabolic rates that required ventilations of 50 to 120 liters/min. The minute ventilation was undoubtedly lower than this on long downhill runs and higher during sustained uphill climbs. During a single day, alveolar ventilation for skiers completing 80 km totalled 30,000 to 50,000 liters. To warm the air from ambient temperature to 37°C required from 400 to 800 kcal and the heat lost through vaporization as the gas was fully saturated at body temperature was from 700 to 1200 kcal (4). Thus, the total heat lost from the respiratory passages was from 1100 to 2000 kcal. This constitutes 9 to 19 percent of the total heat lost during the Marathon.

In 1978, the early morning temperatures on both days was −17°C and the temperature climbed to −8°C at midday and then dropped again by late afternoon. The wind-chill factor was negligible. In 1979, however, a severe Arctic cold wave settled on the Quebec area the week before the Marathon. On Day 1 and 2, early morning lows were −28°C and the highs were −18°C. The wind chill factor was estimated as −55°C. Under these conditions, even the body heat created by the high metabolic demands of the exercise could not, in many cases, compensate for the cooling effects of the environment.

The effect of hypothermic conditions on the performance of all classes of skiers is reflected in the results of the 1979 compared to the 1978 Marathon (Fig. 14-4). The number of preregistered entrants was slightly over 4000 each year but dramatic differences were noted in the number in each category who finished the prescribed distances. In 1978, a negligible number of skiers had problems with frost-bite but in 1979 many skiers terminated the race prematurely because of this problem. In addition to the problem of frost-bite, skiing performance was definitely impaired by the cold. Of the 3 skiers whose physiological data are presented in this study, 2 completed the bronze coureur de bois in 1978. The third completed 80 km on Day 1 and 64 km on Day 2 after breaking a ski at 20 km. In 1979, each of the 3 completed 80 km on Day 1 in approximately 10 hours. On Day 2, 1 skier froze the first digit of his right hand and the third and fourth digits on his right foot during the first section and stopped skiing at 8 AM after sking 16 km. The other 2 could not maintain a touring pace of 8 to 10 km hr^{-1}. At the end of Section 3 (48 km) they stopped skiing

CANADIAN SKI MARATHON

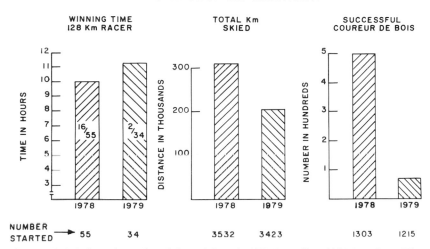

Figure 14-4. Selected results of the 1978 and 1979 Canadian Ski Marathon. The ratios of finishers to starters is inset in the histograms for the racing class. Data on total km skied are from all starters who completed at least one section. Successful coureur de bois are defined as those completing 160 km.

further because each was approximately 60 minutes off the pace necessary to complete the 4 sections by 3 PM.

The cold affected the performance of all classes of skiers. Only 6 percent of the racers finished the 1979 competition compared to 29 percent in 1978. Of the starting coureur de bois, 38 percent finished in 1978 but only 7 percent in 1979. Aside from those who discontinued the event because of frost-bite or discomfort, two factors appear to have reduced the endurance capacity of the skiers. First, the very cold conditions resulted in snow conditions beyond the range of most ski waxes available in eastern Canada and the northeastern United States. Very few skiers had ever skied under comparable conditions, and they did not have wax suitable for the snow conditions. The second factor was the direct effect of cold on physical performance (3, 5). Muscle temperatures are not available for comparable circumstances of metabolic rate and environmental conditions, but certainly superficial, if not deep, muscle temperatures must have been lower than optimal for activity of oxidative enzymes, for excitability of nerves and muscle, and for nerve conduction (6). Definitive data are not available for the effect of low muscle temperatures on endurance performance in cross-country skiing. However, intensive cold appeared to induce an early onset of fatigue. This was evidenced in subjective observations of uncoordinated movements of otherwise skilled skiers, particularly on Day 2.

The heat loss from the respiratory passages was considerably greater in 1979 than in 1978. In spite of this, during the 1979 Marathon the majority of skiers made no attempt to cover their mouths. The few that put wool scarves or ballaclavas over their mouths had difficulty with the accumulation of ice as the water vapor condensed and froze on expiration. In his selective review of cold stress, Buskirk (1) comments on the thermal protection of the upper airways when exercising in the cold. At air temperatures of −10°C, high ventilatory rates can produce pharyngeal temperatures as low as 25°C. Extrapolation of limited data to the condition of the 1979 Marathon could result in pharyngeal temperatures below 20°C. Freezing of the upper airways appears to be unknown even during maximal performance in the cold. Cold-induced pain was reported in the nares and throat and such discomfort during inspiration may serve as a protective mechanism (1).

In summary, the 160 km Canadian Ski Marathon constitutes one of the significant challenges for endurance performance by men and women of all ages. The adverse weather conditions under which the event was conducted in 1979 provided a natural experiment on the endurance performance of highly motivated, well-trained athletes in severe cold. Endurance performance was impaired by frost-bite, snow conditions, and presumably, the direct effect of low temperature on metabolic or neuromuscular pathways, which resulted in greater fatigability of skeletal muscle. Many skiers did not complete the prescribed distance and a significant reduction in performance times was observed for those racers and coureurs de bois who successfully completed the 128 or 160 km course.

REFERENCES

1. Buskirk, E.R.: Cold stress: A selective review. In *Environmental Stress: Individual Human Adaptations,* edited by L.J. Falinsbee et al. New York, Acad Pr, 1978.
2. Christensen, E.H. and Hogberg, P.: Physiology of skiing. *Arbeitsphysiologie, 14*:292, 1950.
3. Clarke, R.S.J.; Hellon, R.F.; and Lind, A.R.: The duration of sustained contractions of the human forearm at different muscle temperatures.

J Physiol, 143:454, 1958.

4. Day, R.: Regional heat loss. In *Physiology of Heat Regulation and the Science of Clothing,* edited by L.H. Newburgh. New York, Hafner, 1968, pp. 240.

5. Edwards, R.H.T.; Harris, R.C.; Hultman, E.; Kaijser, L.; Koh, D.; and Nordesjo, L-O.: Effect of temperature on muscle energy metabolism and endurance during successive isometric contractions, sustained to fatigue, of the quadriceps muscle in man. *J Physiol, 220*:335, 1972.

6. Faulkner, J.A.: Heat and contractile properties of skeletal muscle. In *Heat, Life and Altitude,* edited by M.K. Yousef and S.M. Horvath. Springfield, Thomas, 1980. In press.

7. Grimby, G.; Nilsson, N.J.; and Saltin, B.: Cardiac output during submaximal and maximal exercise in active middle-aged athletes. *J Appl Physiol, 21*:1150, 1966.

8. Hanson, J.S.: Maximal exercise performance in members of the US Nordic Ski Team. *J Appl Physiol, 35*:592, 1973.

9. Maron, M.B.; Horvath, S.M.; Wilkerson, J.E.; and Gliner, J.A.: Oxygen uptake measurements during competitive marathon running. *J Appl Physiol, 40*:836, 1976.

10. Pugh, L.G.C.E.; Edholm, O.G.; Fox, R.H.; Wolff, H.S.; Hervey, G.R.; Hammond, W.H.; Tanner, J.M.; and Whitehouse, R.H.: A physiological study of channel swimming. *Clin Sci, 19*:257, 1960.

11. Taylor, H.L.; Buskirk, E.; and Henschel, A.: Maximal oxygen intake as an objective measure of cardio-respiratory performance. *J Appl Physiol, 8*:73, 1955.

Chapter 15

PHYSICAL ACTIVITY: A PREVENTIVE AND MAINTENANCE MODALITY FOR BONE LOSS WITH AGE

E.L. SMITH, JR.

INTRODUCTION

IT IS ESTIMATED that over 6 million people have excessive bone loss in the 50 and older segment of our population (8). Eighty percent of those 6 million are women. This "normal" involution of bone, without known etiological factors, has been termed postmenopausal, senile, or idiopathic osteoporosis. Largely as a result of bone involution, 300,000 women a year fracture their hips, with 50 percent mortality within 1 year (4). Women on the average begin to lose bone at about 35 years of age and continue to lose bone at .75 to 1 percent per year the rest of their lives (15). Men, on the other hand, do not begin to lose bone until age 55 and do not have significant osteoporosis until their 80s (15). Osteoporotic bone in the aged has been characterized by a decreased bone mineral mass, an enlarged medullary cavity, a normal mineral composition, and no biochemical abnormalities in plasma and urine (13, 16, 15).

The causative factor of senile or idiopathic osteoporosis, other than specific disease states, is multifactorial. Three major factors are (1) changes in estrogen production during female menopause, (2) a decrease of calcium intake and a decline in amounts absorbed across the intestinal tract, and (3) an inadequate level of physical activity. In this text, only physical activity will be considered, realizing the other two factors play a major role in bone changes with age.

MECHANICAL PROPERTIES OF BONE

The physical properties of bone vary slightly from organism to organism with all bone structure affected by genetic and en-

196

vironmental influences. Felts demonstrated that the form of limb bones is inherent, whereas the finer features and internal geometric structure of the bone are related to force dynamics (11). Bone has two main environmental physical forces acting upon it: gravitational force due to the physical mass supported by the bone, and muscular force exerted by the contraction of muscles attached to the bone. These two forces result in a series of stresses on the bone during muscle contraction. The forces resulting from muscular contraction are applied on different areas and at different angles on the bone, causing several combinations of varying lines of stress (1). Gravitational and muscular forces affect the mechanical organization of bone mineral and collagen. The combination of collagen and mineral (hydroxyapatite) forms a two-phase material often compared to fiberglass, having parallel characteristics of lightness and strength (10). The strength of bone has been demonstrated to be similar to cast iron, but with much greater elasticity, while weighing only one-third that of cast iron (10). In general, the elastic properties of bone follow the principle of Hooke's Law, which states that stress is in direct linear proportion to the strain within the elastic limit of the material under study (10). Bell (5) demonstrated that bone follows Hooke's Linear Law until the strain is three-fourths of that necessary to break the bone. With age, the mechanical strength properties of bone have been observed to decline. The cause of this decline may be the changing and decreased environmental stress of muscle contraction and weight bearing in the older, less active adult, which contributes to bone involution. The results of the involutional loss, without the presence of disease, is an osteoporotic bone that exhibits a quantitative reduction in bone mass and thus decreased strength.

In conjunction with the quantitative change in aging bone, there is also a qualitative change. Evans observed that tensile strength of a bone in man is related to the size and number of osteons present in the bone (10). He demonstrated that bone taken from young men, mean age of 41.5, had a greater average tensile breaking load, ultimate tensile strength, and increased density (few spaces in the bone) than bone taken from older men, mean age of 71.0. The older men demonstrated smaller osteons and fragments and an increased number of cement lines than the younger men. Evans suggested this could account for some of the reduced bone strength of the older bone specimens (10). The remaining difference in the strength of the bone may have resulted from the geometric structure of the bone in its distribution per unit area as a response to environmental stress placed upon the bone. This distribution change is observed in increased cell death, which results in regions of devitalized tissue where both lacunae and haversian canals have been found to contain amorphous mineral deposits. Frost has termed these micropetrotic (12). These changes have a clear qualitative effect on the adaptive structure of the aging bone, resulting in an increased probability of fracture.

In women, aged 40 to 54 years, Bauer has reported a sevenfold increase in the annual incidence of fractures of the distal end of the radius (3). He speculates that this rise in fracture incidence in aging women may be associated with a decline in the mechanical quality of the bone as well as the quantity of bone.

BONE DYNAMICS

Human and animal studies have demonstrated bone mineral variations associated with hypodynamics and hyperdynamics (6, 14, 16). Donaldson et al. studied 3 young males during 30 to 36 weeks of bed rest, which resulted in up to 39 percent bone mineral loss of the calcaneus, as measured by photon absorptiometry (9). Upon resumption of ambulation, remineralization of the calcaneus occurred at a similar rate to that of demineralization. All subjects exceeded their initial calcaneus bone mineral content by the week 36 of recovery. Chamay and Tschantz indicated that bone hypertrophy is directly related to physical activity and weight bearing. They removed a section of the radius in dogs and found that the increased stress placed on the ulna resulted in a 60 to 100 percent mineral increase over a 6 month period (6). Dalen found bone hypertrophy in cross-country runners between the ages of 50 and 59. Compared to matched controls of the same age, weight, and height, the cross-country runners had a 20 percent greater bone mineral of both the femora and the humeri (7). Nilsson and Westlin used absorptiometry to measure the bone mineral content of the femur in 64 nationally ranked athletes and 39 age and sex matched controls (16). The bone mineral content of the athletes was significantly greater than the controls. The athletes demonstrated bone hypertrophy in relationship to their specific sport activity. The weight lifters demonstrated the greatest hypertrophy, followed in order by the throwers, runners, soccer players, and swimmers. The control group consisted of an active and an inactive group. The active group participated regularly in physical activity and demonstrated a highly significant greater bone mineral content than the inactive group. Nilsson concluded that it seems possible to increase the bone mineral content above "normal" in man by physical activity, while inactivity will result in bone loss (16).

Few studies have demonstrated that physical activity actually increases bone mineral mass in the osteoporotic aged. E. L. Smith, Jr., however, in an 8 month study, used absorptiometry to measure the radius of 39 subjects. The subjects were placed in one of three groups: a control group (mean age 80), a physical activity group (mean age 75), and a physical therapy group (mean age 82) (18). The physical activity group demonstrated a bone mineral content increase of 2.6 percent ($.05 < p < .1$) while the physical therapy group demonstrated a significant increase of 7.8 percent ($p < .05$). Both groups were different from the control group, which showed no change. The physical therapy group clearly demonstrated bone mineral increase, while a borderline change was observed in the physical activity group. Smith et al. determined *in vivo* bone mineral content by photon absorptiometry on 30 Causasian females age 69–95 (mean age 84). Bone mineral content (BMC) and width of the radius were measured at two sites. The subject population consisted of nursing home volunteers assigned to a control group (N = 18) or physical activity group (N = 12). The groups were matched as to age, weight, and degree of ambulation, and were maintained on similar diets. The control group made no change in their activities of daily living, while the physical activity group participated in a 3 day per week, 30 minute per day exercise program. The null hypothesis for the slope of the bone mineral content equal to zero within the group was tested using the two-tailed *t*-test. No significance for BMC was observed (Table 15-I).

A single-tailed *t*-test was used to compare the groups of the 36 month study. The bone mineral content of the control group declined by 3.28 percent while the physical activity group demonstrated a 2.29 percent increase during the 3 year study. This study showed a significant change in the pattern of bone involution in the aging female. Bone mineral loss was significantly reversed in

TABLE 15-I

THE SUM OF BONE MINERAL CHANGE AT TWO MEASUREMENT SITES OF THE DISTAL RADIUS OVER 36 MONTHS

Study Groups		Mean T_1 GM/CM	Mean T_{10} GM/CM	Calculated Intercept For T_1 GM/CM	Slope	Within Group t-Values	Calculated %Δ	Between Group t-Values Control Slope vs Treatment Slope
Control	$\bar{X}$	0.571	0.556	0.580	-0.0019	1.583	-3.28	
N = 18	SD	0.129	0.144	0.132	0.0054			
	SE	0.009	0.034	0.031	0.0012			
Physical Activity	$\bar{X}$	0.564	0.596	0.567	+0.0013	1.625	+2.29	1.863*
N = 12	SD	0.103	0.121	0.107	0.0030			
	SE	0.030	0.039	0.031	0.0008			

*$p < .05$.

the physical activity group compared to the continued loss by the control group (19).

The observed change in the physical activity group may relate to the hyperdynamic stress placed on the bone, above normal daily use, which resulted in a possible local electrical stimulus as suggested by Bassett (2). Bassett states that the stimulation for bone formation and destruction appears to be largely electrical in nature. He suggests that bone functions as a "Piezoelectric" crystal converting mechanical energy from weight-bearing and muscle contraction to an electric signal. This conversion takes place within the bone structure as the bone crystal is bent, resulting in a concave or convex side to the crystal. The concave side of the crystal produces a negative charge to which calcium is attracted, while the convex side produces a positive charge in which calcium is removed. This results in calcium being laid down in the internal structure of the bone in response to the geometric stress placed on the bone by the external environmental stress. This results in a bone response to the physical stress placed upon it to maintain the skeletal integrity.

One may hypothesize that bone maintenance involves two homeostatic mechanisms. The first mechanism is related to hormonal control, which is primarily concerned with the maintenance of blood calcium levels rather than bone mass. The bone mineral content and structure of the bone are involved in the hormonal homeostatic mechanism because bone functions as a chemical store for various body chemicals, of which calcium is of major concern. The second homeostatic mechanism relates to physical stresses placed on bone by gravity and the muscular system. That physical stresses affect the internal balance of bone accretion and resorption is clear. The reduction in either of these physical stresses results in bone resorption. This can be observed in a limb that is casted or when muscular and gravitational stress no longer acts on the bone. Although the mechanism for bone resorption is the same for all ages, the increased rate of resorption that occurs with aging (30+) may well be the result of decreased activity levels.

REFERENCES

1. Arkin, A.M. and Katz, J.F.: The effect of pressure on epiphyseal growth. The mechanism of plasticity of grow-bone. *J Bone and Joint Surg,* 38-A:1056, 1956.

2. Bassett, C.A.L.: Biophysical principles affecting bone structure. In *The Biochemistry and Physiology of Bone, Vol. III, Development and Growth,* edited by Geoffrey H. Bourne. New York, Acad Pr, 1971.
3. Bauer, G.: Epidemiology of fracture in aged persons. *Clin Orthop, 17*:219, 1960.
4. Beals, R.: Survival following hip fracture: Long follow-up of 607 patients. *J Chron Dis, 25*:235, 1972.
5. Bell, G.H.: Bone as a mechanical engineering problem. In *The Biochemistry and Physiology of Bone,* edited by Geoffrey H. Bourne. New York, Acad Pr, 1956.
6. Chamay, A. and Tschantz, P.: Mechanical influences in bone remodeling: experimental research on Wolff's law. *J Biomechanics, 5*:173, 1972.
7. Dalen, N. and Olsson, K.E.: Bone mineral content and physical activity. *Acta Orthop Scand, 45*:170, 1974.
8. Davis, M.; Lanzl, L.; and Cox: The detection, prevention and retardation of menopausal osteoporosis. In *Osteoporosis,* edited by U.S. Barzel. New York, Grune and Stratton, 1970.
9. Donaldson, C.; Hulley, S.B.; Vogel, J.M.; Hattner, R.S.; Bayers, J.H.; and McMillan, D.E.: Effect of prolonged bedrest on bone mineral. *Metabolism, 19 (12)*:1071, 1970.
10. Evans, F.: Mechanical properties and histology of cortical bone from younger and older men. *Anat Res, 185*:1, May 1976.
11. Felts, W.J.L.: *In vivo* bone implantation as a technique in skeletal biology. *Int Rev Cytol, 12*:243, 1961.
12. Frost, H.: Micreopetrosis. *J Bone Joint Surg, 42A*:144, 1960.
13. Garn, S.W.; Rohmann, C.G.; and Wagner, B.: Bone loss as a general phenomenon in man. *Fed Proc, 26*:1729, 1967.
14. Harris, W.H. and Heaney, R.P.: Skeletal renewal and metabolic bone disease. *N Eng J Med, 280*:193, 253, 303, Jan. 23, 30, Feb. 6, 1971.
15. Mazess, R.B. and Cameron, J.R.: Bone mineral content in normal U.S. whites. *International Conference on Bone Mineral Measurement.* p. 228, Oct., 1973, Washington, D.C., DHEW Publication HIH 75-683.
16. Nilsson, B.E.R. and Westlin, N.E.: Bone density in athletes. *Clin Orthop, 77*:179, 1971.
17. Smith, D.M.; Khairi, M.R.A.; Norton, J.; and Johnston, C.C., Jr.: Age and activity effects of rate of bone mineral loss. *J Clin Invest, 58*:716, 1976.
18. Smith, E.L., Jr.: The effects of physical activity on bone in the aged. *International Conference on Bone Mineral Measurements,* 397, Oct. 1973, edited by R.B. Mazess, Washington, D.C., DHEW Publication No. NIH 75-683.
19. Smith, E.L., Jr. and Reddan, W.: Physical activity, calcium and vitamin D: a modality for bone mineral increase in the aged. In press, *Med. and Sci. in Sports and Ex.*
20. Sweeney, A.W.; Kron, R.P.; and Byers, R.K.: *Mechanical characteristics of bone and its constituents.* Paper presented at The American Society of Mechanical Engineers, Chicago, Il., Nov. 7-11, 1965.

Part 3

EXERCISE IN DISEASE PREVENTION AND THERAPY

PRESIDING: KARL G. STOEDEFALKE

Chapter 16

OBSERVATIONS ON THE HOPE-KELLOGG HEALTH DYNAMICS PROGRAM*

R.A. PETERSON

DESCRIPTION OF PROGRAM

ALTHOUGH KNOWLEDGE of the effects of exercise on health enhancement and/or disease prevention is incomplete, enough information exists to warrant ambitious efforts of a promotional or educational nature. Thus, we have seen the proliferation of program efforts by a wide variety of agencies to many diverse target populations. Such efforts present new challenges for the scientist because the factors of human motivation and educational strategy assume predominant roles. Of course programs must have an accurate factual foundation, but also of importance are the questions of how to present such materials, and to which population strata. Programs also should have a responsible economic base that is cost-effective and financially low-discriminatory. This chapter will describe a health and fitness promotion program already in existence in the setting of a small liberal arts college, as well as to report some short-term observations of that program.

The Hope-Kellogg Health Dynamics Program is an effort at health enhancement education for the students, faculty, and staff of Hope College and for the surrounding community, namely, the environs of Holland, Michigan. The program's major objective is behavioral, i.e. individuals should volitionally adopt and maintain healthful life-styles. Of considerable interest to this program is the determination of approaches or strategies that will work best in reaching the objective over both the short and the long term.

The principle emphasis of the program is directed toward a core curriculum, two sequential semester experience for all

*Funded through a health promotion/disease prevention grant from the W.K. Kellogg Foundation.

freshman students. This experience comprises the complete physical education requirement of the college. Within this experience
are an academic component, an assessment component, an advising component, and an activity component. The purpose of the
academic component is education regarding the relationships
among and between life-style factors such as exercise and diet and
life qualities as, for example, health and fitness. The typical tools
of lecture, discussion, and readings are used. The purpose of the
assessment component is to evaluate current health and fitness, to
assess attitudes and feelings about health and fitness, and to determine behavioral patterns that affect health and fitness. The
advising component provides opportunities for one-to-one interaction with each student, regarding any aspect of personal
health and fitness. Included are such items as an explanation of
the results of their assessments, an exploration of their feelings
about the priority of health and fitness in their value systems,
recommendations for behavioral alterations that seem appropriate, and a response to any questions or concerns they might have.
The activity component provides an organized setting within
which the student experiences physical activity alternatives that
may be effective in promoting health and fitness, that may develop a foundation for a lifetime of healthy exercise, and that are
personally enjoyable, satisfying, and challenging.

The four components described above are designed to com-
plement each other in their impact on the individual. All may be
regarded as sources of information made available to the student
so that decisions regarding health and fitness may have a strong
rational base. After completing the freshman experience, students
are urged to continue their involvement with the program on a
voluntary basis. Provided for such involvement are annual
physiological assessments; individual counselling; seminars, work-
shops, and lectures; health and fitness interest groups; and a variety of physical activity opportunities through classes, intramurals,
and other organized physical activity programs. The same opportunities are provided for faculty, staff, and individuals from the
community.

An interesting and unique feature of the Hope program is the
effectiveness of the integration of several other aspects of the
college into the program. These include the Health Clinic, the
Food Service, and office of the Dean of Students. The physicians

and staff of the Health Clinic screen each student and follow their progress through the program. Interreferrals and interconsultations occur as appropriate. The Food Service provides a nutrition awareness program, a nutrition consultant, and nutrient information on all items served. They also are involved in developing the nutrition education segments of the academic component and convene student food service review committees. The student counselling center and campus activities and residential life offices of the office of the Dean of Students also work closely with the program. An interdepartmental research committee has been formed to originate and carry out research projects from the program base.

The Hope program was implemented in the fall of 1978. Efforts were directed almost exclusively toward the freshman program. Other features will be phased in over time until the total program is operational. Observations that may be of value when considering the potential of such programs in the field of health enhancement were made in the first year of the program. It should be remembered that data reported here are observations made during the conduct of a service program. These should not be considered experimental data such as are generated in the process of controlled empirical investigations.

There are three types of data that will be reported: laboratory data from maximal graded exercise testing and body composition, data about health and fitness-related behavior patterns, and affective data on the feelings, attitudes, and perceptions of the students about such programs in general and about the Hope program as they experienced it this year. The subjects were 350 freshman, about equally divided between males and females.

RESULTS

EXERCISE TESTING: All students were administered a graded exercise test either on a motor-driven treadmill or a mechanically braked bicycle ergometer. By convention, all women began at a workload of 7 METs and all men began at a workload of 9 METs. The workload was increased by one MET each minute until voluntary termination. Heart rate and blood pressure were monitored at rest and during each minute of exercise. Initial testing was conducted at the midpoint of the first semester and final testing was done at the end of the second semester. The results of initial testing are presented in Table 16-I. Tests of statistical difference probabilities seemed inappropriate since this was not a controlled experimental situation. Therefore, only the descriptive data for each observation period are reported. Resting blood pressures, blood pressures at maximal exercise, and 10 second heart rates at maximal or terminal exercise workloads do not appear to differ from what would be expected either for males or females. When examining individual test results of women on the bike test, it appears that some had difficulty achieving expected maximal heart rates. This is not unusual under these circumstances and seems to be related either to local muscle fatigue, poor motivation, or both. For males, maximal MET values of 16 at initial and 17 at final testing appear to be at the upper end of normal when compared to accepted standards. Womens' values of 12.2 and 13 METs respectively are more nearly normal. As will be pointed out later, the exercise habits of these individuals, both as reported to be before encountering the program as well as during the program, are really quite extensive.

BODY COMPOSITION: Body composition was assessed by underwater weighing for both males and females. Those who had difficulty with the technique were also assessed with skinfold methods. The results of body composition testing are presented in Table 16-II. Values for males and females on initial and final testing appear to be quite normal. The result of final testing of the females was of particular interest. Historically, it seemed that Hope women were inclined to gain weight during college, perhaps because the food service operates according to an all-you-can-eat-for-a-meal-ticket system. No particular differences either in body weights or body composition between initial and final testing were noted, however.

HEALTH RELATED BEHAVIORS: Towards the end of the second semester all students were expected to record and file in computer memory certain health related behavior data. These data were recorded daily for one week at a time and for at least two separated weeks in total. A summary of the population data is included as Table 16-III. Average weights and resting heart rates appear normal for this population with the possible exception of average weights for females, which may be somewhat high. In analyzing physical activity data, it soon became obvious that this population of students was quite active. It must be kept in mind,

TABLE 16-I
EXERCISE TESTING OF CARDIOVASCULAR FUNCTION
INITIAL TESTING

Males

	Rest		Max. Ex.	
	Mean	SD	Mean	SD
Systolic BP	130	11.5	194	20.8
Diastolic BP	75	8.2	73	14.2
Heart Rate (10 sec)			32.4	2.55
METs			16.0	1.69

Females

	Rest		Max. Ex.	
	Mean	SD	Mean	SD
Systolic BP	117	12.3	153	29.3
Diastolic BP	70	9.5	71	12.1
Heart Rate (10 sec)			31.0	3.03
METs			12.2	1.64

FINAL TESTING

Males

	Rest		Max. Ex.	
	Mean	SD	Mean	SD
Systolic BP	124	20.8	190	20.0
Diastolic BP	75	7.3	72	8.1
Heart Rate (10 sec)			31.6	1.80
METs			17.0	1.98

Females

	Rest		Max. Ex.	
	Mean	SD	Mean	SD
Systolic BP	114	10.5	158	15.1
Diastolic BP	71	8.4	73	9.1
Heart Rate (10 sec)			31.6	1.70
METs			13.0	1.70

TABLE 16-II
BODY COMPOSITION: PERCENT FAT

	Males		Females	
	Mean	SD	Mean	SD
Initial Test	13.5	5.23	24.2	5.45
Final Test	12.5	5.11	23.2	5.16

however, that these are self-reports of activity and that these data were collected during the spring season of the year, a time when people usually begin to be more active. Even taking these qualifying remarks into account, it was surprising to note that 87 percent of the students reported 4 or more workouts during their record-

TABLE 16-III
HEALTH RELATED BEHAVIOR DATA

Biologic Data:

Average Weight (Kg)	Females 059	
	Males 075	
Average Resting Heart	Females 071	
Rate (Beats/min)	Males 065	

Pattern of Exercise Workouts:

Average number of days with 1 or more workouts—5

Number of people with 4 or more workouts—310

Workout per week

0–1   02%
2–4   019%
3–7   034%
8–   046%

FOR PEOPLE WITH 4 OR MORE WORKOUTS

Consecutive Workout Days		Consecutive Nonworkout Days	
1–2	013%	0–1	079%
3–4	030%	2–3	021%
5–	057%	4–	000%

Ratings of Workouts By Type:

Top 3—No Weighting
  1 Running   0222
  2 Racquetball   0116
  3 Basketball   0080

Top 3—Effectiveness Weighting
  1 Running   0547
  2 Racquetball   0248
  3 Basketball   0167

Intensity-Duration Percents of Workouts:

Low Duration and	Low Intensity	05%
	Med Intensity	18%
	Hgh Intensity	03%
Med Duration and	Low Intensity	08%
	Med Intensity	48%
	Hgh Intensity	12%
Hgh Duration and	Low Intensity	00%
	Med Intensity	03%
	Hgh Intensity	02%

Ratings of Recreation:

Top 3—No Weighting
  1 Dancing: Disco, Rock, Ballroom   0069
  2 Running   0066
  3 Basketball   0049

Top 3—Population Effectiveness
  1 Running   0244
  2 Dancing: Disco, Rock, Ballroom   0229
  3 Racquetball   0177

Top 3—Personal Effectiveness
  1 Floor Hockey   0005
  2 Skiing—Downhill   0005
  3 Circuit Training   0004

Smoking Percents:

Non-Smokers (0)	094%
Light Smokers (1–10)	004%
Moderate Smokers (11–30)	001%
Heavy Smokers (31–)	001%
Non-Pipe Smokers (0)	097%
Pipe Smokers (1–)	003%
Non-Sigar Smokers (0)	097%
Cigar Smokers (1–)	003%

Sleep Percents:

Light (0–5)	10%
Light-Moderate (6–7)	65%
Heavy-Moderate (8–9)	23%
Heavy (10–)	01%

Health Percents:

Low Stress Week (0–4)	20%
Moderate Stress Week (5–7)	59%
High Stress Week (8–)	21%
Illness Week (#Ills > 0 and Ratings > = 3)	011%
Nonillness Week	089%

Population Statistics:

Total Number of Freshman	356
Total Number of Female Freshman	168
Total Number of Male Freshman	188

ing weeks. Almost half said they engaged in 8 or more workouts per week and over half said they worked out on 5 or more consecutive days during those weeks. Running was rated the most frequent form of exercise as well as being the mode from which they felt they gained the most total exercise. Running was followed by racquetball and basketball in each of these categories. Students were asked to estimate average intensities and durations of their workouts. A three by three grid was formed of intensities (low = 1–7 METS; med = 8–12 METS; high = 13+ METS) and durations (low = 0–30 min; med = 31–90 min; high = 91+ min). Almost half felt that their workouts fit into the medium intensity–medium duration category. The other half were spread among the other 8 categories.

Activities engaged in recreationally or incidentally and not used expressly for or considered as workouts were reported separately. Dancing was slightly more popular than running but was also regarded as less strenuous when qualified according to their intensity-duration characteristics. Activities that had the highest reported intensity-duration traits (although not very many people reported engaging in these) were floor hockey, downhill skiing, and circuit training. Health habits, other than physical activity, are reported in the remainder of Table 16-III. Dietary data were not collected during these reporting periods. Only 6 percent of the population reported any cigarette smoking during the reporting period and, of these, 4 percent reported fewer than 10 cigarettes per day. Data on alcohol consumption was not collected because the legal drinking age in Michigan is 21 years, and there was a desire to avoid any potential self-incrimination repercussions. About two-thirds of the population reported getting 6–7 hours of sleep per night. Most felt that their weeks were either low or moderate in perceived stress. Most also reported no significant illness during the recording period. In summary, if the self-reports of health-related behaviors are reasonably accurate, this population may be regarded as quite active and appears to behave responsibly in other health areas. There is a continuing effort to pursue and refine procedures in this important line of investigation.

AFFECTIVE FINDINGS: At the end of the year, the students were asked to anonymously relate their impressions and feelings about this program in particular and about such programs generally. The results of that assessment are recorded in Table 16-IV. As reported earlier, there were several components that comprised the program. The students were asked how they felt about each component. The knowledge component consisted of some lecturing and reading but emphasized discussion and individual analysis. While 88 percent felt that knowledge is a very important ingredient for a personal health enhancement endeavor to flourish, only 54 percent felt that they had "learned something new" in the program. The result was not surprising, because efforts were directed to help the students internalize and act upon their knowledge rather than to overwhelm them. As a result, 65 percent reported that the knowledge component had increased their motivation to live a healthful life-style. This was doubly meaningful since 74 percent had reported high initial motivation to live such a life-style. When asked regarding their feelings about the laboratory assessments, 80 percent reported keen interest in the tests and their results, yet only 55 percent indicated that this component had increased their motivation to live healthy life-

TABLE 16-IV
ATTITUDES ABOUT THE PROGRAM (SUMMARY)

	% Positive responses
Knowledge	
Knowledge is an important part of a health and fitness program.	88
I learned something new in this program.	54
The knowledge component has increased my motivation to live a healthy lifestyle.	65
Laboratory Testing	
I was interested in the tests and their results.	80
The testing component increased my motivation to live a healthy lifestyle.	55
Record Keeping	
A record keeping system is important.	60
The record keeping system of this program has increased my motivation.	15
Physical Activity	
My physical activity class this year has increased my fitness.	78
I enjoyed my physical activity class.	93
I would have liked more skill instruction.	29
The physical activity component has increased my motivation to live an active lifestyle.	74
I am very active outside of class activities.	79
Diet	
My approach to my diet has changed as a result of this program.	44
General Feelings	
This program should continue to be required of freshman students.	77
I would rather have a more typical physical education program.	33
I would like to see most emphasis on physical fitness and skill development.	54
I would like to see most emphasis on a comprehensive health promotion/disease prevention approach.	46

styles. This might be due to the fact that performance on the laboratory tests are very strongly influenced by genetic factors. Therefore, individuals who were living healthy life-styles might display poorer results than those who appeared to bend the guidelines of healthy living practices.

Sixty percent of the students felt that establishing a record-keeping system would be important but only 15 percent felt the system was instrumental in increasing their motivation to live a healthy life-style. The system consisted of filling out a 2 page recording form that summarized weekly physical activity, dietary and other health habits data, and then required the student to file that information in the memory of the college computer. Unfortunately, the computer was not operational much of the time. This frustrated the students and caused much discontent with the system.

The physical activity component was very well received. The major objectives of this component were physiological stimulation and enjoyment. Seventy-eight percent of the students felt that their class had improved their fitness and 93 percent reported that they enjoyed the activity in which they were engaged. Little emphasis was placed on skill instruction yet only 29 percent reported that they wished they had more skill instruction. Seventy-four percent felt that the activity experience had increased their motivation to stay active and fit. Seventy-nine percent reported that they were very active in non–class-oriented physical activities. Among the disappointing findings was the report of only 44 percent who claimed that their approach to their diet had been changed as a result of the program.

There was, initially, concern that significant resistance might occur because the program was required rather than voluntary; however, 77 percent of the students felt it should continue to be required. Only 33 percent felt they would rather experience a more typical physical education program rather than the type offered. When asked whether they would rather have a program principally emphasizing physical fitness and skill development or a program emphasizing a more comprehensive health promotion/disease prevention approach, the students favored the former by a weak 54 to 46 percent margin. Many suggestions were also received for improving several components of the program. The students were very understanding of some of the first year problems and exhibited positive and supportive attitudes.

CONCLUSIONS

Although there are some factors that indicate college freshman are not an ideal target audience for a health fitness approach to physical education, such efforts will be generally well received and can have a significant impact. In order to evaluate the effectiveness of the program, however, it is necessary to know whether the students will have developed active, healthful life-styles 20, 30, and even 40 years from now.

Chapter 17

METABOLIC COSTS AND FEASIBILITY OF WATER SUPPORT EXERCISES FOR THE ELDERLY*

A.D. CLAREMONT, W.G. REDDAN, AND E.L. SMITH

Abstract

WATER SUPPORT was evaluated as a stimulus to increased exercise participation in the elderly by measuring energy expenditures in 5 males ($\bar{X}$ 70.6 ± 6.4 yrs) and 6 females (58.3 ± 4.2 yrs) during constant speed walking at thigh, waist, and chest immersion depths. Oxygen uptakes ($\dot{V}O_2$) and heart rates (HRs) increased with depth for all subjects, females exhibing a slightly higher response at all water levels. HRs in the water were significantly lower ($\bar{X}$ 96.63 ± 15.77) than HRs measured at comparable metabolic demands during treadmill walking ($\bar{X}$ 117.56 ± 21.41). Thus, extrapolation of a HR training intensity guideline from land to water activities requires modification. Despite average energy expenditures (exercise and recovery) of ~ 0.8 l min^{-1} (4 Cal·min^{-1}) body temperature decreased an average of 0.4°C ($p < 0.005$) during 40 minutes exposure to air and water temperatures of 28.5°C and 27.5°C respectively. Advantages of water support exercises for the elderly include (a) providing a sufficient intensity stimulus (66–75% $\dot{V}O_2$max) to promote a training response with lower cardiac costs than comparable metabolic requirements of land exercise; (b) encouraging a greater exercise involvement in movement-restricted individuals through amelioration of inhibitions associated with "fear of falling."

Regression of physical performance capacity with aging necessitates modification of exercise programing for the elderly. Selected activities should be enjoyable, yet of sufficient intensity and duration to promote a desirable level of aerobic conditioning. How-

---
*Financial support for this study was provided by the Marion Laboratories, Inc.

ever, these objectives are often more easily acclaimed than accomplished. Despite appropriate allowances for decrements in strength, coordination, range of motion, and physical working capacity, many elderly restrict their degree of voluntary exercise participation during formal activity classes. This is due to inhibitions associated with a "fear of falling" and possible injury. This attitude is most apparent in the relatively passive and timid motions of individuals with orthopedic or motor coordination limitations. If the apprehension associated with falling could be minimized, many senior citizens might be encouraged to participate more extensively and thus obtain greater physiological benefits from their exercise program. Therefore, a series of walking exercises was conducted including arm movements while partly immersed at different water depths in a swimming pool. The intent was to evaluate the adequacy of this exercise medium relative to (a) encouraging more unrestricted activity participation and (b) providing an environment in which exercise intensities capable of effecting a cardiovascular training response could be safely stimulated.

Methods

Selected characteristics of the subjects are presented in Table 17-I. Five males and 6 females volunteered to undertake a progressive treadmill test and repeat a series of 5 different walking exercises in water at thigh, waist, and chest depths. All were judged sufficiently free of cardiovascular or pulmonary contraindications to vigorous muscular activity based on medical evaluations including a physical exam; a modified Balke treadmill test (2) for assessment of physical working capacity; and resting, exercise, and postexercise electrocardiogram tracings.

TABLE 17-I
SELECTED PHYSICAL CHARACTERISTICS

		AGE YRS	WT. kg	BSA m^2	max $\dot{V}_e$ l BTPS	max $\dot{V}O_2$	
						l	ml/kg/min
MALES	$\bar{X}$	70.8	85.13	1.99	46.47	1.50	17.61
	SD	6.53	7.29	0.05	14.68	0.50	5.15
FEMALES	$\bar{X}$	58.7	67.01	1.69	46.30	1.54	23.34
	SD	4.13	7.68	0.09	9.14	0.26	4.69
COMBINED GROUPS	$\bar{X}$	64.18	72.25	1.83	46.38	1.52	20.64
	SD	8.11	11.85	0.17	11.31	0.36	5.59

Experiments were conducted at a local YMCA swimming pool at the same time of day on 3 occasions separated by 1–3 weeks. Following 10–12 minutes of relaxed sitting, 5 minute resting determinations were made for oxygen ($\dot{V}O_2$) uptake, heart rate (HR), and oral temperature (T_{or}). Body weight and blood pressure (BP) were recorded.

Upon entering the pool at one of three randomly assigned depths, upper thigh (groin), waist (navel), or chest (nipple), the subject donned an expired gas collection assembly consisting of a head frame supporting a one-way low resistance breathing valve with large rubber mouthpiece. An accompanying technician provided above water support for the expired tubing, gas collection bag, and two-way valve. Participants walked across the swimming pool maintaining constant depth at a predetermined speed of 29.26 meters/min (1.1 mph) for a total of 3 minutes (6 crossings). This pace, although arbitrarily determined, represented a preferred work rate selected by the majority of subjects following several preliminary trial crossings on a separate occasion. Speed was maintained with the assistance of a supervisor verbally coordinating pace to arrive at designated locations (e.g. midcrossing, turn) at 15 second intervals. All subjects were able to maintain exercise rates so that they arrived within ± 3 meters of target. Expired gases were collected continuously during the second and third minutes. Exercise HRs were determined by telemetry in 1 subject and by a 10 second carotid or radial pulse count by the technician immediately postexercise in the other 2. This group of subjects then rested out of water while a second group performed. The alternate sequence of exercise-recovery for each of the 5 exercises at each depth occurred in a ratio of 3 minute exercise with 4–6 minutes recovery, totalling 15 minutes exercise and 16–24 minutes recovery. Postexercise BPs were obtained approximately 15–20 minutes following completion of experimental proceedings.

A sequence of 5 exercises was performed at each testing session. Two exercises involved use of the legs only (forward and backward walking) and three included both legs and arms. Arm work involved alternately submerging a flutterboard edgewise and pulling or pushing its broad surface through the water, followed by an airborne recovery. Breaststroke simulated that of the actual swimming stroke. Cyclic arm stroke frequencies were maintained at or slightly faster than walking cadence.

$\dot{V}O_2$ was determined by open circuit methods. Expired gas volumes ($\dot{V}_E$) were measured with a dry gas meter (Parkinson-Cowan) from samples collected in meteorologic balloons. Aliquot samples were drawn from the collection bag into oiled glass syringes for duplicate analysis of O_2 and CO_2 concentration by gas chromatography. Commercially certified reference gases, confirmed by Gallenkamp analysis, were used to calibrate the chromatograph before and following each experiment.

ECG HRs were counted as the distance between R intervals over a 5 second recording strip. BPs were measured by manometric technique, body temperature and weight by standard clinical thermometer and scale, respectively. Responses across conditions were analyzed using paired t tests.

RESULTS

Oxygen Uptake Response During Exercise

As shown in Figure 17-1, the trend for $\dot{V}O_2$ was to increase with water depth for both sexes. Higher oxygen uptakes were associated with those exercises involving both arm and leg work, namely forward and backward walk with flutterboard pull and push respectively and forward walk breaststroke. Chest immersion depth elicited the greatest metabolic demands for both sexes, whereas thigh and waist levels were relatively comparable but considerably lower.

Without exception, metabolic costs for women were higher than for men across exercises and depths (Fig. 17-1, Table 17-II). However, when expressed in terms of percent maximum oxygen uptake, relative work intensities in the water ranged between 68 and 75 percent $\dot{V}O_2$max for men and women, respectively.

Heart Rate

HRs like $\dot{V}O_2$ generally showed a progressive increase with depth (Fig. 17-2). Corresponding to the increased $\dot{V}O_2$ response, HRs for women were consistently higher across exercises and depth than values obtained for men. However, relatively small HR differences and considerable data variability tended to minimize statistical significance between sex differences.

The observation of a pronounced bradycardia ($p < 0.001$) during exercise in the pool was of particular interest. Figure 17-3

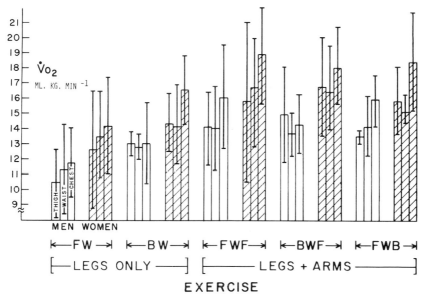

Figure 17-1. Oxygen uptake response for men and women during graded immersion upright exercises. Bars represent mean ± SE of the mean. Symbols: FW = forward walk; BW = backward walk; FWF = forward walk flutterboard pull; BWF = backward walk flutterboard push; FWB = forward walk breaststroke.

clearly shows HR to be consistently above the line of identity or elevated during treadmill versus immersion walking at equivalent levels of oxygen uptake. This response occurred over a $\dot{V}O_2$ range of 0.8 to 1.3 l/min and represented a 21 (19–25) beat/minute reduction in mean HR at the average energy expenditure of 1.0 l/min for water versus land exercises.

Temperature Response

Experiments were conducted at prevailing air and pool temperatures averaging 27.49 ± 2.34 and 28.47 ± 1.0°C respectively. Under these environmental conditions both groups demonstrated an identical 0.4°C decrease in body temperature (T_{or}) over the 31–39 minute experimental session.

DISCUSSION

A primary purpose of this study was to investigate the feasibility of a water support medium to encourage greater exercise participation and hence more physiologically meaningful activity in the

TABLE 17-II
OXYGEN UPTAKE ml·kg⁻¹·min⁻¹ RESPONSE DURING GRADED IMMERSION UPRIGHT EXERCISES

Exercise*		THIGH			WATER DEPTH WAIST			CHEST		
		Male	Female	Sig	Male	Female	Sig	Male	Female	Sig
FW	x̄	10.37	12.67	$p < 0.10$	11.38	13.6	NS†	11.77	14.23	$p < 0.10$
	SE	2.33	3.84	—	2.79	2.83	—	2.33	3.14	—
BW	x̄	13.0	14.43	NS†	12.84	14.26	NS†	13.04	16.57	$p < 0.025$
	SE	0.78	1.91	—	0.81	2.26	—	2.66	2.31	—
FWF	x̄	14.0	15.78	NS†	13.98	16.37	NS†	16.08	18.16	$p < 0.01$
	SE	2.35	5.32	—	2.74	3.56	—	3.44	2.56	—
BWF	x̄	14.87	16.80	NS†	13.60	16.73	$p < 0.025$	14.30	19.05	$p < 0.01$
	SE	3.15	3.21	—	1.45	2.77	—	1.91	3.98	—
FWB	x̄	13.37	15.30	$p < 0.025$	14.12	15.19	NS†	15.90	18.40	$p < 0.10$
	SE	0.45	2.27	—	1.98	0.95	—	1.84	3.31	—

*FW = forward walk
BW = backward walk
FWF = forward walk flutterboard pull
BWF = backward walk flutterboard push
FWB = forward walk breaststroke
†NS: $p > 0.10$

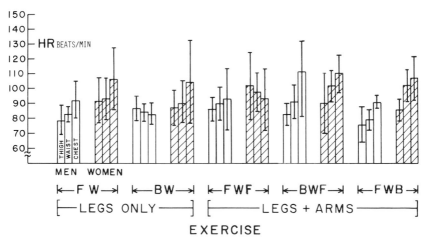

Figure 17-2. Heart rate response for men and women during graded immersion exercises. Symbols: FW = forward walk; BW = backward walk; FWF = forward walk flutterboard pull; BWF = backward walk flutterboard push; FWB = forward walk breaststroke.

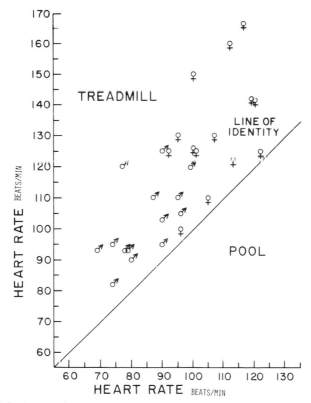

Figure 17-3. Comparison of treadmill and pool heart rate responses at equivalent $\dot{V}O_2$ ranging from 0.8 to 1.3 $l \cdot min^{-1}$.

aged. The graded immersion exercises consistently ranged from 3 to 4.5 METS. These elevated activity levels were most likely attributable to a diminution of the "fear-of-falling" dry land inhibition minimized in the security of the water environment.

The reason for increased absolute energy expenditures for females over that of the males (Fig. 17-1, Table 17-II) was not resolved. It is possible the women's breasts may have contributed to higher O_2 costs of arm work by virtue of shorter horizontal stroking with higher cyclic frequencies observed during flutterboard and breaststroke actions. However, this does not account for the elevated $\dot{V}O_2$ occurring during leg exercise only, which would tend to suggest possible sex differences in walking efficiency in the water. At chest depth in particular, the added buoyancy of breast immersion might be expected to contribute an increased vertical elevation of the body's center of gravity with each step, partially compensating the horizontal force component. Female subjects most frequently indicated difficulty in maintaining traction with the pool bottom during push-off at this level. Increased efforts to maintain the prescribed work rate are reflected in the higher oxygen uptakes for women over men at this depth (Table 17-II). However, because of the higher $\dot{V}O_2$max of the female subjects (23 ± 4.69 versus 17.41 ± 5.15 ml·kg^{-1}·min^{-1}), relative work intensities were comparable and ranged between 68 and 75 percent $\dot{V}O_2$max for both groups. At these intensities, intermittent bouts of 3 minute exercise with 4–6 minutes recovery for 30 minutes or more have been shown to place sufficient demands on aerobic processes to stimulate a cardiovascular training response (1, 3, 5, 7, 8). The remaining ingredient necessary to achieve a desirable state of fitness is regular participation at frequency of at least 3 days per week (7).

Since there is a linear relationship between heart rate and levels of energy expenditure, individualized prescription of training threshold heart rates is a feasible and practical guide for determining desired work intensities. Training levels between 50 and 70 percent of $\dot{V}O_2$max corresponding to 65 to 80 percent of HRmax are considered within a range adequate to demonstrate a substantial conditioning response while at the same time minimizing the inherent dangers of too high intensities (10). However, to avoid undue risk to elderly participants, many of whom exhibit ECG abnormalities, it is necessary to strongly caution against extrapolating a training HR from land to water activity. The results of Craig (4) and of this study show the HR:$\dot{V}O_2$ relationships shifted to the right during exercise-immersion; that is, a lower pulse rate response occurs in the water than on dry land at comparable O_2 uptakes. For example at the mean $\dot{V}O_2$ of 1.04 l/min, HR averaged 96 beats/minute (70% HRmax) during immersion walking compared to 117 beats/minute (84% HRmax) during treadmill walking. However, this 21 beat/minute bradycardia may be a double-edged sword with potentially beneficial or deleterious effects. The physiologic advantage is that myocardial efficiency is generally considered improved (i.e. lower myocardial O_2 consumption demands) if a given cardiac output ($\dot{Q}$) can be maintained with a low HR and large stroke volume (SV) (12). Exercise immersion studies by Rennie (9) and McArdle (6) clearly demonstrate the major adjustment to a decrease in HR is an increase in SV. These investigators further showed the $\dot{Q}$-$\dot{V}O_2$ relationship to be quite similar in air and water over a range (18–33°C) of water temperatures. Thus, the inherent danger in recommending exercise intensities in the water at HRs similar to land values would be to impose excessively high metabolic demands. Indeed, O_2 uptakes approaching maximum aerobic capacity would have been required to achieve equivalent land-water HR responses by the elderly participants of this study. Such high intensities are unnecessary for promoting an optimal training response; rather, they constitute an unwarranted health hazard.

A final precaution is indicated. Immersion bradycardia is largely an effect of water temperature rather than a hydrostatic effect per se. In thermoneutral water (35–35.5°C) cardiovascular responses are similar in air or water (6). At lower temperatures an increased central blood volume, reduced HR, and augmented SV are largely attributable to a cold-induced increase in peripheral and cutaneous vasoconstriction. However, the relationship is not necessarily linear (6). A prediction response is therefore unreliable and underlines the need to identify the decrease in HR with a specific water temperature.

For practical reasons, it is recommended that pool temperatures be regulated, if possible, slightly above 28°C. Most subjects, although adequately insulated by virtue of being overweight, experienced a decrease of 0.4–0.5°C in body temperature during the 31–39 minute experimental period. Despite being in the water about 40 to 50 percent of the time, complaints of cold sensations became increasingly frequent after 20–25 minutes. Slightly warmer water temperatures would still provide for a cardiovascular training response, and lessened cold sensations would encourage regular attendance.

SUMMARY

Metabolic costs of water support exercises were measured in 11 elderly subjects at a preferred constant walking rate in thigh, waist, and chest water levels. Oxygen uptakes ranged between 68 and 75 percent $\dot{V}O_2$max, while HRs averaged $\sim$ 20 beats/minute lower than HRs at comparable $\dot{V}O_2$ demands during treadmill walking. These voluntarily selected exercise intensities in the water are sufficient to promote a training response with less cardiovascular stress than similar training intensities on dry land. However, to avoid unduly taxing individuals in the water it is necessary to modify the HR training intensity guideline from land to water according to the degree of bradycardia experienced in the water. It is recommended that ambient and pool temperatures be maintained slightly above 28°C for thermal comfort. With these factors considered, partial immersion upright exercise involving dynamic big muscle activities are highly recommended for safely stimulating increased activity levels in the elderly.

REFERENCES

1. Astrand, P.O. and Rodahl, K.: Circulation. In *Textbook of Work Physiology,* 2nd ed. New York, McGraw-Hill, pp 154, 1970.
2. Balke, B. and Ware, R.W.: An experimental study of physical fitness of Air Force personnel. *US Armed Forces Med J, 10*:675, 1959.
3. Barry, A.J.; Daly, J.W.; Pruett, E.; Steinmetz, J.R.; Birkhead, N.C.; and Rodahl, K.: The effects of physical conditioning on older individuals. I. work capacity, circulatory-respiratory function and work electrocardiogram. *J Gerontol, 21*:182, 1966.
4. Craig, A.B. and Dvorak, M.: Comparison of exercise in water of different temperatures. *Med Sci Sports, 1(3)*:124, 1979.
5. deVries, H.A.: Physiological effects of an exercise training regimen upon men 52 to 88. *J Gerontol, 25*:325, 1970.
6. McArdle, W.; Magel, J.; Lesmes, G.R.; and Pechar, G.S.: Metabolic and cardiovascular adjustments to work in air and water at 18, 25, and 33°C. *J Appl Physiol, 40*:85, 1976.
7. Pollock, M.; Miller, H.S., Jr.; Linnerund, A.C.; and Casper, K.H.: Frequency of training as a determinant of cardiovascular function and body composition of middle-aged men. *Arch Phys Med Rehabil, 56*:141, 1975.

8. Pollock, M.; Ward, A.; and Ayres, J.: Cardiorespiratory fitness: response to differing intensities and durations of training. *Arch Phys Med Rehabil, 58*:467, 1977.

9. Rennie, D.W.; DiPrampero, P.; and Cerretelli, P.: Effects of water immersion on cardiac output, and stroke volume of man at rest and during exercise. *Med Dello Sport, 24*:223, 1971.

10. Wilmore, J.H.: Exercise prescription: Role of the physiatrist and allied health professionals. *Arch Phys Med Rehabil, 57*:315, 1976.

Chapter 18

THE NATIONAL EXERCISE AND HEART DISEASE PROJECT*

THE NATIONAL Exercise and Heart Disease Project (NEHDP) is a 5 center clinical trial sponsored by the Rehabilitation Services Administration (now the National Institute for Handicapped Research of the Department of Education), of the Department of Health, Education and Welfare, to determine the effects of medically prescribed, regularly performed physical activity on selected outcomes of cardiac rehabilitation. The project was funded initially in June, 1972, with the prospect that it would be a definitive clinical trial in which up to 4300 myocardial infarction subjects would be studied in a randomized manner for as few as 5 and as many as 7 years. However, funding limitations and a major agency policy change made in June, 1973, mandated a study of much smaller scale. The project investigators recognized from the outset that the crucial question of the effect of exercise on mortality and morbidity probably could not be answered by the trial, but that other important questions concerning exercise testing, the rehabilition process, and the effects of physical activity on selected physiological, psychosocial, and vocational outcomes could be determined. Therefore, the investigators agreed to pursue a more limited 5 center† trial. The work was coordinated with the Biostatistical Center located in Bethesda, Maryland and the Electrocardiographic Center in Washington, D.C.

Prepared for the Project Staff by John Naughton.
*Presented to the workshop on Physical Conditioning and Cardiac Rehabilitation sponsored by the National Heart, Lung and Blood Institute, Bethesda, Maryland, May 15-16, 1979.
†University of Alabama, Birmingham, Alabama; Case-Western Reserve University, Cleveland, Ohio; Emory University, Atlanta, Georgia; George Washington University, Washington, D.C.; Lankenau Hospital, Philadelphia, Pennsylvania. Coordinating Centers: George Washington University, Washington, D.C. and SUNY-Buffalo, Buffalo, New York.

PROJECT DESIGN

FIRST EVALUATION: The project was designed as a randomized trial in which male survivors of one or more myocardial infarctions were referred to each collaborating center for an initial evaluation (E_1). This evaluation included a complete history and physical examination, standard chest x ray, 12-lead plus Frank X, Y, and Z lead ECG recorded at supine rest, measurement of plasma cholesterol and triglyceride levels, pulmonary function testing, and completion of a number of psychosocial questionnaires including the Minnesota Multiphasic Personality Inventory (MMPI). Plasma HDL was measured on subjects from 2 of the centers. The spouses completed the Katz Adjustment Scale (KAS). Each subject performed a standardized, multistage exercise test (MSET) on a motor-driven treadmill.

PREP: Subjects who satisfactorily completed E_1 were admitted to a 6 week prerandomization exercise program (PREP) in which each subject was required to attend 14 of 18 consecutively scheduled sessions within a period of 6 weeks before proceeding to the second evaluation (E_2). A total of 12 weeks was allowed for the completion of this requirement. PREP was designed as a program in which patients would become familiar with the activity requirements of the randomized treatment phase of the project, patients could decide on their commitment to the study, and adherence would be promoted. It was thought desirable from the outset that such a program would permit subjects to drop out early without damaging the randomization process; the likelihood of drop-out during the actual trial would be reduced. Since the investigators did not wish to dilute the effects of therapy, PREP was conducted as a low-level, nonconditioning program in which subjects peak activity heart rates were not permitted to exceed 85 percent of the peak heart rate level reached at the first MSET. For those subjects who reached 85 percent APHR (age predicted heart rate), this meant that the PREP exercise heart rate could not exceed 72 percent APHR. In other words, the lower the activity heart rate during PREP, the better.

PREP sessions were conducted 3 times a week. Subjects exercised on 6 different machines: arm-wheel, hand crank, rowing machine, treadmill, bicycle ergometer, and steps. Each subject performed at each station for 4 minutes. Heart rate level was controlled with a cardiotachometer to which the patient was attached via hard-wire cable. Each activity was interspersed by 2 minutes of rest.

SECOND EVALUATION: A second evaluation (E_2) was completed at the completion of PREP. This evaluation was comparable to E_1 with the exception that during the second exercise test, subjects were permitted to work to the 100 percent age-predicted heart rate level (APHRL) in the absence of symptoms or abnormal signs instead of being arbitrarily terminated at 85 percent APHR, as was the situation for E_1.

RANDOMIZATION: The subjects were randomly assigned to either an exercise treatment group (ETG) or to a nontreatment group (NTG) by the Biostatistical Center. Of the 931 subjects initially referred for study, 651 completed the requirements of E_1, PREP, and E_2, and of these 323 were assigned to ETG and 328 to NTG.

Once assigned, subjects were considered members of that group until the completion of the project regardless of whether they adhered to the treatment assignment, had surgery, or dropped-out.

POSTRANDOMIZATION PROGRAM: Subjects assigned to ETG were given an updated physical activity prescription at each evaluation. For the first 8 weeks postrandomization (Post-R), they met in the same facilities used for PREP and the activity was conducted in the same manner except that all subjects were permitted to work to 85 percent of the peak heart rate measured at the second MSET. All subjects were reevaluated 8 weeks post-R, and subsequently, at 6 month intervals post-R until the completion of the trial.

The ETG subjects were entered into a gymnasium program after the first post-R evaluation. This program also met 3 times a week, but the format included games, walking-jogging, calisthenics, and swimming. It was supervised by project staff, but no attempt was made to monitor the exercising heart rates with the precision and accuracy employed during PREP and the first 8 week period post-R.

The NTG subjects were treated as controls. Project staff were advised not to counsel the NTG subjects about physical activity nor to encourage an activity not considered a part of their daily routine. These subjects were reevaluated on the same schedule as the ETG subjects.

DURATION OF FOLLOW-UP: All subjects were followed for at least 2.5 years, and 70 percent were followed for 3 years.

SUBJECT CHARACTERISTICS

The subjects ranged from age 30 to 64 years with a mean of 51.8 years. Six percent were under age 40, 78 percent from 40 to 59, and 16 percent were 60 to 64.

All subjects were men. Seventeen percent had sustained more than one myocardial infarction (MI). Forty-seven percent earned $20,000 or more dollars per year. Ninety-four percent were white. Twenty percent entered NEHDP from 2 to 6 months post-MI, 37 percent from 7 to 12 months, and 43 percent from 13 to 36 months postevent.

The mean measurements and standard deviations for the 651 subjects were determined for several categories: height, 179.7 ± 0.4 cm; weight, 79.4 ± 0.4 kg; body fat, 20.6 ± 0.6 percent; plasma cholesterol, 221 ± 1.6 mg/dl; plasma triglycerides, 185.9 ± 7.8 mg/dl; total forced expiratory ventilation, 3.7 ± 0.8 l; and timed forced expiratory ventilation, 2.9 ± 0.6 l (78%).

SELECTED OBSERVATIONS

The NEHDP completed the clinical trial on May 31, 1979. The data analysis period will consume the major portion of a project year, and a final report together with appropriate publications will be submitted on behalf of the project staff and the subjects who contributed so much of their time and talent. Therefore, for this report only selected observations are available. Among them are observations that relate to the desirability of an 85 percent versus a 100 percent APHR limited exercise test; the effects of 6 weeks of low level physical activity on performance capacity; the prognostic value of an exercise test; and the effects of long-term training on performance capacity.

Observations of an 85 Percent Heart Rate Limited Exercise Test and of a 100 Percent Limited Procedure

The 651 subjects performed two MSETs approximately 7 weeks apart. The procedures were identical with the exception that the first was terminated at 85 percent APHR in the absence of abnormal symptoms or signs and the second at 100 percent APHR. The investigators selected this methodology at the first MSET because of the uncertainty of how many early recovery patients would be referred for study and because they desired to insure patient safety. In addition, they were concerned about quality control had the full-scale study been implemented as initially visualized.

One of 8 stopping codes was used to terminate an MSET: symptoms, physical signs, ischemic ST-T changes in the ECG, ventricular arrhythmias, systolic blood pressure in excess of 225 mmHg, diastolic blood pressure increase of 20 mmHg or more above rest, and a subjective sense that the subject could proceed no further.

The findings from the two MSETs quite clearly established the 100 percent APHR procedure as the preferred approach. At the first MSET, 54 percent of the 651 subjects reached the 85 percent APHR in the absence of overt cardiovascular abnormality. At the second MSET, only 15 percent of the subjects reached 100 percent APHR. Thus, the 100 percent APHR precipitated or aggravated more overt cardiovascular limitation, and at the same time, provided an improved determinant of the actual level of aerobic work capacity. Since both procedures were performed without precipitating a major cardiovascular event, both were judged as safe.

Since exercise testing has not been applied to such a large population sample in a consistently rigorous manner among a group of collaborating centers, the data provided meaningful standards concerning levels of aerobic work capacity among patients. At the 100 percent MSET, the mean aerobic work capacity was 7.9 METs. There was a relationship of work capacity to end points observed; subjects capable of reaching the higher heart rate levels had a mean work capacity of 9.5 METs compared to a capacity of 7.6 METs for symptom-limited subjects and 7.2 METs for the sign-limited subjects. Although the latter 2 values do not differ significantly, the sign-limited subjects were consistently lower in performance capacity across all ages.

The second MSET provided valuable physiological observations concerning the adaptation of systolic blood pressure and heart rate to graded levels of exercise. These parameters were evaluated in relation to level of work capacity attained, reasons for stopping MSET, and age. For purposes of these analyses, the end points were grouped into 3 classifications as follows: symptom-limited (overt symptoms, a subjective sense that subject could proceed no further), sign-limited (ECG changes, physical signs, blood pressure abnormality), and heart rate-limited (100% APHR reached in the absence of symptoms or signs).

The findings indicated a close correlation between level of work capacity achieved and level of peak heart rate reached. In other words, the lower the aerobic threshold, the lower the mean peak heart rate response. This relationship was confirmed by the finding of lower peak heart rates among the symptom-limited and sign-limited subjects and higher mean peak heart rates among the subjects who reached the high APHR levels. As expected, in part because of the employment of the 100 percent APHR criteria, the mean peak heart rate decreased with age. On the other hand, mean peak systolic blood pressure was not related to these variables in the same way. Mean peak systolic pressure did not differ significantly according to reason for stopping MSET or by virtue of age. Only for the subjects with significantly reduced aerobic thresholds (i.e. ≤ 6 METs) was the mean peak value significantly lower than for the other variables.

The above findings suggest that of the two variables, heart rate is the principal determinant used for meeting the myocardial oxygen requirements of exercise in MI subjects. Thus, changes in double product (SBP × HR × 10^{-2}) among these variables reflect mainly the contribution of heart rate and not of SBP.

The Effects of PREP

The findings at the second MSET were confounded by the slight change in protocol; therefore, a special analysis was required to discern the relative contribution of protocol change and of the low level physical conditioning program to the differences in aerobic threshold measured at the second procedure.

A major part of the analysis was accomplished by determining the changes in heart rate and systolic blood pressure at that workload at the first procedure at which the highest heart rate was measured for each subject. Using this approach the findings indicated that at the second MSET the subjects attained mean aerobic threshold due to conditioning 0.57 ± .04 METs higher, that the mean peak heart rate decreased 9.2 bpm, and that the mean peak systolic blood pressure decreased 7.4 mmHg. The absolute mean difference in work capacity between the two protocols was 1.6 METs. The mean difference ascribed to the methodological change approximated 1.0 MET and to physical conditioning approximated, 0.57 METs.

These findings indicated clearly that as few as 14 exercise sessions, even though of a low degree of intensity, were sufficient to produce a significant cardiovascular training effect.

Prognostic Value of Exercise Testing

The results recorded at the 100 percent APHR were evaluated to determine if subsequent mortality and morbidity have any relationship to selected outcomes. A total of 39 deaths and 40 recurrent MIs were documented for the 36 months following this exercise test. The relationship of mortality and morbidity to level of aerobic capacity, peak systolic blood pressure, peak heart rate, and ST-T segment depression on the Frank lead X were determined.

The findings indicated a significant relationship of mortality to all 4 variables, with the highest relationship being to level of aerobic capacity and peak systolic blood pressure. Subjects with an aerobic threshold of 6 METs or less had 4.5 times the mortality rate experienced by subjects with aerobic capacity levels of 7 METs or more. The event rate for subjects with peak systolic blood pressures of 140 mmHg or less was 3 times that of subjects who exceeded 140 mmHg. Subjects who did not exceed 85 percent APHR had twice the mortality experience of those who exceeded the 85 percent APHR level; subjects who had 1.0 mm (0.1MV) or more ST-T depression on lead X with exercise had 2.5 times the mortality experience of those who did not. Morbidity bore no relationship to any of these variables.

Since some investigators have emphasized the importance of a low peak heart rate response to exercise, the data were analyzed in terms of high (> 7 METs) and low (≤ 6 METs) work capacity levels and by degree of peak heart rate achieved, i.e. < 85% or ≥ 85% APHR. The findings indicated no significant relationship of level of mean peak heart rate reached to mortality, a finding that suggests aerobic capacity and not level of peak heart rate is the important determinant of future fatal events. Thus, the concept of chronotropic incompetence, the inability to achieve a high heart rate response, obviously deserves more critical physiological and clinical appraisal.

On the other hand, the relationship of a low peak systolic blood pressure to subsequent mortality was of almost equal importance to level of aerobic capacity. These findings suggest that this group of subjects have probably lost the greatest amount of myocardial integrity and thus were not able to increase their cardiac outputs commensurate with the level of external work imposed during the testing.

The above findings do not invalidate the concept that cardiac subjects as a group cannot attain the same peak heart rate thresholds observed in presumably healthy subjects. Rather, they confirm the finding of other investigators and lend credance to the concept of "heart rate impairment" (HRI). For those 555 subjects incapable of reaching 100 percent APHR, the mean degree of HRI was 17.5 percent, while for subjects of 6 METs or less it was 24.7 percent and for subjects of 7 METs or more 13.9 percent. The data were analyzed by age and it was determined unequivocally that HRI related to the level of aerobic capacity achieved and not to age.

The Effects of Long-Term Training

The postrandomization MSETs were used to determine the changes in the ETG and NTG subjects. At randomization, ETG had a mean aerobic capacity of 7.8 METs and for NTG of 8.0 METs. Eight weeks later the ETG subjects had experienced a significant increase to 8.6 METs while the NTG subjects remained essentially unchanged.

From 6 months to 1 year post-R, the ETG subjects experienced only an additional modest increase in aerobic capacity while the NTG subjects decremented slightly. From 1 year post-R to the completion of the trial, both groups decremented with ETG experiencing a more dramatic change than NTG from 18 to 24 months post-R.

These findings indicate that the trial was effective in inducing a physiological training effect but that it was not sustained throughout the course of the trial. These data are being evaluated to determine if factors such as compliance and adherence have a relationship, or if factors of selection for training (sick subjects, no; well subjects, yes) explain the difference.

SUMMARY AND CONCLUSIONS

The NEHDP is a 5 center clinical trial designed to determine the effects of medically prescribed, regularly performed physical activity on selected outcomes of the cardiac rehabilitation process. In many respects it is a feasibility trial that will provide meaningful data and experiences should a larger scale, definitive trial of exercise and heart disease be necessary. In size and scope it is comparable to the trials reported by Sanne in Sweden and investigators in Ontario. In contrast to those trials it has attempted to deal more specifically with a range of rehabilitation issues including the value of the stress test, exercise testing methodology, and physiological, psychosocial and vocational outcomes.

To date the investigators have established the feasibility of conducting such a trial. The cooperation of the subjects has been good and each collaborating center staff has worked intact throughout the course of the trial. The findings have provided new insights into testing methodology, the prognostic value of an exercise test, the physiological adaptation to low-level and high-level physical conditioning and to the long-term training process. The definitive results in mortality and morbidity will be available in mid-1980.

REFERENCES

1. Naughton, J. et al. (for the Project Staff): The National Exercise and Heart Disease Project: Development, recruitment, and implementation. *Cardiovascular Clinics, 9*:205-222, 1978.
2. Naughton, J. et al. (for the Project Staff): The National Exercise and Heart Disease Project: The pre-randomization exercise program. Report No. 2. *Cardiology, 63*:352-367, 1978.
3. Naughton, J. (for the Project Staff): The National Exercise and Heart Disease Project. In *Heart Disease and Rehabilitation,* edited by Michael L. Pollock and Donald H. Schmidt, pp. 330-340, 1979.
4. The Project Staff: *Adaptations to Sub-Maximal and Near-Maximal Multiple Stage Exercise Tests* (In Preparation).
5. The Project Staff: *The Physiological Effects of a Low-Level Physical Activity Program of Six Weeks Duration* (In Preparation).
6. The Project Staff: *Predictors of Mortality form a Near-Maximal Exercise Test* (In Preparation).

Chapter 19

INTERPRETATION OF DIAGNOSTIC GRADED EXERCISE TESTS ON THE BASIS OF ELECTROCARDIOGRAPHIC, HEMODYNAMIC, AND SYMPTOMATIC RESPONSES

G.H. PORTER AND T.J. ALLEN

DESPITE SOME limitations, graded exercise testing (GXT) has become a well-established and valuable tool that can have several applications in evaluating the functional capacity of the cardiovascular system in health and disease (18). One of the important uses of GXT in the clinical setting is to assist in the evaluation of the presence or absence of significant coronary artery disease (CAD). This diagnostic utilization of GXT is predominantly a qualitative approach to CAD detection through indentification of an ischemic myocardial response from the exercise test responses of a patient (19). Transient upward or downward deviation of the ST segment of the electrocardiogram (ECG), specifically during or following exercise, has been the traditional crite rion for evaluating the presence of myocardial ischemia. However, the diagnostic usefulness of exercise electrocardiography has been challenged by Borer et al. (2). The challenge was made because false negative responses are frequent in patients with documented CAD and false positive responses are frequent in asymptomatic patients. The occurrence of these false responses has stimulated efforts to examine other aspects of the exercise responses in addition to the presence or absence of exercise-induced ST segment displacement, in an attempt to increase the diagnostic utility of the graded exercise test (14, 15).

We gratefully acknowledge the contribution of cardiologists A. Brailey, M.D., J. Edgett, M.D., R. Evans, M.D. and R. Green, M.D., who supervised the exercise tests and/or performed coronary angiography.

The current "gold-standard" diagnostic test for the evaluation of CAD is the coronary angiogram. The diagnostic interpretation of the graded exercise test responses has been compared to the results of the coronary angiogram in a Latin square fashion (Table 19-I). From this Latin square diagram the definitions for sensitivity, specificity, and predictive value of positive and negative graded exercise tests can be derived. These measures of test accuracy can be influenced by several known factors that include (1) screening criteria, (2) test population, and (3) method of GXT.

Recently, interest has been generated in trying to predict the severity of CAD or trying to quantitate the degree of disease present from the responses to a graded exercise test (5). This approach assumes that the severity of CAD is the major determinant of the severity of myocardial ischemia, and the myocardial ischemia is in turn reflected in the exercise responses of the patient. The variables that appear to be most useful in predicting the severity of CAD may be grouped into electrocardiographic, hemodynamic, and symptomatic responses (7). The electrocardiographic responses include magnitude, duration, configuration, and time of onset of ST segment depression, ST elevation, and significant exercise-induced arrhythmias. The hemodynamic responses include the appropriateness of the systolic blood pressure and heart rate responses. Chest pain is the major symptomatic response.

TABLE 19-I

LATIN SQUARE TABULATION ILLUSTRATING DERIVATION OF
SENSITIVITY, SPECIFICITY, AND PREDICTIVE VALUE

Exercise Test	Cineangiogram			
	Disease	No Disease		
Positive	True Positives (a)	False Positives (c)	a + c	Predictive Value (+) $\frac{a}{a + c}$
Negative	False Negatives (b)	True Negatives (d)	b + d	Predictive Value (−) $\frac{d}{b + d}$
	a + b Sensitivity $\frac{a}{a + b}$	c + d Specificity $\frac{d}{c + d}$		

In an attempt to improve upon the diagnostic usefulness of GXT in predicting the presence and severity of CAD, the traditional ST segment criterion has been supplemented by incorporating the other electrocardiographic, hemodynamic, and symptomatic variables mentioned above. These different variables have been brought together in a quantitative manner by computing a treadmill score for each patient based on his or her responses to a standard diagnostic graded exercise (DGXT) protocol. A recent investigation by Cohn et al. (5) reported on this type of approach. The previous investigation used discriminant function analysis to determine the treadmill score (TMS) formula. The present study has attempted to devise a TMS formula by empirically assigning numerical point values to the responses found to be significantly related to CAD in the present test population.

METHODS

Eighty-five consecutive patients (65 males and 20 females, mean age 53.8 yrs, range 33 to 72 yrs) who presented to Gundersen Clinic, Ltd., La Crosse, Wisconsin, were subjects for this investigation. The patients were evaluated with both a DGXT and subsequent (3 months or less after the DGXT) selective coronary angiography. None of the patients were previously known to have documented CAD. The patients did not stop taking medications, if previously prescribed, before performing the DGXT. Patients with complete bundle branch block on the ECG were excluded from the study.

The DGXT utilized was a Sheffield modification of the standard Bruce protocol. The modification included a beginning stage of 1.5 mph at a 5 percent grade for 3 minutes duration. The standard Bruce procedure was followed thereafter. The DGXT was terminated upon the presence of significant symptoms, signs, or the attainment of 90 to 100 percent of the patient's age-predicted maximal heart rate. The preexercise protocol included recording at rest a supine, standing, and posthyperventilation 12-lead ECG. All ECGs recorded during exercise were recordings using the Mason-Likar modification of the standard ECG lead placements. Arm-cuff blood pressures were recorded during the first and third minutes of each stage of the DGXT. Blood pressures and ECGs were recorded at 2 minute intervals for at least 6 minutes during a recovery period. Any symptomatic responses of the patients were recorded.

Coronary angiograms were made using the standard Judkins technique with the catheters being inserted by use of a Seldinger percutaneous method. All coronary vessels were visualized in at least 2 planes, which were at right angles to each other. The angiograms were interpreted by the cardiologist who performed the angiography, and a team of 3 or 4 cardiologists later reviewed the angiograms to determine if the patient had significant CAD. Vessel narrowing of the luminal diameter of ≥ 50 percent was considered obstructive and indicated the presence of significant CAD.

The minimum criterion for having a positive DGXT was defined as one showing 1 mm ST segment elevation or depression for a period of .08 second after the end of the QRS complex anytime during exercise or recovery. A negative DGXT was one in which the ST segment displacement did not meet the minimum requirement defined above. The graded exercise tests were then classified as true positive (TP), false negative (FN), false positive (FP), or true negative (TN) on comparison with the angiographic findings. Sensitivity, specificity, predictive value of a positive test, and predictive value of a negative test were calculated as illustrated in Table 19-I. In addition, the correct classification rate, the ratio of TP + TN/number of patients, was also determined.

Patients with CAD were grouped into the following exclusive (separate, not overlapping) categories: (1) single vessel disease, (2) moderate to severe disease, or (3) advanced disease. Single vessel disease involved any one coronary artery (excluding the left main coronary artery) with a stenosis of ≥ 50 percent. Moderate to severe disease consisted of (1) ≥ 50 percent stenosis in 2 of the 3 major (right, circumflex, or left anterior descending) coronary arteries (left main excluded), (2) the left main coronary artery with ≥ 50 percent stenosis, or (3) triple vessel disease, provided the left main had < 50 percent stenosis and the left anterior descending had < 90 percent stenosis. Advanced disease consisted of either (1) ≥ 90 percent stenosis of the left main along with an obstructed right coronary or (2) triple vessel disease with ≥ 50 percent stenosis of the left main and/or ≥ 90 percent stenosis of the left anterior descending artery. An additional subgrouping included those patients with ≥ 50 percent stenosis of the left main, regardless of the disease in other coronary arteries.

In an attempt to bring together the different variables from the DGXT, a quantitative scale for computing a treadmill score (TMS) was developed. The electrocardiographic, hemodynamic, and symptomatic exercise responses were examined independently, and empirically a point value from 1 to 6 was assigned to those responses that appeared most useful in predicting the presence and severity of CAD. Subsequently, a single TMS was calculated for each patient's DGXT. Theoretically, the larger the TMS, the greater the probability of the presence and severity of CAD. Inspection of the derived treadmill scores for the patients with and without CAD resulted in the decision to call any TMS ≥ 5 units as positive for CAD. A TMS ≤ 4 units was called negative for CAD.

The positive and negative DGXTs based on the TMS method were than classified as TP, FN, FP, or TN. Sensitivity, specificity, predictive value of a positive test, predictive value of a negative test, and correct classification rate were calculated. The mean TMS for each of the following subgroups was calculated: (1) no CAD, (2) any/all CAD, (3) single vessel CAD, (4) moderate to severe CAD, (5) advanced CAD, and (6) left main CAD.

Statistical analyses utilized to compare the usefulness of the TMS method to the traditional ECG method of predicting presence and severity of CAD included (1) chi-square analysis, (2) a one-tail test for differences between proportions, and (3) non-paired
student's *t*-tests. The .05 level of significance was used to reject all null hypotheses.

RESULTS AND DISCUSSION

Coronary angiography revealed that 61 of the 85 patients (72%) had ≥ 50 percent stenosis of at least 1 coronary artery. Sixteen patients (19%) had single vessel CAD, 26 (31%) had moderate to severe CAD, and 19 (22%) had advanced CAD as defined in the present study. Thirteen (15%) had a significant obstruction of the left main coronary artery. The prevalence of CAD found in the population in the present study was the same as that reported by Cohn et al. (5) who have published the only other study that has attempted to develop a treadmill score to predict presence and severity of CAD.

Several variables were numerically quantified based on their ability to distinguish those patients with CAD from those without

CAD. Initially those patients with angiographic documented CAD were examined to determine which, if any, abnormal exercise-induced responses separated TP from FP responses. The abnormal responses were empirically assigned a numerical value in an attempt to reclassify a FN as a TP test. This approach was also taken in an attempt to separate FP from TN tests. The variables included were symptoms (chest pain), systolic blood pressure responses, as well as the resting and exercise characteristics of the ECG. The method devised to calculate the treadmill score (TMS) is shown in Table 19-II. The rationale for including each of the specific variables in the calculation will be explained in the following discussion.

Exercise-induced chest pain has been documented to indicate a poorer prognosis and an increased probability of having CAD (3, 6, 17). The onset of chest pain during the DGXT was reported by 6 of the patients classified as having a FN test (based on the ST segment only). Figure 19-1 indicates that a greater percentage of those patients with CAD reported chest pain during the DGXT (p < .01). In addition, there was a tendency for the percentage of symptomatic responses to increase with the severity of CAD. All patients with left main CAD reported chest pain during the DGXT. Thus, those patients with CAD constitute a greater percentage of the patients with chest pain symptoms, and in patients with severe CAD the chest pain usually presents itself at a lower

TABLE 19-II
CALCULATION OF THE TREADMILL SCORE*

ST Segment	Systolic Blood Pressure
0 = normal	0 = normal increase with exercise
1 = 1-1.9 mm after 4 METS	3 = flattened or plateaued
3 = 1-1.9 mm before 4 METS	5 = drop ($\geq$ 10 mmHg)
4 = $\geq$ 2 mm after 4 METS	
5 = 1-1.9 mm before 4 METS,	
$\geq$ 2 mm after 4 METS	Premature Ventricular Contractions
6 = $\geq$ 2 mm before 4 METS	0 = none
	1 = occasional
ST Segment Configuration	3 = significant ($\geq$ 8 per minute,
1 = horizontal or upsloping	bigeminy, trigeminy)
3 = downsloping	
Chest Pain	Resting Electrocardiogram
0 = no pain	0 = normal
2 = chest pain after 4 METS	2 = inverted T waves
5 = chest pain on or before 4 METS	

*Numbers shown are the point values given for each response within a category.
Treadmill score equals the sum of the point values given for each of the six categories.

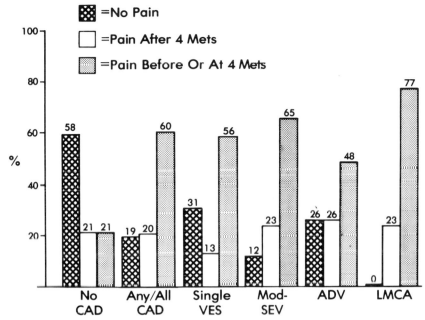

Figure 19-1. Relationship between the time of onset of chest pain and the severity of coronary artery disease. The number at the top of the bar is the calculated percentage of patients in each subgrouping. CAD = coronary artery disease; Single Ves = single vessel disease; Mod-Sev = moderate to severe disease; Adv = advanced disease; LMCA = left main disease.

MET level. It should be noted, however, that 42 percent of the patients without CAD subjectively reported "chest discomfort" during the exercise test.

The type of systolic blood pressure (SBP) response to exercise significantly ($p < .02$) distinguished between those patients with and without CAD (Fig. 19-2). There was approximately a fourfold increase in the percentage of flattened or hypotensive SBP responses in those patients with CAD. Ten of 12 (83%) patients with exercise-induced hypotension (≥ 10 mmHg decrease in SBP) had CAD. Seventeen of 18 (94%) patients having a flattened SBP response to exercise (< 10 mmHg increase and < 10 mmHg decrease in SBP over the last 3 readings) had documented CAD. It can be observed (Fig. 19-2) that there was a tendency for those patients eliciting a flattened or hypotensive SBP response to have advanced or left main CAD. The present findings are in general agreement with previously reported results (11, 13, 16).

Exercise in Health and Disease

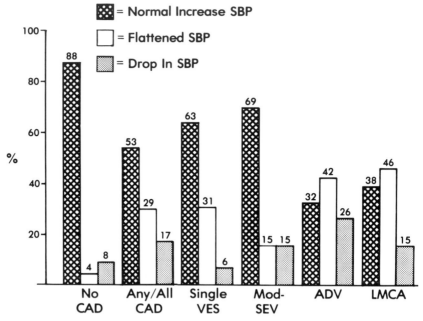

Figure 19-2. Relationship between the type of systolic blood pressure response to graded exercise testing and the severity of coronary artery disease. The number at the top of the bar is the calculated percentage of patients in each subgrouping. CAD = coronary artery disease; Single Ves = single vessel disease; Mod-Sev = moderate to severe disease; Adv = advanced disease; LMCA = left main disease.

As had been hypothesized (4, 9, 10, 12), the ECG provided the most significant information regarding the presence and severity of CAD. Specifically, ST segment displacement, configuration, and time of onset of ST segment displacement, exercise-induced ventricular arrhythmias, and resting inverted T waves were studied. The magnitude and configuration of ST segment displacement significantly ($p < .01$) differentiated between the CAD and non-CAD groups. Eleven of the patients (85%) with significant left main CAD had ≥ 2 mm ST segment depression before or equal to the 4 MET exercise level. ST segment configuration was also useful in correctly differentiating a positive from a negative DGXT (Fig. 19-3). Of the 44 patients with horizontal or upsloping ST segment depression, 34 (77%) had documented CAD. In contrast, 58 percent without CAD had no ST segment depression, and none of the patients without CAD had downsloping ST segment depression during the DGXT. Figure 19-3 illustrates an inverse relationship between severity of disease and the percent of patients without ST segment depression. The FP rate was 23 percent for the horizontal and upsloping ST configurations combined and 0 percent for the downsloping configuration. Goldschlager et al. (10) have reported a FP rate of 47 percent and 1 percent for the horizontal upsloping and downsloping configurations respectively.

The frequency of exercise-induced premature ventricular contractions (PVCs) has been shown to separate patients with and without CAD (5). The present findings indicated that 15 percent of those patients with CAD had frequent PVCs (≥ 8 per minute, bigeminy, trigeminy) as opposed to only 4 percent of the patients without CAD. The absence of PVCs was observed in 79 percent of those patients with CAD and 83 percent of those patients without CAD. Resting inverted T waves on the ECG have also been shown

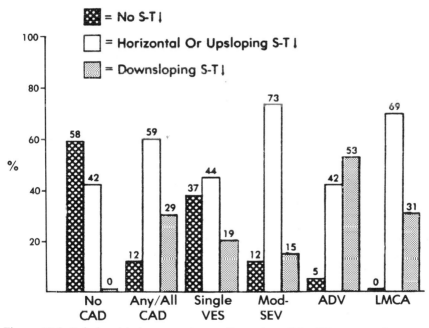

Figure 19-3. Relationship between the configuration of the ST segment depression and the severity of coronary artery disease. The number at the top of the bar is the calculated percentage of patients in each subgrouping. CAD = coronary artery disease; Single Ves = single vessel disease; Mod-Sev = moderate to severe disease; Adv = advanced disease; LMCA = left main disease.

to be useful in predicting the presence of CAD (8). In the present study, inverted T waves at rest were found in 15 percent of the patients with CAD and in 8 percent of the patients without CAD.

Other hemodynamic variables such as the maximal heart rate and rate pressure product were not included in the present study because of the fact that several patients (26 of 85) were taking beta-adrenergic blocking medication at the time of the DGXT. Although including attained maximal heart rate and rate pressure product has been shown to increase test sensitivity (1), the presence of CAD in the present study was not disguised by medications taken by the patients. This was indicated by the fact that no FN test was found in a patient who had been taking medications prior to the DGXT.

The independent examination of each of the variables discussed above resulted in the empirical assignment of a point value from 1 to 6 to each of the components of a given variable. This resulted in the development of a quantitative method (Table 19-II) that could be used to assign a TMS to each patient's DGXT. The developed method allowed for a possible range of scores from 0 to 24 units. Inspection and comparison of the TMSs for those patients with and without CAD resulted in the empirical decision to interpret a DGXT with a TMS $\leq$ 4 units as negative for CAD. A TMS of $\geq$ 5 units was interpreted to be positive for CAD.

The TMS method of interpreting the DGXT for the presence of CAD resulted in 18 negative and 67 positive tests. Fifty-eight of the 67 positive tests were TP. Figure 19-4 illustrates the complete breakdown of the study group into TP, FN, FP, and TN exercise tests. The percentage of patients in each subcategory, expressed as a percentage of the number of patients in the previous category, is also indicated. All 3 of the FN tests were patients with single vessel CAD. Nine patients were found to have FP exercise tests.

Based on the diagnostic interpretation of the ECG response (ST segment) alone, sensitivity, specificity and correct classification rate were 84, 58, and 76 percent, respectively. The predictive value of a positive and negative DGXT was 84 and 58 percent, respectively (Fig. 19-5). Following reinterpretation and reclassification of the DGXTs (on the basis of the TMS method), sensitivity, specificity, and correct classification rate increased to 95, 63, and 86 percent, respectively. The predictive value of a positive and negative DGXT was increased to 87 and 83 percent, respectively

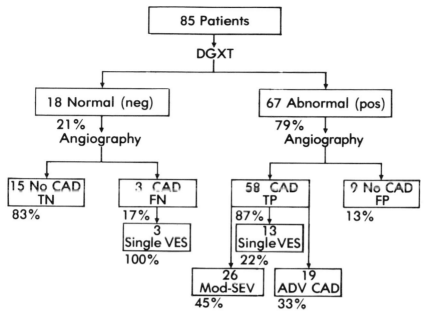

Figure 19-4. The study group, illustrating the separation of patients on the basis of the treadmill score and angiography. Comparison of the treadmill interpretation and the angiographic interpretation results in the classification of the patients as true negative, false negative, true positive, or false positive. Those with coronary artery disease are grouped into single vessel disease, moderate to severe disease, and advanced disease. Percentages are the number of patients in a given category divided by the number of patients in the previous category. DGXT = diagnostic graded exercise test; Neg = negative treadmill test; Pos = positive treadmill test; TN = true negative exercise test; FN = false negative exercise test; FP = false positive exercise test; TP = true positive exercise test; CAD = coronary artery disease; Single Ves = single vessel disease; Mod-Sev = moderate to severe disease; Adv = advanced disease.

(Fig. 19-5). The observed increases were statistically significant for sensitivity ($p < .03$), correct classification rate ($p < .03$), and predictive value of a negative test ($p < .04$). The values found in the present study for sensitivity, specificity, correct classification rate, and predictive value of a positive and negative test, when the TMS method was used, are very similar to the values reported by Cohn et al. (5) who used discriminant function analysis to derive a treadmill score also based on several exercise test responses. The improvement in sensitivity means that the number of FN tests was reduced (10 to 3). Only a small improvement in specificity resulted because the number of FP tests was only reduced from 10 to 9 by

Exercise in Health and Disease

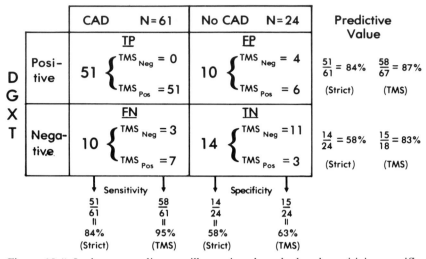

Figure 19-5. Latin square diagram illustrating the calculated sensitivity, specificity, and predictive value when the ST segment criterion is compared to the treadmill score method. The large numerals in the blocks are the number of patients classified on the basis of the ST segment only. The smaller numerals in the blocks are the number of patients classified on the basis of the treadmill score method. TMS = treadmill score; Strict = calculation based on the ST segment only; DGXT = diagnostic graded exercise test; CAD = coronary artery disease; TP = true positive exercise test; FP = false positive exercise test; FN = false negative exercise test; TN = true negative exercise test.

applying the TMS method. The DGXT may be FP for CAD, yet TP for other types of coronary heart disease (19). Upon closer examination of the angiographic data of the 9 FP tests, 2 patients had documented aortic stenosis, 1 had dextrocardia, and 2 had abnormally elevated left ventricular end diastolic pressures. If these 5 FP tests were reclassified as TP for coronary heart disease, then specificity, predictive value of a positive test, and correct classification rate would be improved from 63, 87, and 86 percent to 79, 94, and 91 percent, respectively.

Figure 19-6 illustrates the differences among the TMSs of those patients with and without CAD. The TMS increased with increased severity of CAD. The highest TMS was for the group of patients with left main CAD. The left main patients are known to have the poorest prognosis and survival rate. The mean TMSs

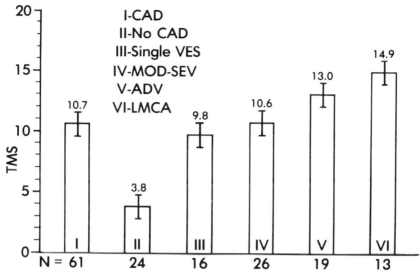

Figure 19-6. Relationship among the calculated mean treadmill scores and the severity of coronary artery disease. The values at the top of the bars are the group means (± SEM). N = number of patients in each category; TMS = the calculated treadmill score value; CAD = coronary artery disease; Single Ves = single vessel disease; Mod-Sev = moderate to severe disease; Adv = advanced disease; LMCA = left main disease.

were significantly different between the groups with (1) CAD and no CAD ($p < .01$), (2) single vessel disease and advanced disease ($p < .02$), (3) single vessel disease and left main disease ($p < .01$), and (4) between moderate to severe disease (excluding those with left main disease) and left main disease ($p < .01$). All other paired mean differences were not statistically significant ($p > .05$).

CLINICAL IMPLICATIONS

Based on the results of this investigation, it would appear that the concept of using the TMS or quantitative approach to interpreting DGXTs enhances the probability of predicting the presence and severity of CAD. The TMS approach supplements the traditional interpretation based only on the ST segment of the ECG and considers additional variables from the exercise test, which have also been shown to predict the presence and severity of CAD. The TMS method appears to significantly reduce the number of FN tests while not increasing the number of tests considered FP for CAD. The quantitative aspects of the TMS approach enables the method to predict the presence of the more severe types of CAD. The higher the TMS, the more likely that the test reflects CAD, and the greater the probability of severe CAD being present.

It should be made quite clear that the TMS calculation developed in this study resulted from empirical judgments and the empirical assignment of point values to various types of exercise-induced responses. In addition, all results are dependent on the (1) population being studied, (2) DGXT protocol utilized, (3) use of medications by the patients, (4) interpretation of the coronary angiograms, and (5) any other methods and procedures that might influence the specific data being collected. The derived score may only be useful in one specific setting. The TMS calculation that was developed from the present data needs to be applied to subsequent DGXTs in this institution for the purpose of cross-validating the results reported in this chapter. Further improvement in the present results might be found if the present data are analyzed with discriminant function analysis. In conclusion, the concept of using a TMS approach seems to have merit, and others are encouraged to apply this type of approach in their diagnostic graded exercise testing.

REFERENCES

1. Berman, J.L.; Wynne, J.; and Cohn, P.F.: A multivariate approach for interpreting treadmill exercise tests in coronary artery disease. *Circulation,* 58:505, 1978.
2. Borer, J.S.; Brensike, J.F.; Redwood, D.R.; Itscoitz, S.B.; Passmani, E.R.; Stone, N.J.; Richardson, J.M.; Levy, R.I.; and Epstein, S.E.: Limitations of the electrocardiographic response to exercise in predicting coronary artery disease. *N Engl J Med, 293*:367, 1975.
3. Chaitman, B.R.; Waters, D.D.; Bourassa, M.G.; Tubau, J.F.; Wagniart, P.; and Ferguson, R.J.: The importance of clinical subsets in interpreting maximal treadmill exercise test results. *Circulation, 59*:560, 1979.
4. Cheitlin, M.D.; Davia, J.E.; de Castro, C.M.; Barrow, E.A.; and Anderson, W.T.: Correlation of critical left coronary artery lesions with positive submaximal exercise tests in patients with chest pain. *Am Heart J, 89*:305, 1975.
5. Cohn, K.; Kamm, B.; and Feteih, N.: Use of treadmill score to quantify ischemic response and predict extent of coronary disease. *Circulation, 59*:286, 1979.
6. Cole, J.P. and Ellestad, M.H.: Correlation of chest pain during treadmill exercise electrocardiography and coronary events. *Circulation, 54 (Suppl 2)*:206, 1976.

7. Cooke, B.M., Jr. and Ellestad, M.H.: Using stress testing to identify the severity of coronary artery disease. *J Cardiovasc Pul Tech, 6(6)*:14, 1979.
8. Ellestad, M.H.: The false positive stress test: Multivariate analysis of 215 subjects. *Circulation, 56 (Suppl 3)*:7, 1977.
9. Goldman, S.; Iselos, S.; and Cohn, K.: Marked depth of ST segment depression during treadmill exercise testing: Indication of severe coronary artery disease. *Chest, 69*:729, 1976.
10. Goldschlager, N.; Selzer, A.; and Cohn, K.: Treadmill stress tests as indicators of presence and severity of coronary artery disease. *Ann Intern Med, 85*:277, 1976.
11. Irving, J.B.; Bruce, R.A.; and DeRoven, T.A.: Variations in and significance of systolic pressure during maximal exercise testing. *Am J Cardiol, 39*:841, 1977.
12. McNeer, J.F.; Margolis, J.R.; Lee, K.L.; Kisslo, J.A.; Peter, R.H.; Kong, Y.; Behar, V.S.; Wallace, A.G.; McCants, C.B.; and Rosanti, R.A.: The role of the exercise test in the evaluation of patients for ischemic heart disease. *Circulation, 57*:64, 1978.
13. Morris, S.N.; Phillips, J.F.; Jordan, J.W.; and McHenry, R.L.: Incidence and significance of decreases in systolic blood pressure during graded treadmill testing. *Am J Cardiol, 41*:221, 1978.
14. Selzer, A.; Cohn, K.; and Goldschlager, N.: On the interpretation of the exercise test. *Circulation, 58*:193, 1978.
15. Sheffield, L.T.; Reeves, T.J.; Blackburn, H.; Ellestad, M.H.; Froclicher, V.F.; Roitman, D.; and Kansal, S.: The exercise test in perspective. *Circulation, 55*:681, 1977.
16. Thomson, P.D. and Keleman, M.H.: Hypotension accompanying the onset of exertional angina. *Circulation, 52*:28, 1975.
17. Weiner, D.A.; McCabe, C.; Hueter, D.; Hood, W.B.; and Ryan, T.: The predictive value of chest pain as an indicator of coronary disease during exercise testing. *Circulation, 54 (Suppl 2)*:10, 1976.
18. Wilson, P.K.: Application for exercise testing in diagnosis; sports medicine; and prevention, intervention and rehabilitation exercise programs. In *Coronary Heart Disease, Exercise Testing and Cardiac Rehabilitation,* edited by W.E. James and E.A. Amsterdam. Miami, Symposia Specialists, 1977.
19. Zohman, L.R. and Kattus, A.A.: Exercise testing in the diagnosis of coronary heart disease. *Am J Cardiol, 40*:243, 1977.

Chapter 20

DROPOUT AND POTENTIAL COMPLIANCE—IMPROVING STRATEGIES IN EXERCISE REHABILITATION*

N.B. OLDRIDGE

DESPITE EXTENSIVE investigation into the clinical, physiological, and psychological effects of regular physical activity in apparently healthy subjects (4, 11) and patients with coronary heart disease (4, 5, 9), few studies on the long-term effects of exercise are available, if long-term is defined as participation for 12 months or more. This may be because investigators perceive the short-term exercise study to be more productive, i.e. more data in a given time, or because they are consciously or unconsciously deterred from launching long-term exercise studies on account of the intuitive concern about the problem of dropout and possibly lower productivity in terms of data generated.

One of the major problems in medicine today is the low compliance or adherence rate, or alternatively the high dropout rate, which is particularly evident in extended treatment regimens and life-style modifications. Adherence and compliance should be considered as being synonymous in this paper. The exercise dropout curve is similar to that observed in other programs or studies involving adoption and adherence with health behavior changes (2, 6, 8). Dropout rates in exercise rehabilitation programs of more than 12 months duration generally follow an exponential curve with the early dropout rate considerably greater than the later dropout (14). Exercise therapy programs for patients with heart disease are both extended and involve life-style modifications. Reports on both adherence rates and the identification of characteristics of dropouts in cardiac rehabilitation exercise

*This work has been partially supported by Grant #PR 263 (Ontario Department of Health) and Grant #6606 (National Health and Research Development Program, Health and Welfare Canada).

programs are largely nonexistent. What information is available has recently been reviewed (14) and gives some insight into the magnitude of the problem as well as some tentative identification of the potential dropout.

Strategies to improve adherence with exercise therapy programs may include those initiated either on entry into a program or at some time during the program. A recent report by Reid and Morgan (17) on the adherence of healthy firefighters to prescribed exercise shows that while health education at the start of the program improved short-term adherence, the long-term situation was not affected by either the health education or by self-monitoring techniques during the 6 month exercise program. No published information has been located on the effect of alternative compliance improving strategies initiated at entry into or during cardiac exercise rehabilitation programs. This chapter outlines alternative strategies proposed for use with coronary artery disease patients on entry into an exercise rehabilitation based on present knowledges. It describes a stratified randomization into the strategy and control group and gives some interim data on the characteristics of the first 59 patients allocated to either of the 2 groups.

BACKGROUND

A review of the determinants of compliances by Haynes (8) suggests that few studies have demonstrated an association between demographic features and compliance, between features of the disease and compliance, or between features of the therapeutic source and compliance. Therapeutic regimens requiring passive cooperation are more likely to have a high compliance rate, while those requiring changes in personal habits are more likely to have a high dropout rate. The complexity of the regimen appears to increase the dropout rate, as does an increasing duration of treatment. However, Haynes (8) points out that "overshadowing the complexity of the regimen, the degree of behavioral change required, the level of supervision and the convenience of the clinic operation as determinants of compliance are those features of patients that fall into the sociobehavioral realm."

From the sociobehavioral perspective, the Health-Belief Model derived by Becker (1) from previous work outlined by Rosenstock (18) may help to identify elements of an individual's health behavior by relating perceptions of illness, the efficacy of treatment received, and the cues that promote both adoption and adherence with health behavior changes. However, it is possible that health behavior change may in fact be the result rather than the cause of compliance. While there appears to be little relationship between compliance of myocardial infarction patients and other measures of health behavior prediction such as locus of control, it is felt that a lack of measures of the perceived value of health might account for this finding (10). Sackett (19) suggests that goal achievement may be attained with either a high or a low compliance. Whether this is true in exercise rehabilitation or not remains to be determined, although the attitude generally taken is that optimal benefit requires regular participation. An important area of concern at this time for exercise rehabilitation is that of long-term compliance with behavior change. Just because subjects drop out of a supervised exercise program does not automatically mean that they have dropped out of regular exercise; they may in fact be exercising on their own. Just because they attend exercise sessions does not automatically mean that they are achieving a training effect. The most meaningful sign of the subject's success is evidence of extended behavior change in an unsupervised situation where safe and appropriate exercise is undertaken.

With the increasing patient population being referred to supervised exercise programs, and the inescapable increasing number of dropouts, it is essential that factors related to adoption of and adherence with health behavior changes, such as increasing exercise habits, be identified. Why do some patients decide to adopt health behavior changes while others do not? Why, once having adopted the change, do some adhere for a short term and others for a long term? Can we identify the potential dropout? Can we offer alternative strategies to individuals on entry into, or during, the program? Can the program design be altered so as to meet individual as well as group needs? With answers to some or all of these questions, we should be able to offer exercise programs more likely to meet individual needs, so potentially reducing the high dropout rate in exercise rehabilitation programs.

Information on the characteristics, either single or in matrix form, of the dropout is scanty in long-term cardiac exercise rehabilitation studies. Nye and co-workers (12) in an on-going exercise "club" for postinfarction patients state that "there is a suggestion from the data that non-smokers may be better adherers to the exercise program than smokers, although further data would be needed to establish this for certain." To our knowledge no further evidence has been forthcoming to confirm or reject this observation. Bruce et al. (3) have noted that the "initial homegeneity of these two groups (active participants and dropouts) with respect to age, predominant medical diagnosis, and particularly to physical characteristics and functional performance of the cardiovascular system in the first test of maximal exercise, is notable." The present author agrees with this observation on the basis of the analysis of the Ontario Exercise Heart Collaborative Study (15, 16). However, Bruce and his co-workers (3), while not specifically reporting on sociobehavioral data, do observe that there are considerably fewer active participants who are unemployed than dropouts who are unemployed, a finding also observed in the Ontario Study (15). Sanne and Rydin (20) have reported that 54 percent of their subjects stated that they found training was "difficult to perform." Most commonly, these were associated with the inconvenience of the training session scheduling and the travelling costs. Other emotional factors reported by the participants in the same study (20) were the "aversion to the hospital" and a "dislike of physical training." The authors remark that "we found it more serious that the training per se gave an increased feeling of illness." Without identifying any specific individual characteristics relative to dropout, they state that "adherence and attendance rates will vary with several factors. This renders comparisons difficult."

Two separate analyses of the characteristics that identify the potential dropout in the Ontario Exercise Heart Collaborative Study (15, 16) have been completed. The first study was carried out on the 1 year experience in the McMaster cohort (16); specific characteristics were identified with the dropout at 1 month and 12 months; more than one previous myocardial infarction, A-type behavior pattern, and inactive leisure habits. In addition, the 1 month dropout, but not the 12 month dropout, was more likely to be smoking on entry into the program than either having quit or never having smoked. When all 751 subjects in the study were analyzed for both early (≤ 3 months) or late (≤ 23 month) dropout, the characteristics most likely to be identified with dropout at both times were smoking, blue collar work classification, and inactive leisure habits. In addition, the early dropout was also likely to have had more than one previous infarction (15). The fact that in both studies the early dropout is similarly characterized suggests that there is a consistent pattern for dropout and at least for smoking. This has been tentatively confirmed in similar patients in New Zealand (12).

While it may not be possible to generalize from these data, it appears intuitively safe to suggest that the person who does not change other important health behavior patterns (smoking) following a myocardial infarction, who is a blue collar worker with the suggestion of a lower educational level (21), possibly with less understanding of the disease process or poorer communication between themselves and health care workers (7), and in addition who has inactive leisure habits is more likely to be a dropout than an adherer. In addition, individual concern about activity levels after 2 or more previous infarctions is probably not likely to increase long-term adherence in a program where progress is often slow. In summary, the characteristics identifying the potential dropout in the Ontario Exercise Heart Collaborative Study are not surprising and probably are also reflective of persons who generally would not have good adherence behavior in other similar programs of long-term therapy.

FUTURE DIRECTIONS

The original hypothetical model developed to explain dropout contained two elements, i.e. those of Becker (1) and Sackett (19). With the observations made in the Ontario Exercise Heart Collaborative Study (15, 16), the model was expanded to include its present elements (13). It is hypothesized that a model combining the health-belief model and other information such as knowledge of locus of control with a checklist of relevant characteristics may help to identify the potential dropout at entry into an exercise program. If this were true such identification might lead to more appropriate strategies being incorporated into the individual's exercise plan, thus improving the individual adherence outlook and potential for clinical benefit.

Before it is possible to attempt to reduce the comparatively high dropout rate in exercise programs designed for patients with documented coronary artery disease, information about potential compliance-improving strategies needs to be collected, analyzed, and assessed. One such strategy may be patient education: dissemination of information about changing health-related behaviors, specifically information about the role of physical activity following myocardial infarction or bypass surgery. Another possible compliance-improving strategy may be "contracting" or "goal-setting" on entry, regular diary recording of achievement or nonachievement, and discussion of the success or nonsuccess in the contract and possible solutions for the latter.

At McMaster University, the two alternatives discussed above are being reviewed. As we feel that withholding the educational information from one group is perhaps unethical and certainly not warranted, the following study is being carried out. Patients with documented coronary artery disease, either a previous myocardial infarction or bypass surgery, are stratified and randomly allocated to a control or strategy group; the stratification is based on the 4 following characteristics previously shown to be identified with dropout at McMaster University (16) and in the Ontario Study (15): blue collar status, inactive leisure habits, smoking, and more than one previous infarction. Both groups receive the education program but only one group, the strategy group, is involved in the "contracting" or "goal-setting." The areas for "contracting" are determined by the subject and the contract is then worked out in conjunction with the prescriber. The areas of "contracting" include one or more of the following: smoking, diet, weight loss, physical activity, and where necessary referral to a psychological counsellor. For example, a recruit into the study chooses a goal or goals from the five alternative areas; a smoker may choose a goal anywhere from continuing his present consumption to complete abstinence. Let us suppose he chooses to cut smoking by half (say, from 30 to 15 per day) during the next three months; the prescriber, however, may feel a more desirable and yet achievable goal during the next three months is to cut down to below 5 per day. The discrepancy is discussed, the importance of smoking cessation reemphasized, and a goal agreed on by both the participant and prescriber. A standard is thus set for the coming 3 months and is regularly assessed and reevaluated. Compliance with this standard and other goals or contracts can be measured at the end of the program.

The exercise program consists of the following activities for both control and strategy groups. Each session is divided into two phases, a formal and an informal phase. Activity is prescribed on the basis of a functional capacity test carried out on referral to the program. The formal phase consists of prescribed physical activity with regular monitoring of heart rate. When appropriate, ECG and blood pressure may be also monitored during exercise in this phase. Treadmill walking, bicycle ergometry, arm cranking, walking, walking/jogging, or jogging type activities form the basis for this phase. The informal phase consists of games and other activities such as flexibility exercises, noncompetitive relays, swimming, and dual activities. Monitoring of heart rate is routinely carried out by the patients and regularly checked by the exercise specialists.

The major outcome measure in this study is the determination of compliance with the activity program, compliance being defined as the degree of adherence with the protocol. In other words, will the "contracting" or "goal-setting," whether successful or not, have any effect on improving the compliance rate with the activity program? Interim entry data show that, at this time (June, 1979), 59 subjects have been entered into the program, with referral being made for the following reasons: MI (n=43), bypass (n=8), and angina (n=8). There are 30 subjects in the strategy group and 29 in the control group; the mean age of the former group is 50.9 years (28–68) and the latter group 49.8 years (29–66). The mean maximum power output of the strategy group is 850 kpm·min^{-1} and that of the control group 865 kpm·min^{-1}. The number of persons in each cell of the stratified randomization is given in Table 20-I. While there are more than twice as many inactive individuals as active individuals, and inactive nonsmokers are equally likely to be blue or white collar workers, the following observations can be made: (1) the majority (2.9:1) of blue and white collar workers are nonsmokers; (2) inactive white collar workers are more likely to be nonsmokers than smokers (6.5:1) in comparison to inactive blue collar workers (1.6:1); (3) inactive smokers are more likely (4.5:1) to be blue collar workers than white collar workers. These initial observations on an admittedly small population tend to reinforce and extend the report by Hackett and Cassem (7) about the problems that blue collar workers have in the coronary care unit regarding communication about such things as the coronary care unit, medications, the concept of infarction and repair, and long-term behavior changes following discharge.

TABLE 20-I
NUMBER OF SUBJECTS IN EACH CELL FOLLOWING
RANDOMIZED STRATIFICATION

		< 1 M.I.		> 1 M.I.	
		ACTIVE	INACTIVE	ACTIVE	INACTIVE
SMOKING	BLUE	2	9	0	1
	WHITE	1	2	0	1
NON-SMOKING	BLUE	6	14	0	2
	WHITE	8	13	0	0

SUMMARY

Little information is available on compliance with cardiac rehabilitation programs. The literature would suggest that approximately 35 percent of the subjects will be dropouts within 6 months of entry into such programs. Limited information from 1 long-term exercise rehabilitation study suggests that the dropout is likely to be a blue collar worker, be inactive in his leisure time, be a smoker, and have had more than one previous infarction. Whether this dropout rate can be reduced by introduction of compliance-improving strategies—such as (1) education material, vis-à-vis the need for health behavior change and specifically the role of physical activity and coronary artery disease and (2) "contracting" or goal-setting" techniques—is unclear. Reduction of dropout rate is an important issue in the design of future exercise cardiac rehabilitation programs.

REFERENCES

1. Becker, M.H.: Sociobehavioral determinants of compliance. In Sackett, D.L., and Haynes, R.B. (Eds): *Compliance with Therapeutic Regimens.* Baltimore, Johns Hopkins, 1976.
2. Blackwell, B.: Treatment adherence. *Br J Psychiatr, 129*:513, 1976.
3. Bruce, E.G.; Frederick, R.; Bruce, R.A.; and Fisher, L.D.: Comparison of active participants and dropouts in CAPRI cardiopulmonary rehabilitation programs. *Am J Cardiol, 37*:53, 1976.
4. Clausen, J.P.: Circulatory adjustments to dynamic exercise and effect of physical training in normal subjects and in patients with coronary artery disease. *Prog Cardiovas Dis, 43*:459, 1976.
5. Detry, J-M.R.: *Exercise Testing and Training in Coronary Heart Disease.* Baltimore, Williams & Wilkins, 1973.
6. Dunbar, J.M. and Stunkard, A.J.: Adherence to diet and drug regimens. In Levy, R.; Rifkind, B.; Dennis, B.; and Erust, N. (Eds): *Nutrition, Lipids, and Coronary Heart Disease.* New York, Raven, 1979.

7. Hackett, T.P. and Cassem, N.H.: White-collar and blue-collar responses to heart attack. *J Psychosom Res, 20*:85, 1976.

8. Haynes, R.B.: A critical review of the "determinants" of patient compliance with therapeutic regimens. In Sackett, D.L. and Haynes, R.B. (Eds): *Compliance with Therapeutic Regimens.* Baltimore, Johns Hopkins, 1976.

9. Haskell, W.L.: Mechanisms by which physical activity may enhance the clinical status of cardiac patients. In Pollock, M.L. and Schmidt, D.H. (Eds): *Heart Disease and Rehabilitation.* Boston, Houghton-Mifflin, 1979, pp. 276-296.

10. Marston, M.V.: Compliance with medical regimens: A review of the literature. *Nurs Rev, 19*:312, 1970.

11. Nagle, F.J.: Cardiovascular effects of exercise. In Wilson, P.K. (Ed): *Adult Fitness and Cardiac Rehabilitation.* Baltimore, Univ Park, 1976.

12. Nye, G.R. and Poulsen, W.T.: An activity programme for coronary patients: A review of morbidity, mortality and adherence after five years. *NZ Med J, 79*:1010, 1974.

13. Oldridge, N.B.: Compliance in exercise rehabilitation. *Phys Sportsmed, 7*:94, 1979.

14. Oldridge, N.B.: Compliance with exercise programs. In Pollock, M.L. and Schmidt, D.H. (Eds): *Cardiac Rehabilitation: State of the Art.* New York, HM, (in press).

15. Oldridge, N.B.; Andrew, G.M.; and Sangal, S.: Identification of the drop-out from a cardiac rehabilitation program. Submitted to *Am J Cardiol.*

16. Oldridge, N.B.; Wicks, J.R.; Hanley, C.; Sutton, J.R.; and Jones, N.L.: Non-compliance in an exercise rehabilitation program for men who have suffered a myocardial infarction. *Can Med Assoc J, 118*:361, 1978.

17. Reid, E.L. and Morgan, R.W.: Exercise prescription: A clinical trial. *Am J Pub Health, 69*:591, 1979.

18. Rosenstock, I.M.: Why people use health services. *Milbank Mem Fund Q, 44*:94, 1966.

19. Sackett, D.L.: The magnitude of compliance and noncompliance. In Sackett, D.L. and Haynes, R.B. (Eds): *Compliance with Therapeutic Regimens,* Baltimore, Johns Hopkins. 1976.

20. Sanne, H. and Rydin, C.: Feasibility of a physical training program. *Acta Med Scand [Suppl], 551*:59, 1973.

21. Weinblatt, E.; Ruberman, W.; Goldberg, J.D.; Frank, C.W.; Shapiro, S.; and Chavdhary, B.S.: Relation of education to sudden death after myocardial infarction. *N Engl J Med, 299*:60, 1978.

Chapter 21

PREDICTION OF ADHERENCE TO HABITUAL PHYSICAL ACTIVITY

R.K. DISHMAN

THE RECENT upsurgence in public attention to the potential health benefits of vigorous physical activity has fortunately been accompanied by a growing research literature that generally supports a beneficial role for exercise in maintaining wellness (15, 19). Available evidence typically confirms many traditional beliefs held by both the lay and professional communities regarding the efficacy of exercise in the control of tension (8, 9), anxiety (16), depression (12, 20), and certain risk factors associated with coronary heart disease (3, 5). This is *fortunate* since exercise is currently being actively marketed to the American public in a "Madison Avenue" approach ironically similar to that previously employed in the commercialization of tobacco.

The emergent theme of the research literature on the consequences of exercise appears to focus on the role of physical activity in man's adaptation to stress—either from an indirect standpoint as a strategy for coping with psychological stressors or more directly from a standpoint of specific biological adaptations to increased metabolic demands (11). Since it has been estimated that between 30 and 70 percent of the patients treated by physicians in general practice suffer from disorders stemming from excessive unrelieved stress (4), and that 60 million Americans per annum manifest symptoms of either anxiety, depression, or cardiovascular disease (23, 21, 14), exercise therapeutics apparently represents an effective alternative solution to several major health problems of society.

However, since it is apparent that such adaptations *result from* participation, a more fundamental problem relates to *adherence* to exercise prescription—a problem seemingly analogous to that of ensuring patient compliance in a variety of medical treatment settings. While guidelines have been advanced regarding minimal frequency, duration, and intensity of exercise necessary to evoke physiological adaptations to exercise stress (24), similar information about optimal "dosages" required for psychological change is not available. However, it is clear that in order for exercise-induced alterations to endure, exercise involvement must be habitual in nature. Yet, in programs designed to prescribe and supervise exercise therapeutics, it is a typical clinical observation that roughly 50 percent of those individuals participating drop out within 6 months of initial involvement (18, 29). This dropout or attrition rate is remarkably similar over time to that observed in a wide range of medical treatment programs (10) and, as mentioned, represents a major social problem in itself. Habitual exercise apparently is an effective agent in adapting to stress-related disorders, yet a majority of Americans who might benefit are unable to adhere to an exercise program.

From a very pragmatic standpoint of adherence faciliation, the initial identification of the dropout-prone participant would appear to offer a distinct advantage. Such a prediction would permit careful monitoring of the likely dropout, subsequent attention to specific individual "needs," and nonrandom implementation of a variety of facilitation strategies that might enhance adherence.

A review (29) of literature dealing with medical compliance, exercise science, and theoretical psychology has indicated that specific factors relating to patient symptomatology, motivation, and treatment expectations might best enhance such a prediction by discriminating between eventual adherers and dropouts at the outset of exercise involvement. Thus, it is reasonable to expect that participants who are more symptomatic with regard to coronary disease or risk or who manifest a biological profile indicative of low physical working capacity may tend to adhere in order to reduce coronary risk factors such as obesity or hypertension or to increase the functional capacity of the cardiorespiratory system. Furthermore, individuals who perceive physical activity as having instrumental values relating to health and feel they are responsible for their health status might tend to adhere, as might individuals who are attracted to physical activity and possess a high degree of self-motivation or perseverance.

This chapter will summarize a series of investigations concerned with determining predictors of adherence to habitual physical activity. Specific data will be discussed regarding biological, psychological, and behavioral factors that may influence adherence. More detailed accounts of these studies may be found in related papers (10, 30, 31).

RETROSPECTIVE STUDY

The initial investigation involved a retrospective analysis of medical and biological profiles of 362 adult male participants in the Biodynamics Exercise Program at the University of Wisconsin–Madison, over a 5 year period from June, 1972, to July, 1977. Aside from attendance records, information was available from a standardly employed patient screening protocol, which includes a medical history and a substandard Balke exercise tolerance treadmill test. Specific variables of interest included age, height (cm), weight (kg), percent body fat (28), resting and maximum exercise heart rates and blood pressures, and metabolic capacity (mets). In addition, data were available regarding previous incidents of myocardial infarction, present status relative to coronary heart disease risk during exercise, and previous exercise behavior prior to program enrollment.

Classification systems were adopted for both adherence and coronary risk in order to provide greater discrimination among participants. Adherence was categorized discretely according to the following groups: (1) continuous for less than 1 month, (2) continuous from 1 to 3 months, (3) continuous from 3 to 5 months, (4) continuous from 5 to 12 months, (5) continuous for more than 12 months, (6) discontinuous for less than 5 months, (7) discontinuous for more than 5 months. Inspection of attendance patterns for these subjects indicated that participants appeared to cluster into these groups and subsequently, the adopted criterion groups seemed most meaningful.

Since, as mentioned, coronary disease symptomatology was anticipated as being an influence upon adherence, patients were also categorized according to coronary risk during exercise. The classification system employed incorporated risk criteria standardly used in the Biodynamic's program and is based upon exercise tolerance, cardiovascular examination, and medical history. This system provides for the following groups: (A) normal, nonrisk, (B) normal risk with suspected heart disease, (C) normal risk with established heart disease, (D) high risk—supervision indicated

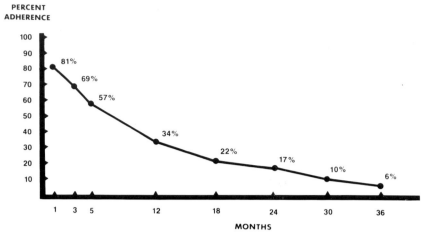

Figure 21-1. Dropout curve representing adherence to the Biodynamics Exercise program over a 5 year period. Adherence rates at time points >18 months are necessarily underestimates since individuals who entered the program later than July, 1974 were mathematically prevented from adhering for the entire 36 month period.

with no geographical limits, (E) high risk—supervision indicated with definite geographical limits.

Analysis

An initial analysis was conducted to determine if the biological variables assessed could discriminate between adherence groups. A subsequent analysis of coronary risk groups was designed to determine if differences observed between adherence groups would also replicate on the basis of coronary risk—thus adding support for the influence of symptomatology on adherence behavior. For each analysis, a random sample (N=181) was selected from the initial sample (N=362) of patient profiles for the purpose of discriminant analysis and group contrasts. The remaining observations (N=181) were used as a holdout sample for external classification and validation of the derived discriminant function prediction equations. Discriminant analysis was employed to provide the weighted linear combination of standardly assessed exercise screening information that could best discriminate between participants. In a practical sense, an attempt was made to provide a statistical means for making *a priori* decisions about adherence group membership that could be applied in an exercise prescription setting.

Results

MANOVA and stepwise multiple discriminant analysis as a *post hoc* test indicated that percent body fat, body weight, and metabolic capacity discriminated (p < .05) among criterion adherence groups and metabolic capacity and body weight subsequently discriminated (p < .05) among coronary disease risk groups.

Multiple regression of these discriminating variables on dummy contrast variables (26) indicated that comparisons of individuals who adhered for less than 1 month with those adhering for more than 1 month and with those adhering more than 12 months, and comparison of individuals adhering more than 12 months with those adhering less than 12 months, best accounted for between groups variance in adherence. Similarly, comparison of patients diagnosed as "risk-free" and as "normal risk with suspected heart disease" with remaining patients manifesting established heart disease best accounted for separation among coronary risk groups.

These results suggest that individuals with greater adherence to exercise prescription tended to manifest lower values on each of the discriminating variables and were also more symptomatic with regard to coronary disease. Furthermore, in a more direct test of

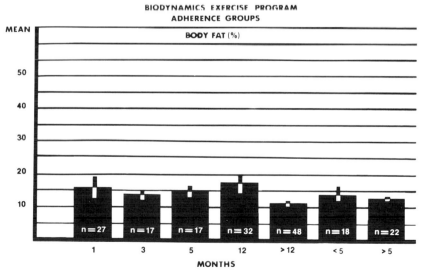

Figure 21-2. Discriminating biologic variables for adherence groups in retrospective study.

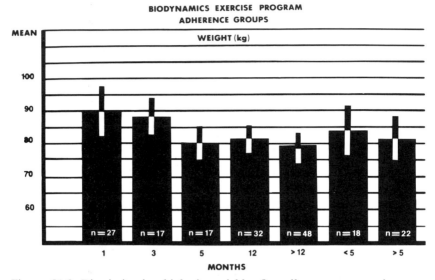

Figure 21-3. Discriminating biologic variables for adherence groups in retrospective study.

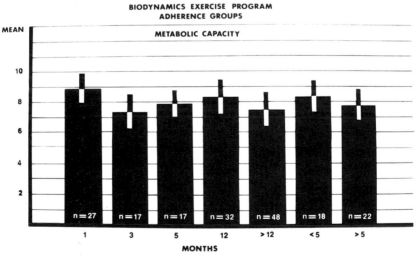

Figure 21-4. Discriminating biologic variables for adherence groups in retrospective study.

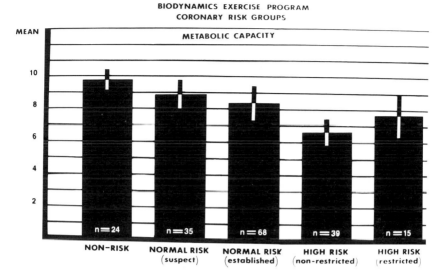

Figure 21-5. Discriminating biologic variables for coronary disease risk groups in retrospective study.

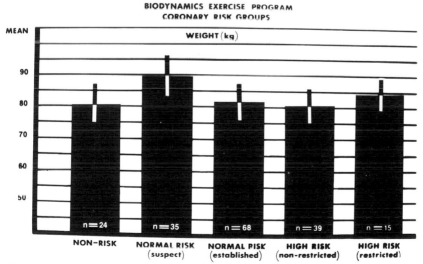

Figure 21-6. Discriminating biologic variables for coronary disease risk groups in retrospective study.

this hypothesis, adherence was found to be significantly related to coronary risk ($p < .05$). However, the magnitude of this relationship was minimal (Rho = .123), and adherence was found to be not associated (using a Chi-square test of independence, $p > .05$) with the incidence of myocardial infarction.

Behavioral self-reports of exercise involvement prior to the Biodynamic's prescription indicated no relationship between program adherence and previous exercise intensity, frequency, and duration ($r = .05$). Also, previous athletic experience was not associated with adherence ($X^2, p > .05$).

Discussion

These findings seemed to support the influence of symptomatology on exercise adherence. Due to functional impairment of the cardiovascular system coincident to coronary disease, symptomatic patients may be disposed to greater adherence in attempts to alleviate or retard heart disease symptoms or risk factors. In this regard, it is noteworthy that metabolic capacity discriminated between coronary risk groups and adherence groups as well. For the most part, between group variance in this separation indicated that metabolic capacity decreased with increasing exercise risk. Although in a more direct test coronary risk was not observed to be substantially associated with adherence, this association could have been masked by attrition at either extreme of the symptom continuum, that is, participants might have discontinued due to early relief of minor symptoms or may have suffered from intense symptoms and "given up" on treatment. Partial support for this explanation was provided by the relatively large percentage (70%) of moderately symptomatic participants who became long term adherers (> 5 months).

In summary, these results suggest that the decision to adhere or drop out of a therapeutic exercise program may be significantly dependent upon body composition, metabolic capacity, and coronary disease symptomatology. The implications of these findings are rather straightforward in their suggestion that standardly assessed exercise screening information may statistically enhance the initial diagnosis of individuals who have a low probability of adhering to exercise prescription. However, in the present population the low "hit rate" of 25 percent [using the derived discriminant function equation to classify unknown observations (N=181)

TABLE 21-I

MEANS AND STANDARD DEVIATIONS FOR THE BIOLOGICAL VARIABLES WITH
CLASSIFICATION ON ADHERENCE DURING THE RETROSPECTIVE STUDY

Biological Variables		Adherence Groups (N = 181)						
		1 (n = 27)	2 (n = 17)	3 (n = 17)	4 (n = 32)	5 (n = 48)	6 (n = 18)	7 (n = 22)
Age (yrs.)	$\bar{x}$	45.37	48.12	48.65	48.91	51.35	49.33	48.82
	s.d.	9.01	7.63	7.42	7.64	7.?1	6.95	8.62
Height (cm)	$\bar{x}$	178.17	179.26	175.14	178.03	175.41	178.11	174.06
	s.d.	6.76	5.48	6.53	4.92	5.72	8.53	7.44
Weight (kg)	$\bar{x}$	90.72	88.04	80.44	82.80	78.27	84.79	82.63
	s.d.	15.36	11.53	10.14	8.03	9.40	15.74	13.01
Body Fat (%)	$\bar{x}$	16.77	14.00	14.90	17.00	12.41	14.23	13.44
	s.d.	6.06	3.65	5.42	6.12	2.30	5.31	2.11
Resting Heart Rate (bpm)	$\bar{x}$	76.52	78.41	78.18	77.72	81.17	78.67	81.68
	s.d.	10.72	12.50	13.18	9.57	13.27	11.72	14.86
Resting Systolic Blood Pressure (mmHg)	$\bar{x}$	135.56	139.76	136.29	133.28	136.94	138.56	141.50
	s.d.	14.58	16.88	25.60	16.11	16.27	20.40	16.62
Resting Diastolic Blood Pressure (mmHg)	$\bar{x}$	91.44	90.35	92.06	89.38	90.19	89.17	94.36
	s.d.	10.39	13.42	13.34	13.54	11.28	9.73	9.15
Maximum Exercise Heart Rate (bpm)	$\bar{x}$	164.00	155.71	158.06	161.03	152.73	157.94	158.73
	s.d.	20.92	21.78	18.64	18.82	21.71	21.79	19.79
Maximum Exercise Systolic Blood Pressure (mmHg)	$\bar{x}$	205.89	192.18	194.29	189.44	188.00	206.39	193.64
	s.d.	30.49	3?.28	25.09	23.47	27.05	30.56	30.70
Maximum Exercise Diastolic Blood Pressure (mmHg)	$\bar{x}$	92.52	90.41	94.08	91.85	91.98	88.67	92.82
	s.d.	16.81	12.23	12.22	14.44	13.63	12.22	16.04
Metabolic Capacity (mets)	$\bar{x}$	8.98	7.46	7.92	8.31	7.56	8.31	7.76
	s.d.	1.92	2.34	1.75	2.13	2.16	2.06	2.02

TABLE 21-II

MEANS AND STANDARD DEVIATIONS FOR THE BIOLOGICAL VARIABLES WITH
CLASSIFICATION ON CORONARY DISEASE EXERCISE RISK DURING THE RETROSPECTIVE STUDY

Biological Variables		Coronary Risk Groups (N = 181)				
		1 (n = 24)	2 (n = 35)	3 (n = 68)	4 (n = 39)	5 (n = 15)
Age (yrs.)	x̄	46.17	45.83	49.88	51.85	49.07
	s.d.	5.54	10.05	7.10	7.46	6.44
Height (cm)	x̄	177.89	178.54	175.80	176.16	179.48
	s.d.	7.73	5.66	5.87	6.36	7.86
Weight (kg)	x̄	80.70	89.36	82.29	80.54	84.18
	s.d.	12.62	13.75	11.57	11.02	10.73
Body Fat (%)	x̄	13.76	15.95	14.90	13.88	12.83
	s.d.	3.49	6.69	4.79	4.05	2.49
Resting Heart Rate (bpm)	x̄	77.00	78.69	80.29	78.59	79.80
	s.d.	9.37	11.66	13.48	13.18	9.96
Resting Systolic Blood Pressure (mmHg)	x̄	127.33	140.37	135.09	142.18	139.87
	s.d.	13.25	15.74	15.91	21.57	16.67
Resting Diastolic Blood Pressure (mmHg)	x̄	84.54	93.71	90.41	92.00	94.07
	s.d.	9.48	12.58	10.53	11.91	12.68
Maximum Exercise Heart Rate (bpm)	x̄	172.75	166.31	159.24	139.03	157.60
	s.d.	12.58	16.72	18.39	15.66	26.39
Maximum Exercise Systolic Blood Pressure (mmHg)	x̄	201.54	202.86	192.15	184.62	199.13
	s.d.	21.70	31.98	24.32	32.93	28.59
Maximum Exercise Diastolic Blood Pressure (mmHg)	x̄	85.25	93.34	90.16	95.15	98.07
	s.d.	12.27	15.46	12.96	12.80	17.36
Metabolic Capacity	x̄	9.75	8.79	8.28	6.47	7.54
	s.d.	1.29	1.79	2.04	1.57	2.67

into actual adherence groups] limits the clinical significance of this discrimination.

Considering this of limited clinical importance, a second, prospective investigation was designed to determine the replicability of the initial findings of the retrospective study and to consider conceptually relevant psychological influences as well. Not only are there theoretical reasons to expect a significant role for psychological factors in adherence (1, 29) but "psycho-social" factors have commonly been implicated by exercise clinicians (6, 22). Moreover, an abundant literature supports the efficacy of multivariate inquiry (17), and it was reasoned that a psychobiologic model might offer greater predictive power.

PROSPECTIVE STUDY

The prospective study involved 66 adult males in medically prescribed and supervised programs of either muscular or cardiovascular endurance training 3 days per week for 20 weeks. Participants were involved in 1 of 3 organized exercise programs: Biodynamics Exercise Program (N=16); LaCrosse Exercise Programs, University of Wisconsin-LaCrosse (N=16); and the Institute for Aerobics Research, Dallas, Texas (N=34).

Following informed consent, assessment was made of specific biologic variables [body weight (kg), percent body fat (28), and metabolic capacity (2, 7)] and selected psychological variables relating to treatment expectations and motivation [attraction to physical activity and self-perceptions of physical ability (PEAS; 25); instrumental values of physical activity (ATPA; 13); health locus of control (HLC; 27); and self-motivation (SMo; 32)]. Although each of the psychological variables have been theoretically linked to exercise adherence, only self-motivation has been demonstrated to have an empirical relationship with adherence (10), and subsequently it was of particular interest for the prospective study.

Results

MANOVA revealed a significant ($p < .01$) overall difference between dropouts and adherers on the biological and psychological variables. Application of stepwise multiple discriminant analysis as a *post hoc* test indicated that only percent body fat, self-motivation, and body weight made a significant ($p < .05$)

contribution to this group separation. Furthermore, these variables permitted accurate classification of participants into actual adherence or dropout groups for approximately 80 percent of all cases. Group means for the discriminating variables revealed that adherers possessed lower values for both percent body fat and body weight but had higher self-motivation scores.

Stepwise multiple regression analysis yielded similar results in that percent body fat, self-motivation, and body weight entered the regression equation consecutively and were the only variables that significantly ($p < .05$) enhanced the prediction of adherence. In fact, nearly 50 percent of the variance in adherence behavior could be accounted for by the derived regression equation.

Discussion

In summary, these findings seem to support a significant influence of symptomatology upon exercise program adherence. Functional capacity of the cardiovascular system discriminated between participants both on the basis of adherence and coronary risk with long term adherers (> 12 months) and symptomatic patients manifesting lowest metabolic capacities. However, this discriminative power appears to offer little clinical significance in view of the limited classification success. Furthermore,

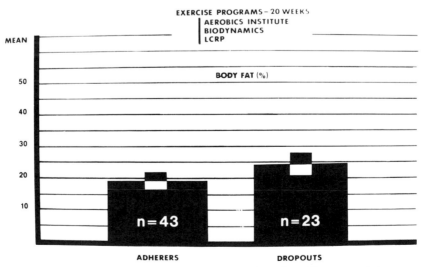

Figure 21-7. Discriminating psychobiologic variables for adherers and dropouts in prospective study.

only a slight relationship between adherence and coronary risk was observed.

These findings do, however, support a substantial influence of body composition on adherence. Transportation of a lighter, leaner mass would offer certain advantages in terms of both

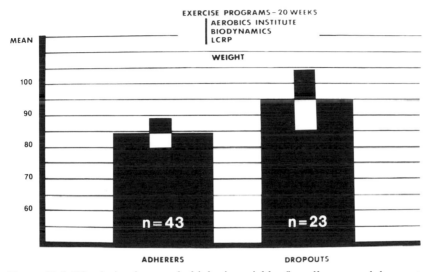

Figure 21-8. Discriminating psychobiologic variables for adherers and dropouts in prospective study.

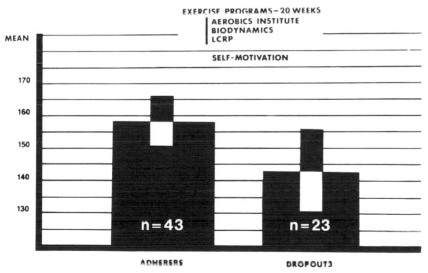

Figure 21-9. Discriminating psychobiologic variables for adherers and dropouts in prospective study.

TABLE 21-III
MEANS AND STANDARD DEVIATIONS FOR THE PSYCHOLOGICAL
AND BIOLOGICAL VARIABLES WITH CLASSIFICATION ON
EXERCISE ADHERENCE DURING THE PROSPECTIVE STUDY

Variables		Adherers (N = 43)	Dropouts (N = 23)
Body Fat (%)	x̄	19.07	24.09
	s.d.	5.08	7.88
Self-Motivation	x̄	158.65	143.78
	s.d.	16.41	26.46
Body Weight (kg)	x̄	84.34	94.03
	s.d.	9.51	19.02
Health Locus of Control	x̄	29.81	34.04
	s.d.	7.20	7.38
Aesthetic Experience	x̄	41.47	43.22
	s.d.	8.40	7.54
Catharsis	x̄	39.12	37.91
	s.d.	6.57	8.82
Social Experience	x̄	43.16	43.30
	s.d.	6.04	6.00
Health and Fitness	x̄	43.49	39.70
	s.d.	7.56	8.40
Ascetic Experience	x̄	37.40	33.83
	s.d.	8.58	9.99
Attraction	x̄	37.72	33.13
	s.d.	8.77	11.24
Estimation	x̄	22.65	19.13
	s.d.	6.80	10.35
Persuit of Vertigo	x̄	37.51	34.17
	s.d.	8.85	11.01
Metabolic Capacity (mets)	x̄	10.81	9.56
	s.d.	2.52	2.85

metabolic and perceptual efficiency and intuitively should increase the attractiveness of endurance-type exercise. However, exercise prescription typically is made on the basis of relative intensities, which should negate the influence of differential work capacities. Moreover, low body weight and body fat might also be indicative of previous exercise behavior or a vigorous life-style that might be perpetuated in a formal exercise setting. However, as mentioned, no association between self-reports of antecedent exercise behavior and actual program adherence was observed. This is surprising, since the best logical predictor of behavior should be previous behavior.

Replication of body weight and ability of percent body fat to discriminate in the prospective study adds considerable support to the influence of body composition on adherence. When combined with self-motivation scores in a psychobiologic prediction model, these variables appear to be of considerable clinical importance in assisting in the initial identification of likely dropouts.

The inability of psychological constructs such as attitude toward physical activity and locus of control to predict adherence, although inconsistent with certain theoretical notions, *is* in agreement with earlier research (18). The relationship between exercise adherence and self-motivation is notable not only due to its substantial nature ($r = .44, p < .05$) and the fact that it provided for considerably better prediction than did any of the remaining psychological factors but also because it provides additional empirical support for what previously has been largely only a conceptual link between motivation and adherence to exercise therapeutics.

CONCLUSIONS

The major findings of these investigations seem to be quite straightforward in their implications for the administration of exercise programs of a therapeutic or preventive medicine nature. They initially suggest that the decision to drop out or adhere to an exercise prescription may be influenced in large part by participants' body composition and self-motivation.

The clinical significance of these findings are particularly striking in view of the fact that these characteristics are easily assessed at the outset of exercise involvement and appear to be quite effective in enhancing the prediction of adherence.

Since self-motivation is conceptually a trait-like behavioral disposition (test-retest $r = .86$ over 20 weeks) that is situationally invariant, individuals diagnosed as likely adherers may be only slightly influenced by the dynamics of the exercise setting (e.g. exercise mode, exercise leader, or interpersonal relations with other participants). Subsequently, initial identification of the probable adherer would permit more direct attention to "needs" of dropout-prone individuals and nonrandom implementation of possible strategies for adherence facilitation.

Furthermore, since self-motivation assessment is based upon self-perceptions of perseverant behavior, it is theoretically possible that this construct might be altered as a function of an exercise experience. In this regard, an individual who initially possesses low self-motivation but who is somehow able to maintain involvement beyond what appears to be the critical 3–5 month period may subsequently make a self-attribution of increased self-motivation, which might then perpetuate adherence independent of further administrative intervention. Of course, this conjecture awaits empirical support.

At any rate, these initial findings suggest that self-motivation scores used in conjunction with measures of body fat and body weight may considerably enhance the prediction of exercise adherence.

REFERENCES

1. Baekeland, F. and Lundwall, L.: Dropping out of treatment: A critical review. *Psychol Bull, 82*:738, 1975.
2. Balke, B. and Ware, R.: The status of physical fitness in the Air Force. *School Aviat Med.* USAF, 1959.
3. Blackburn, H.: Physical activity as primarily preventive in coronary disease. In *Proceedings of the International Congress of Physical Activity Sciences,* edited by F. Landry and W. Orban. New York, Symposia Special, 1978.
4. Blythe, P.: *Stress Disease.* New York, St. Martin, 1973.
5. Boyer, J.L. and Kasch, F.W.: Exercise therapy in hypertensive men. *JAMA, 211*:1668, 1970.
6. Bruce, E.H.; Frederick, R.; Bruce, R.A.; and Fisher, C.D.: Comparison of active participants and dropouts in CAPRI cardiopulmonary rehabilitation programs. *Am J Cardiol, 37*:53, 1976.
7. Bruce, R.A.; Kusumi, F.; and Hosmer, I.: Maximal oxygen intake and nomographic assessment of functional aerobic impairment in cardiovascular disease. *Am Heart J, 85*:546, 1973.
8. Byrd, O.E.: The relief of tension by exercise and a survey of medical viewpoints and practices. *J School Health, 43*:238, 1963.
9. deVries, H.A.: Immediate and long term effects of exercise upon resting muscle action potential level. *J Sports Med, 8*:1, 1968.
10. Dishman, R.K.; Ickes, W.; and Morgan, W.P.: Self-motivation and adherence to habitual physical activity. *J Appl Soc Psychol, 10*:115, 1980.
11. Falls, H.; Baylor, A.; and Dishman, R.K.: *Essentials of Fitness.* Phildelphia, Saunders, Holt, Rinehart, and Winston, 1980.
12. Greist, J.H.; Klein, M.H.; Eischens, R.R.; and Faris, J.W.: Antidepressant running: Running as a treatment for non-psychotic depression. *Behav Med, June*:19, 1978.
13. Kenyon, G.S.: Six scales for assessing attitude toward physical activity. *Res Q, 39*:566, 1968.
14. Kolata, G.B. and Marx, J.L.: Epidemiology of heart disease: Searches for causes. *Science, 194*:509, 1976.
15. Milvy, P. (Ed): The marathon: Physiological, medical, epidemiological, and psychological studies. *Ann NY Acad Sci, 301*: 1977.
16. Morgan, W.P.: Anxiety reduction following acute physical activity. *Psychiatr Ann, 9*:3, 1979.

17. Morgan, W.P.: Efficacy of psychobiologic inquiry in the exercise and sport sciences. *Quest, 20*:39, 1973.
18. Morgan, W.P.: Involvement in vigorous physical activity with special reference to adherence. In *Proceedings of the College Physical Education Conference, Orlando, Florida,* p. 235, 1977a.
19. Morgan, W.P.: Psychological consequences of vigorous physical activity and sport. In *The Academy Papers,* edited by M. Gladys Scott. Iowa City, Am Acad Physical Educ, 1977b.
20. Morgan, W.P.; Roberts, J.A.; Brand, F.R.; and Feinerman, A.D.: Psychological effect of chronic physical activity. *Med Sci Sports, 2*:213, 1970.
21. National Institute of Mental Health, *Statistical Report, 1977.* Bethesda, Md, NIMII, 1977.
22. Oldridge, N,B,: Compliance of post M.I. patients to exercise programs. In *Proceedings of the American College of Sports Medicine Conference on Coronary Artery Disease—Prevention, Clinical Assessment, and Rehabilitation.* Tulsa, Okla, Oral Roberts U, 1977.
23. Pitts, F.N.: The biochemistry of anxiety. *Sci Am, 220*:69, 1969.
24. Pollock, M.L.: The quantification of endurance training programs. In *Exercise and Sport Sciences Review,* Vol. 1, edited by J.H. Wilmore. New York, Acad Pr, 1973.
25. Sonstroem, R.J.: Attitude testing examining certain psychological correlates of physical activity. *Res Q, 45*:93, 1974.
26. Stevens, J.P.: Four methods of analyzing between variation for K-group MANOVA problem. *Multivar Behav Res, 7*:499, 1972.
27. Wallston, B.S.; Wallston, K.A.; Kaplan, G.D.; and Maides, S.A.: Development and validation of the health locus of control (HLC) scale. *J Consult Clin Psychol, 44*:580, 1976.
28. Yuhasz, M.S.: *Physical Fitness and Sports Appraisal Laboratory Manual.* University of Western Ontario, 1965.
29. Dishman, R.K.: Adherence to habitual physical activity: A review in Sachs, M., and Buffone, G. (eds.), *The Psychology of Exercise and Running: Therapeutic and Practical Applications,* in press.
30. Dishman, R.K.: Biologic influences on adherence to habitual physical activity. Manuscript submitted for publication, 1979.
31. Dishman, R.K. and Gettman, L.R.: Psychobiologic influences on adherence to habitual physical activity. *J Sport Psychology,* in press.
32. Dishman, R.K. and Ickes, W.: Self-motivation and adherence to therapeutic exercise. *J Behav Med,* in press.

Chapter 22

THE PSYCHOLOGICAL RESPONSES
OF POSTHOSPITALIZED
PSYCHIATRIC PATIENTS
TO EXERCISE STRESS TESTING*

M.A. ROSS AND S.J. LEVIN

CURRENTLY, there does not appear to be a universally accepted course of treatment for individuals with affective or psychiatric disturbances. While considerable progress has been made in the treatment of emotional disorders, specifically depression (1), the diversity of psychotherapeutic techniques renders the judgment of comparative treatment outcomes problematic. During the past decade, the field of mental health has moved away from long-term hospitalization toward community involvement for patients with chronic mental disorders. Communities, however, have been ill-equipped to assist patients in the transition from prolonged hospitalization to community living.

Attention to the field of community health has led to the growth of the Social Rehabilitation Clinic (SRC), which provides a structured daily program for posthospitalized psychiatric patients. Besides providing individual and group psychotherapy, the SRC offers a variety of ancillary activities, such as dance and art therapy, meditation, and structured work groups, which are thought to be rehabilitative. These adjunctive treatments may help to involve the patient in concrete tasks that might otherwise not be sought out. Psychiatric patients with schizophrenic disorders, for instance, upon discharge from hospitalization spend the majority of their time watching television (15).

The majority of patients attending the SRC have some type of schizophrenic disorder as either the primary or secondary diagnosis. Schizophrenia is an illness manifested by characteristic

*The authors wish to acknowledge the Post Gradute Center for Mental Health, New York, New York, and the YMCA of Greater New York for supporting this research.

276

disturbances in thinking, mood, and behavior. According to the Diagnostic and Statistical Manual of the American Psychiatric Association:

> Disturbances in thinking are marked by alterations of concept formation which may lead to misinterpretation of reality and sometimes to delusions and hallucinations, which frequently appear psychologically self-protective. Corollary mood changes include ambivalent, constricted and inappropriate emotional responsiveness and loss of empathy with others. Behavior may be withdrawn, regressive and bizarre (American Psychiatric Association, 1977, p. 33).

Schizophrenia thus represents a self-protective coping mechanism to remove the individual from painful realities.

Psychiatric patients, in general, appear to be characterized by hyperponetic states and high muscular tension levels (49). Impairments in psychomotor function, usually associated with inattention, echo-phenomena, fear of destruction, and defects in self-object discrimination have been observed in schizophrenic patients (14). Chronic schizophrenic patients have also been found to have sensory (19) and neuromuscular dysfunction (29), including elevated resting levels of creatine phosphokinase (30) and abnormalities in muscle structure (28). Schizophrenics appear to suffer from disturbances of perception and loss of ground figure discrimination (8, 9) and may also lack the ability to accurately process sensations of physical exertion (35).

Within the past few years, the awareness of the beneficial effects of vigorous physical activity on mental health (36) has led to the adoption of exercise somatotherapy as an adjunctive psychotherapeutic treatment (46, 21). To date, however, there appears to be a paucity of research documenting the psychological responses of chronic schizophrenics to exercise stress. Since these patients have apparently led a sedentary existence, as reflected by low levels of muscular strength, endurance (17), and physical work capacity (23, 43, 32), the prescription of exercise requires an assessment of their exercise tolerance and cardiovascular health.

Based on the description of schizophrenic symptomatology, there appears to be sufficient reason to support the expectation that schizophrenics and other highly disturbed patients might not have a favorable reaction to exercise itself, or exercise stress examinations. As part of a larger study designed to assess the effects of exercise on schizophrenic patients (22), the psychometric characteristics and psychophysical responses of a group of schizophrenics to exercise stress testing were examined. The following five hypotheses were tested:

H_1: Schizophrenic patients would score within clinical ranges on selected psychological states and traits.

H_2: Schizophrenic patients would be categorized by low physical work capacities.

H_3: Schizophrenic patients would subjectively underestimate their level of physical fitness.

H_4: Schizophrenic patients and normals would differ in ratings of perceived exertion.

H_5: Schizophrenic patients would respond to exercise stress testing with high levels of anxiety.

METHOD

SUBJECTS AND DESIGN: The subjects in this investigation were adult male (n=21) and female (n=14) psychiatric outpatients attending the SRC, Post Graduate Center West, New York, New York. All subjects had a previous history of hospitalization for psychiatric disturbances. Of the sample, 43 percent had a high school education and 54 percent had one or more years of college experience. Subjects ranged in age from 19 to 54 years, with a mean of 31.2 years.

With the cooperation of the group counselors and administrative staff of the SRC, patients were initially informed of the opportunity to participate in a YMCA affiliated study concerning physical activity and mental health. An informal presentation (slide show), followed by a question and answer period, was given at the SRC to inform patients about the nature and requirements of the research. Patients expressing an interest in participating in the study were instructed to leave their names with their group counselor.

Patients who volunteered to participate in the study signed a consent form, which stated that it would be necessary to respond to 2 short series of questionnaires, designed to measure various mood states, and to complete an Exercise Tolerance Test (ETT), designed to assess physical fitness and cardiovascular health status. The first series of questionnaires was completed at the SRC one week prior to the administration of the ETT. Subjects completed the second series of questionnaires shortly after their arrival at the YMCA for their ETT.

PSYCHOLOGICAL MEASURES: In order not to overwhelm the subjects with an excessive amount of questionnaires to be completed in a single session, the measurement of selected psychological states (situational responses) and traits (enduring responses) was accomplished in two sessions. The first series of questionnaires (T_1) was completed at the SRC one week prior to the administration of the ETT and the second series of questionnaires (T_2) was completed upon arrival at the YMCA for the ETT.*

T_1: The psychological tests in the first battery consisted of the Profile of Mood States (POMS) (27), to measure tension, anger, depression, vigor, fatigue, and confusion; State-Trait Anxiety Inventory (STAI) (48), to measure state anxiety (STAI X_1) and trait anxiety (STAI X_2); SCL 90 Symptom Check List (10) to measure the states of psychoticism, somatization, obsessive-compulsiveness, interpersonal sensitivity, depression, anxiety, hostility, phobic anxiety, and paranoid ideation.

T_2: The psychological tests in the second battery consisted of the Eysenck Personality Questionnaire (EPQ) (12), to measure the traits of extroversion-introversion, neuroticism-stability, psychoticism, and response distortion (lie scale); Physical Estimation and Attraction Scale (PEAS) (47) to measure estimation (EST) and attraction (ATT) toward physical activity; and state anxiety (STAI X_1) (48).

PROCEDURE

EXERCISE TOLERANCE TEST APPOINTMENT SCHEDULE: Patients were scheduled in groups of 5 or 6 for their ETT appointment. All testing was completed within a 4 day period. To facilitate traveling to the YMCA from the SRC, one author (S.L.) met the patients at the SRC and escorted them to the YMCA. Upon arrival at the YMCA, the patients completed medical and physical activity history forms in addition to the second series of psychological tests.

ETT PREPARATION: Subjects were prepared for their ETT in pairs. The remaining subjects were attended by an SRC staff

---

*The SCL-90 Symptom Checklist was administered as part of the design of one study (22) to assess the effects of an aerobic exercise training program on psychiatric symptoms in schizophrenic out-patients.

member while waiting in a room adjoining the exercise testing laboratory. The waiting room contained an ample supply of magazines, and a radio was provided. Preparation for the ETT involved the following sequence of events:

1. recording of height and weight
2. drawing of blood
3. electrode attachment (skin abrasion)
4. physician examination.

ETT PROTOCOL: Immediately after preparation for the ETT, three 12-lead electrocardiograms (ECG) were recorded under conditions of supine rest, standing, and hyperventilation. All exercise testing was conducted in accordance with the American College of Sports Medicine Guidelines for ETT and a cardiologist was present throughout the testing procedure. A modified Balke Treadmill Test (4) was administered with progressive increments of 2.5 percent every 2 minutes and a constant speed of 3 mph for the first 10 minutes of the test, followed by progressive increments of 2 percent and a constant speed of 3.5 mph. Resting measures of blood pressure and heart rate were recorded immediately before the start of the ETT. An accommodation period of 3 minutes preceded the diagnostic phase of the ETT. During the last 15 seconds of each exercise level, ECG tracings were recorded on a Marquette Series 8400 cardiogram and blood pressure was obtained by auscultation. The following criteria were used as end-points for the ETT: attainment of the age-predicted maximum heart rate, failure to maintain adequate pulse pressure, detection of significant electrocardiographic abnormalities, or the patient's desire to stop.

STATE ANXIETY RESPONSE TO THE ETT: A 4 item modified State Anxiety Inventory (48) was administered pre- and postexercise. Subjects were asked to rate how they felt at the moment 5 minutes before and 5 minutes after exercise. This short form of the STAI (X_1) has been substantially correlated with the longer version.

RATINGS OF PERCEIVED EXERTION: The patients' subjective rating of perceived exertion (RPE), in conjunction with measures of heart rate and blood pressure, were obtained during the last 15 seconds of each exercise stage. Perceived exertion was measured with Borg's revised psychophysical category rating scale (6). The perceived exertion scale ranges from 6 to 20 and is presented in quarto format with the lower boundary of the scale (7) anchored by the description Very, Very Light and the upper boundary of the scale (19) anchored by the description Very, Very Hard. Each odd number between these boundaries is anchored by the following descriptions: (9) Very Light, (11) Fairly Light, (13) Somewhat Hard, (15) Hard, (17) Very Hard.

Patients rated their degree of perceived exertion according to a standardized instructional set:

> Throughout your exercise test we want you to rate how you feel. That is, we want you to judge your degree of perceived exertion. By perceived exertion we mean the total amount of exertion and physical fatigue, combining all sensations and feelings of physical stress, effort and fatigue. As you make your ratings, don't concern yourself with any one factor such as leg pain, shortness of breath, or the work intensity, but try to concentrate on your *total, inner* feeling of exertion. Try to estimate as honestly and objectively as possible. Don't overestimate the degree of exertion you feel, but don't underestimate it either. Just try to estimate as accurately as possible (39).

RESULTS AND DISCUSSION

The majority of subjects in this investigation were classified as schizophrenic.* Although the Diagnostic Manual of the American Psychiatric Association lists 19 subcategories of schizophrenic disorders (2), these subcategories have not been differentiated in this paper for purposes of data analyses. Inspection of the SRC intake records revealed schizophrenia as the primary diagnosis for 74 percent of the cases and the remaining 26 percent of the cases were diagnosed as possessing other psychiatric illnesses. Table 22-I contains demographic and resting physiological characteristics of the sample.

While psychiatric diagnosis contains nosological difficulties, the psychometric characteristics of this patient sample substantiates their clinical pathology. Whereas, in mentally adjusted samples, 10 percent of the subjects may fall within clinical ranges, more than 30 percent of the patients scored a standard deviation above the mean on neuroticism, state anxiety, trait anxiety, and depression.

---

*The subcategories of schizophrenia diagnoses were schizophrenia, paranoid type; schizophrenia, schizo-affective type; schizoid personality; schizophrenia, simple type; schizophrenia, chronic undifferentiated; schizophrenia, latent type; and acute schizophrenic episode.

Exercise in Health and Disease

TABLE 22-I

SELECTED DEMOGRAPHIC AND RESTING PHYSIOLOGICAL
CHARACTERISTICS OF THE PATIENT SAMPLE (N = 35)

Variable	Mean	SD
Age (yrs)	31.20	9.26
Height (cm)	171.11	9.70
Weight (kg)	73.11	16.11
Resting Heart Rate (bpm)	75.17	11.10
Resting Systolic Blood Pressure (mmHg)	116.20	16.44
Resting Diastolic Blood Pressure (mmHg)	76.77	11.45

TABLE 22-II

MEANS AND STANDARD DEVIATIONS FOR THE PATIENT SAMPLE
(N = 35) ON SELECTED PSYCHOLOGICAL STATES AND TRAITS
COMPARED TO NORMATIVE DATA

Variable	Patients		Norms	
	Mean	SD	Mean	SD
State Anxiety	46.17	10.02	36.35	9.67
Trait Anxiety	48.30	9.02	37.68	9.69
Tension	15.51	7.50	12.9	6.8
Depression	19.48	12.31	13.1	10.3
Anger	14.68	10.37	10.1	7.8
Vigor	13.22	6.14	15.6	6.0
Fatigue	9.50	7.27	10.4	6.2
Confusion	9.9	4.46	10.2	11.3
Psychoticism	4.58	2.12	3.7	3.09
Extraversion	11.57	4.93	12.19	4.91
Neuroticism	14.80	5.26	9.83	5.18
Lie	8.97	3.80	6.8	4.14
Attraction	30.51	8.16	40.00	5.00
Estimation	15.51	6.50	25.00	5.00

Conversely, less than 5 percent of the patients scored a standard deviation below the mean on these psychological states and traits. Table 22-II and Figure 22-1 compares the patients' scores with normative values for selected psychological states and traits.

Due to the emotional lability of the patients, most of the group counselors at the SRC "intuitively" felt that the procedures involved for the preparation (blood sampling and skin abrasion) and administration of the exercise stress test would constitute a threatening and aversive experience. In other words, the SRC

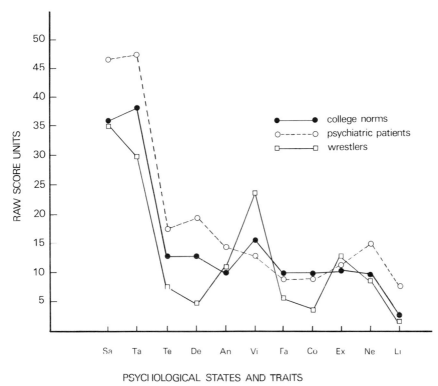

PSYCHOLOGICAL STATES AND TRAITS

Figure 22-1. Comparison of psychiatric patients with college norms and elite wrestlers for the following psychological states and traits: state anxiety (Sa); trait anxiety (Ta); tension (Te); depression (De); anger (An); vigor (Vi); fatigue (Fa); confusion (Co); extroversion (Ex); neuroticism (Ne); and conformity (Li).

staff was quite concerned whether these schizophrenic patients had sufficient defense mechanisms to cope with exercise stress test procedures. Since schizophrenics are characterized by distorted perceptions of reality and body image (3), the SRC staff thought that the anxiety associated with the preparatory procedures might cause some patients to decompensate. In point of fact, only 2 patients were unable to complete the exercise stress test: one patient became acutely paranoid and asked to leave; the other patient became extremely anxious. Both patients, however, had already completed the electrode placement procedures.

The expectation of an aversive psychological reaction to the stress testing procedures was not confirmed at both an observational and empirical level. Although the patients were characteristically functioning at a high level of trait anxiety ($\overline{X}$= 48.30; SD = 9.02), their degree of state anxiety remained fairly constant from 1 week prior to the test ($\overline{X}$= 47.14; SD = 1.73) to the day of their test ($\overline{X}$= 46.17; SD = 1.69). Since scores on the modified STAI range from a low of 4 to a high of 16, the mean score of the patients (8.4; SD = 2.46), recorded several minutes within the start of the exercise stress test, indicates that anticipation of the stress test did not cause an undue rise in anxiety states. Also, this state of emotional arousal was not accompanied by physiological manifestations of elevated resting heart rate or resting blood pressure (*see* Table 22-I). However, the patients were somewhat more anxious in anticipation of their test than a sample of adult males examined under similar circumstances (45).

Examination of the maximum aerobic capacities and maximum physiological responses of the patients to exercise stress demonstrates that their level of cardiovascular fitness compares favorably with published norms (44). Table 22-III shows that a functional maximum aerobic capacity of 10.9 METS was achieved with a corresponding mean maximum heart rate of 172 bpm and mean maximum blood pressure of 160/72 mmHg. The lack of an association between psychopathology and physical fitness is noteworthy since there is sufficient evidence to suggest that psychiatric patients possess low physical work capacities (23, 26, 43, 32). However, the patients attending the SRC may represent a distinct population (13). It may well be that these posthospitalized outpatients are in better physical condition than their hospitalized counterparts. Indeed, psychiatric patients with higher degrees of muscular endurance have been reported to experience shorter hospitalization (33) and (15) suggest that the physically active psychiatric patient has a better prognosis than sedentary patients.

TABLE 22-III
MAXIMUM PHYSIOLOGICAL RESPONSES OF THE PATIENT SAMPLE (N = 35)

Variable	Mean	SD
Maximum Heart Rate (bpm)	172.26	19.08
Maximum Systolic Blood Pressure (mmHg)	160.69	25.53
Maximum Diastolic Blood Pressure (mmHg)	72.29	15.06
Maximum Physical Work Capacity (METS)	10.90	1.93

While physical activity has been demonstrated to contribute towards positive mental health by reducing levels of anxiety (38, 42) and depression (7, 16), as well as increasing estimations of physical self-esteem (40), physically active individuals are not protected from psychiatric disturbances. Morgan (42) noted that physical activity can be a form of negative addiction, and Little (24, 25) reported that overevaluation of physical prowess can lead to psychological deterioration for individuals sustaining disabling injuries. Therefore, it was not surprising that a subsample of 7 high fit patients, with an average aerobic capacity of 13.4 METS, scored a standard deviation above the mean on measures of neuroticism, state anxiety, trait anxiety, and depression. However, all the high fit patients were males and a comparison of fitness level by sex ($F_{1,33}$ = 5.55, $p < .05$) revealed the females to possess a lower aerobic capacity than the males. At any rate, a causal relationship between exercise and mental health has not been demonstrated (41), and the psychological benefits of physical activity may be due to its diversional qualities (5).

Of particular relevance to this schizophrenic sample is the observation by Sonstroem (47) that feelings of security may be more related to how fit or healthy you *think* your body is as opposed to how fit or healthy your body *actually* is. It is thus interesting that despite having aerobic capacities similar to nonschizophrenic sedentary controls, the patients' estimation of their physical abilities was lower than that reported for samples of college students (11), prisoners (40), and police officers (37). Similarly, the patients' attraction toward physical activity was also lower than reported for these samples. Since a significant correlation (.32, $p < .05$) between self-estimation of physical ability and maximum aerobic capacity was found, the patients tended either to underestimate or distort their true performance capacities. This viewpoint concurs with Morgan's (31) conclusion that the psychiatric patients' physical condition may be more related to affective states than to actual physiological capacity. Table 22-IV compares the schizophrenics' scores for attraction toward physical activity and estimation of physical ability with values for the samples of college students, prisoners, and police officers.

Although schizophrenics may tend to distort estimates of their physical work capacity, their ability to read and process somatic cues regarding their level of exertion does not appreciably differ

TABLE 22-IV

PHYSICAL ESTIMATION AND ATTRACTION TOWARD
PHYSICAL ACTIVITY SCORES OF PSYCHIATRIC PATIENTS (N = 35),
MALE (N = 30) AND FEMALE (N = 30) COLLEGE STUDENTS,
PRISONERS (N = 54), AND POLICE OFFICERS (N = 77)

| | Estimation | | Attraction | |
Sample	Mean	SD	Mean	SD
Psychiatric Patients	15.51	6.50	30.51	8.16
Male College Students	25.40	5.26	41.13	5.12
Female College Students	26.13	5.39	41.13	5.14
Prisoners*	22.70	5.40	37.51	6.10
Police Officers	21.48	5.92	39.30	6.79

*Scores for the prisoners reflect the average of several subgroups reported by Morgan and Pollock (40).

from normals. The comparison of the schizophrenic patients' ratings of perceived exertion with a sample of nonschizophrenic controls was made with Ross's (45) study of adult males possessing behavior patterns Type A and Type B. A two-way repeated measures ANOVA failed to reveal group differences between patients and controls for their judgments of perceived exertion. Figure 22-2 shows, however, that a significant group by trials interaction ($F_{4,260} = 8.57, p < .05$) was obtained. While the patients initially rated their degree of exertion to be higher than the controls, subsequent ratings of perceived exertion were lower than control values as the exercise intensity increased. Post hoc analysis with Tukey's HSD test (20) demonstrated that differences in mean perceived exertion ratings were significant ($p < .05$) only for the initial stage of the stress test. This is apparent by the overlap of the standard error bands in Figure 22-2 for the remaining stages of the test. The difference in perceived exertion, at the beginning of the test, may have been due to the patients' inattention. With progressive work, however, the increased metabolic requirements, associated with increased ratings of perceived exertion ($F_{4,260} = 170.91, p < .05$) may have caused the patients to pay more attention to feedback from their bodies.

In view of the perceptual and cognitive distortion characteristic of schizophrenics (8, 9) as well as the likelihood of somatic delusions (18), these results are noteworthy. These findings suggest that psychopathology does not interfere with the judgment of perceived exertion and conflict with the expectation that psychiatric patients might distort ratings of perceived effort (35). An accurate perception of physical exertion suggests the possibility of a conflict-free area of ego functioning related directly to physiologi-

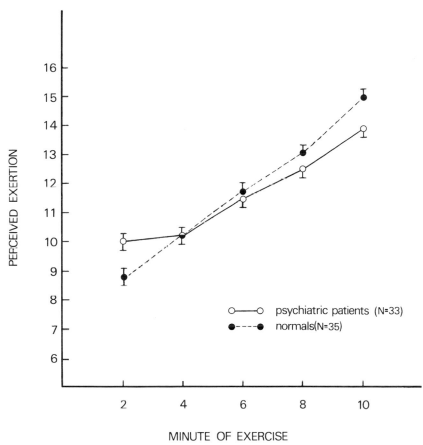

Figure 22-2. Mean (± SEM) perceived exertion ratings of psychiatric patients and normals.

cal stimuli, which is uncontaminated by cognitive disturbances. The implication of this data for treatment should be explored in further research.

REFERENCES

1. Akiskal, H.S. and McKinney, W.T.: Overview of recent research in depression. *Arch Gen Psychiatr, 32*:285, 1975.
2. American Psychiatric Association. *Diagnostic and Statistical Manual*–II. Washington, D.C., Am Psychiatric, 1978.
3. Arieti, S.: *Interpretation of Schizophrenia.* New York, Basic, 1974.
4. Balke, B. and Ware, R.W.: An experimental study of physical fitness of Air Force personnel. *US Armed Forces Med J, 10*:675, 1959.
5. Bahrke, M.S. and Morgan, W.P.: Anxiety reduction following exercise and meditation. *Cognitive Ther Res, 2*:323, 1978.

6. Borg, G.V. (Ed.).: Physical work and effort. In *Proceedings of the First International Symposium.* New York, Pergamon, 1977.
7. Brown, R.: The prescription of exercise for depression. *Phys Sportsmed, 6*:34, 1978.
8. Burnham, D.L.: Autonomy and activity passivity in the psychotherapy of a schizophrenic man. In H. Burton (Ed.): *Psychotherapy of the Psychoses.* New York, Basic, 1961.
9. Chapman, J.; Freeman, T.; and McGhie, A.: Clinical research on schizophrenia. *Br J Med Psychology, 32*:75, 1959.
10. Derogatis, L.R.: *Manual for the SCL-90 Symptom Checklist.* Baltimore, Md, John Hopkins U School Med, 1977.
11. Dishman, R.K.: Aerobic power, estimation of physical ability, and attraction to physical activity. *Res Q, 49*:285, 1978.
12. Eysenck, H.J. and Eysenck, S.B.: *Manual for the Eysenck Personality Questionnaire.* San Diego, Calif. Ed Industrial Testing Serv, 1975.
13. Fairweather, G.W.; Sanders, D.M.; Haywnard, H.; and Cressler, D.L.: *Community Life for the Mentally Ill: An alternative to community care.* New York, Aldine, 1969.
14. Freeman, T.: Symptomatology, diagnosis and clinical course. In L. Bellak and L. Loeb (Eds.): *The Schizophrenic Syndrome,* New York, Grune, 1979.
15. Gordon, H.L.; Rosenberg, D.; and Morris, E.E.: Leisure activities of schizophrenic patients after return to the community. *Ment Hygiene, 50*:452, 1966.
16. Griest, J.H.; Eischens, R.R.; Klein, M.H.; and Faris, J.W.: Antidepressant running. *Psychiatr Ann, 9*:23, 1979.
17. Hodgdon, R.E. and Reimer, D.: Some muscular strength and endurance scores of psychiatric patients. *J Assoc Physical Mental Rehab, 14*:38, 1960.
18. Jacobsen, E.: "Depersonalization." *J Am Psychoanal Assoc, 7*:581, 1959.
19. Jorstad, V.; Wilbert, D.E.; and Wirrer, B.: Sensory dysfunction in adult schizophrenia. *Hosp Community Psychiatry, 28*:280, 1977.
20. Kirk, R.E.: *Experimental Design: Procedures for the behavioral sciences.* Belmont, Wadsworth, 1978.
21. Kostrubala, T.: *The Joy of Running.* New York, Lippincott, 1976.
22. Levin, S.J. and Ross, M.A.: The effects of an aerobic exercise training program on psychiatric symptoms in schizophrenic outpatients, 1979 (in preparation).
23. Linton, J.M.; Hamelink, M.H.; and Hoskins, R.G.: Cardiovascular system in schizophrenia studied by the Schneider method. *Arch Neurol Psychiatry, 32*:712, 1934.
24. Little, J.C.: The athlete's neurosis—a deprivation crisis. *Acta Psychiatr Scand, 45*:187, 1969.
25. Little, J.C.: Neurotic illness in fitness fanatics. *Psychiatr Ann, 9*:50, 1979.
26. McFarland, R.A. and Huddelson, J.H.: Neurocirculatory reactions in the psychoneurosis studies by the schneider method. *Am J Psychiatr, 93*:956, 1936.
27. McNair, D.M.; Lorr, M.; and Droppleman, L.F.: *Manual for the Profile of Mood States.* San Diego, Calif, Industrial Testing Serv, 1971.

28. Meltzer, H.Y. and Engel, W.K.: Histochemical abnormalities of skeletal muscle in acutely psychotic patients, Part II. *Arch Gen Psychiatr, 23*:492, 1970.

29. Meltzer, H.Y.: Neuromuscular dysfunction in schizophrenia. *Schizophr Bull, 2*:106, 1976a.

30. Meltzer, H.Y.: Serum creatine phosphokinase in schizophrenia. *Am J Psychiatr, 133*:192, 1976b.

31. Morgan, W.P.: Selected physiological and psychomotor correlates of depression in psychiatric patients. *Res Q, 39*:1037, 1968.

32. Morgan, W.P.: A pilot investigation of physical working capacity in depressed and nondepressed psychiatric males. *Res Q, 40*:859, 1969.

33. Morgan, W.P.: Physical fitness correlates of psychiatric hospitalization. In G.S. Kenyon (Ed.): *Contemporary Psychology of Sport.* Chicago, Athletic Inst, 1970.

34. Morgan, W.P.: Psychological factors influencing perceived exertion. *Med Sci Sports, 5*:97, 1973.

35. Morgan, W.P. and Borg, G.V.: Perception of effort in the prescription of physical activity. In *The Humanistic and Mental Health Aspects of Sports, Exercise and Recreation,* Craig, T., ed., Chicago: AMA, 1976, p. 126.

36. Morgan, W.P.: Psychological consequences of vigorous physical activity and sport. In M.G. Scott (Ed.): *The Academy Papers.* Iowa City, Am Acad Physical Ed, 15, 1976.

37. Morgan, W.P.: *Influence of chronic physical activity on selected psychological states and traits of police officers* (Technical Report). Paper presented at International Association of Chiefs of Police, Inc., Gaithersburg, Md., 1976.

38. Morgan, W.P. and Horstman, D.H.: Anxiety reduction following acute physical activity. *Med Sci Sports, 8*:62, 1976.

39. Morgan, W.P.: Perception of effort in selected samples of Olympic athletes and soldiers. In G.V. Borg (Ed.): *Physical Work and Effort: Proceedings of the first international symposium.* New York, Pergamon, 1977.

40. Morgan, W.P. and Pollock, M.L.: Physical activity and cardiovascular health: Psychological aspects. In *Physical Activity and Human Well-Being,* Landry, F. and Orban, W., eds. Miami: Symposium Special, 1978, pp. 163-181.

41. Morgan, W.P.: Anxiety reduction following acute physical activity. *Psychiatr Ann, 9*:36, 1979.

42. Morgan, W.P.: Negative addiction in runners. *Phys Sportsmed,* 1979b.

43. Nadel, E.R. and Horvath, S.M.: Physiological responsiveness of schizoid adolescents to physical stress. *Int J Neuropsychiatr, 3*:191, 1965.

44. Nagle, F.J.: Physiological assessment of maximum performance. In *Exercise and Sport Sciences Review.* J. Wilmore, ed., New York, Acad Pr., 1972.

45. Ross, M.A.: The perception of effort in adult males possessing either the Type A or Type B behavior pattern. Unpublished dissertation, U. of Wis., 1977.

46. Solomon, E.G. and Bumpus, A.K.: The running meditation response: An adjunct to psychotherapy. *Am J Psychother, 32*:583, 1978.

47. Sonstroem, R.J. Physical estimation and attraction scales: Rationale and research. *Med Sci Sports, 10*:97, 1978.

48. Spielberger, C.D.; Gorsuch, R.L.; and Luschene, R.E.: *Manual for the State-*

Trait Anxiety Inventory. Palo Alto, Calif, Consulting Psychologists Press, 1970.

49. Whatmore, G.B. and Ellis, R.M.: Some neurophysiologic aspects of depressed states: An electromyography study. *Arch Gen Psychiatry, 1*:70, 1959.

Chapter 23

ALTERATIONS IN ANXIETY FOLLOWING EXERCISE AND REST

M.S. Bahrke

ANXIETY IS widely recognized as a major underlying cause for many physical and psychological illnesses. It has been reported that nearly 50 percent of all patients currently visiting their physician are doing so as a result of various kinds of stress (10). In addition, about 15 percent of the nation's adult population will consume a tranquilizer this year (9). Various therapies, such as biofeedback, drugs, hypnosis, meditation, exercise, and quiet rest have been employed in an attempt to cope with this stress. The question arises as to whether one procedure is more effective than another in reducing anxiety. In a recent investigation by Bahrke and Morgan (2) it was reported that acute physical activity, noncultic meditation, and quiet rest were all equally effective in reducing anxiety. However, an equally important question is that while the *quantity* of the decrement may be similar, the *quality* of the change may differ among the therapies. In other words, one procedure may reduce anxiety for a longer period of time than another.

It has been hypothesized that daily exercise results in anxiety reduction that is followed by a growth in anxiety across the subsequent 24 hour period (7). Hence, one of the major psychological benefits of exercise would be its ability to maintain a desired tension state. To this end, a recent investigation was conducted by Seemann (11) in order to assess the changes in anxiety following exercise over the ensuing 24 hour period. Seemann demonstrated a significant decrement in anxiety following exercise, followed by a gradual increase in anxiety that eventually returned to preexercise levels by the fifth hour following exercise. However, while Seemann was able to demonstrate anxiety reduction for a limited period following exercise, it may be possible that other therapies are similarly effective in reducing tension for a period of time following treatment. Therefore, the purpose of this investigation was to compare the time course of state anxiety across a 48 hour period following both acute exercise and quiet rest.

METHOD
Subjects

The subjects consisted of 30 regularly exercising adult male and female volunteers. Subjects' ages ranged between 22 and 65 years with a mean of 40.1 years. The mean height and weight of this sample were 172.7 cm (SD=7.8) and 73.6 kg (SD=14.6), respectively. The participants in the study were members of the University of Kansas Morning Adult Fitness Program.

Procedure

The experimental protocol was explained to each subject with the understanding that random assignment would be to either the exercise or the rest treatment. An informed consent document was signed and a 24 hour history dealing with consummatory behavior and activity during the previous day as well as general state of health was completed by each subject. Prior to being randomly assigned to a treatment, anxiety was assessed by completion of the 4 item STAI, the state scale of the complete STAI, and the trait scale of the STAI (12). The subjects completed the 4 item STAI immediately following each experimental treatment. The subjects were also instructed to complete a series of state anxiety inventories over the next 48 hour period. An envelope containing 7 state scales was given to each subject. Subjects were instructed to complete these forms (1) 30 minutes, (2) 2 hours, (3) 4 hours, (4) 8 hours, (5) 15 hours, (6) 24 hours, and (7) 48 hours following each experimental session. These forms were to be completed in a quiet environment free of distractions.

Treatment Conditions

Subjects in the rest group (N=15) sat quietly for 20 mintues in a comfortable rocking chair and were provided a current issue of the *Reader's Digest* to read during this period if they so desired. Heart rate was recorded using a HP-7712 Recorder with the final 15 seconds of each minute used to determine cardiac frequency. Electrodes for monitoring and recording heart rate were placed in a lead II position. Systolic and diastolic blood pressure were also measured before and following the session.

The exercise group (N=15) walked for 20 minutes on a motor-driven treadmill at 75 percent of their age-predicted maximal heart rate following 3 minutes of warm-up. Seventy-five percent of age-predicted maximal heart rate was based upon data compiled by Londeree and Moeschberger (3). A 3 minute cooldown followed each exercise bout. Heart rate was continuously monitored and recorded. As in the rest treatment, blood pressure was obtained prior to and shortly after the completion of exercise.

Means, standard deviations, and standard errors were computed for each variable. A series of 2 way repeated measures ANOVAs for state anxiety (4 item STAI and STAI X-1) across the 48 hour period, heart rate, and blood pressure was performed. The Newman-Keuls (13) procedure was employed where significant F ratios ($p < .05$) were observed.

RESULTS

Inspection of the data in Figure 23-1 indicates that state anxiety decreased immediately following both exercise and rest. However, a 2 way repeated measures ANOVA (13) demonstrated no significant decrease ($p < .05$) in state anxiety across time ($F=1.92$). No significant differences ($p < .05$) were demonstrated between groups ($F=0.29$) or for the interaction between time and group ($F=0.56$).

When both groups were combined and subjects were divided into high (N=7) and low (N=7) anxious categories based upon their initial level of trait anxiety, mean state anxiety values decreased but not significantly ($p < .05$) in both the high trait (8.0 to 7.7) and in the low trait anxious (5.0 to 4.4) subjects across time. In addition, evaluation of state anxiety responsivity in high (N=7) and low (N=7) state anxious subjects revealed that state anxiety decreased slightly for the high anxious (9.3 to 9.1) subjects and increased for the low anxious subjects (4.6 to 5.1). However, neither change was significant ($p < .05$).

The primary purpose of the present investigation was to compare the time course of state anxiety across a 48 hour period following acute physical activity and quiet rest. This represented a replication and extension of earlier research by Seemann (11). As illustrated in Figure 23-2, a small increase in state anxiety oc-

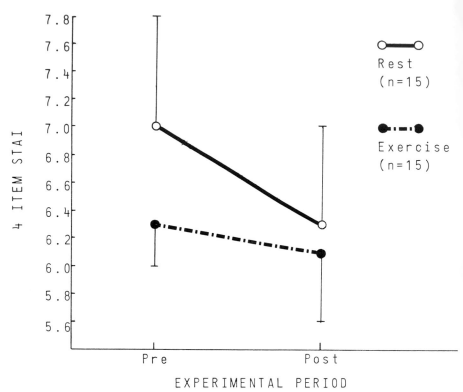

Figure 23-1. Four-item STAI scores before and immediately following exercise and rest.

curred 30 minutes following both exercise and rest. A nonsignificant increase in state anxiety took place over the next 15 hours following exercise, while a small increase took place at 2 hours following rest, and a nonsignificant decrease occurred by hour 15 following rest. This in turn was followed by a return to slightly below initial baseline values at 24 hours for both exercise and rest groups. Data are presented for only 6 subjects from the exercise group and 11 subjects from the rest group at 48 hours, owing to a decision by some subjects to exercise prior to this final assessment. A two-way repeated measures ANOVA failed to demonstrate a significant difference ($p < .05$) between the groups ($F=0.00$). Also, no significant differences were demonstrated across time ($F=0.49$) or for the interaction of time and group ($F=1.43$).

The response of heart rate to the two treatments is illustrated in Figure 23-3. A relatively constant heart rate occurred in each

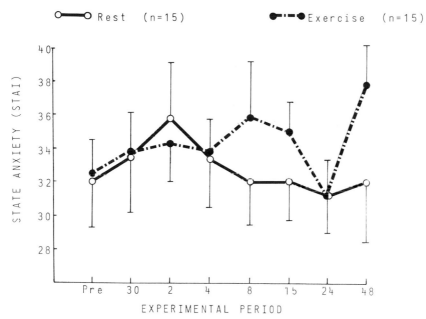

Figure 23-2. State anxiety before, ½ hour, 2 hours, 4 hours, 8 hours, 15 hours, 24 hours, and 48 hours following exercise and rest treatments.

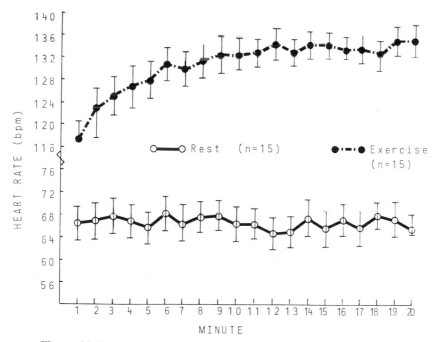

Figure 23-3. Heart rate in beats per minute during exercise and rest.

Exercise in Health and Disease

treatment. A 2 way repeated measures ANOVA demonstrated a significant difference ($p < .05$) between the 2 groups ($F=239.55$). A significant difference ($p < .05$) was also demonstrated across time for the 2 groups ($F=38.94$), and for the interaction of time and group ($p < .05$). This change across time and interaction was due to the increase in heart rate during the first 6 minutes for the exercise group. As noted in Figure 23-3, the exercise group achieved a steady state after the fifth minute of exercise. Heart rate in the rest group remained virtually unchanged during the rest period.

DISCUSSION

It has been demonstrated in a number of investigations that vigorous physical activity is followed by a decrease in state anxiety (1, 2, 4, 5, 8, 11). The results of the present study tend to support this expectation. Likewise, a reduction in anxiety following quiet rest was also seen. However, neither of these decreases were significant.

It is also important to note that high anxious individuals did not experience a significant reduction in state anxiety. This finding contrasts with results reported by Morgan (2, 5–8), which indicate a reduction in state anxiety not only for those falling within the normal range of anxiety but for those classified as high anxious as well. One possible explanation for these findings would be that the exercise intensity might need to be more vigorous in order to significantly reduce anxiety. In addition, the rest treatment may not have been conducive to deep relaxation. However, the heart rate response would support the notion that treatment was satisfactory in both groups. The exercise stimulus employed in the present study did require a vigorous level of activity (75% of age-predicted maximal heart rate). Furthermore, this workload was similar to that used by Bahrke and Morgan (2), a workload that resulted in a significant anxiety decrement. This issue has been discussed previously (2, 6, 7). A second possibility is that the average preexercise anxiety level was 0.5 standard deviation below the norm for both state and trait anxiety; therefore, it might be unreasonable to expect a significant shift in anxiety in those who were already low anxious.

State anxiety responsivity to exercise and rest over the following 48 hour period in the present study does not support the findings of Seemann (11). Seemann reported a significant decrease in state anxiety immediately following exercise with a gradual increase in anxiety to preexercise level by the fifth hour following exercise, remaining asymptomatic for the ensuing 24 hour period. Although a decrease in anxiety did occur immediately following exercise in the present investigation (although not significant), state anxiety *increased* during the next 30 minutes to 2 hours following both exercise and rest. Anxiety continued to increase following exercise over the next 15 hours, while anxiety decreased following rest over the same period of time. Both groups did return to pretreatment levels at 24 hours. It would probably be unwarranted to expect a significant shift in anxiety following treatment since the anxiety decrement immediately following both treatments was not significant.

It has been suggested that perhaps just taking "time out" or simple rest breaks may be effective in the management of anxiety. Moreover, it is possible that certain individuals unknowingly and routinely incorporate some type of diversional activity into their daily schedule, thus employing anxiety-reducing techniques throughout the course of the day. For example, the 4 hour time trial took place at approximately noon, lunchtime, or break time from the daily routine for most of the subjects. It is at this point that we see a small shift towards reduced anxiety levels. One subject related the solving of a complex laboratory problem during the course of the day, with the result being an appreciable reduction of his anxiety. On the other hand, the anxiety level of another subject was understandably elevated when informed during the day of a serious illness in his family. As a result it appears to be quite difficult to accurately assess the time-course of anxiety following exercise and rest since so many outside factors appear to be operating that influence the level of anxiety.

In the present study both the quantitative and qualititative aspects of anxiety reduction following exercise and rest were examined. The present data support the view that acute physical activity and quiet rest are associated with a reduction of state anxiety. However, the underlying cause for the reduction of anxiety following exercise and rest remains unanswered. Further, the results of the present inquiry indicate that exercise and rest have very little influence on state anxiety over the ensuing 48 hour period. In addition, anxiety levels following both rest and exercise did not differ significantly at any point during this same 48 hour period.

REFERENCES

1. Bahrke, M.S.: Exercise, meditation and anxiety reduction: a review. *Am Corr Ther J, 33*:41, 1979.
2. Bahrke, M.S. and Morgan, W.P.: Anxiety reduction following exercise and meditation. *Cognitive Ther Res, 2*:323, 1978.
3. Londeree, B.R. and Moeschberger, M.L.: Effect of age and other factors on maximal heart rate. (In press).
4. Mitchum, M.L.: *The effect of participation in a physically exerting leisure activity on state anxiety level.* Master's Thesis, Florida State University, 1976.
5. Morgan, W.P.: Influence of acute physical activity on state anxiety. In *Proceedings of the National College Physical Education Association for Men.* January, 1973. Minneapolis: National College Physical Education Association for Men, pp. 113-121.
6. Morgan, W.P.: Anxiety reduction following acute physical activity. *Psychiatric Annals, 9*:36, 1979.
7. Morgan, W.P.: Use of exercise as a relaxation technique. In *Proceedings of the Second National Conference on Emotional Stress and Heart Disease.* Hendricks, J.H., ed., Columbia, S.C.: South Carolina Heart Association, 1979, pp. 596-601.
8. Morgan, W.P. and Horstman, D.H.: Anxiety reduction following acute physical activity. *Med Sci Sports, 8*:62, 1976.
9. New and refill prescriptions. *Pharmacy Times, 44*:41, April, 1978.
10. Pitts, F.N.: The biochemistry of anxiety. *Sci Am, 220*:69, 1969.
11. Seemann, J.C.: *Changes in state anxiety following vigorous exercise.* Master's Thesis, University of Arizona, 1978.
12. Spielberger, C.D.; Gorsuch, R.L.; and Lushene, R.E.: *Manual for the State-Trait Anxiety Inventory.* Palo Alto, Calif, Consulting Psychologists Press, 1970.
13. Winer, B.J.: *Statistical Principles in Experimental Design.* New York, McGraw, 1971.

Chapter 24

PSYCHOLOGICAL BENEFITS OF PHYSICAL ACTIVITY

W.P. MORGAN

INTRODUCTION

THIS CHAPTER will review the existing literature dealing with the psychological benefits of physical activity. Special attention will be paid to the potential role of exercise in prevention and restoration of psychopathologic states where possible. Prior to beginning the general discussion of this topic, it would appear necessary to delimit the review. First, personality is usually taken to mean the sum or totality of an individual's psychological states and traits. The distinction between state and trait psychology with special reference to exercise and sport has been reviewed extensively in several recent papers (36–38, 40), and therefore, this matter will not be discussed in the present chapter. The actual review, however, will deal primarily with affective measures such as anxiety and depression and, to a far lesser degree, with psychological traits—the primary reason for this decision is that traits are regarded as relatively enduring features of one's personality structure and, as such, not readily amenable to change.

It will also be necessary to delimit the topic of exercise since it is possible to include various activities under the exercise rubric. Physical activities performed at various metabolic costs (e.g. light, moderate, or heavy) such as (i) walking, cycling, swimming, and running, (ii) competitive or noncompetitive recreational activities (e.g. bowling, golf or tennis), and (iii) highly competitive team or individual sports (e.g. football, baseball, or track and field athletics) can all be subsumed under the rubric of exercise. These exercises can also be approached from the standpoint of age, which brings into consideration such seemingly diverse activities as "little league" or "age group" baseball, football, soccer, and

299

swimming, as well as "master's competition" in various sports. The psychological consequences of sport have been reviewed in several papers (20, 32, 36, 38–40); therefore, this topic will not be addressed in the present chapter.

The existing research involving the psychological consequences of physical activity per se has utilized either young or middle-aged adults as subjects. Indeed, research involving the psychological benefits of exercise on the elderly is almost nonexistent. The present review, therefore, will deal primarily with the influence of noncompetitive physical activity on selected psychological states of young and middle-aged adults. Occasional reference will be made to psychological traits and sport per se where necessary, but these particular topics have intentionally not been addressed in detail since they have been covered in other reviews.

Much of the research conducted in this area of inquiry has been characterized by statistical and design inelegancies. First, much of the work has been cross-sectional rather than longitudinal, and this has eliminated causal attribution. Second, most of the available investigations did not employ control groups, much less placebo groups (35), and these are simply imperative in order to quantify Hawthorne effects (i.e. any treatment versus no treatment).

METHODOLOGICAL CONSIDERATIONS

Prior to proceeding directly to a review of the literature dealing with the psychological beneficence of physical activity it would appear appropriate to first comment on selected methodological considerations, which must be considered in evaluating the available literature. The intent of this brief section is to highlight some of the more fundamental or basic considerations.

It is imperative that control groups be employed in research dealing with the psychologic effects of exercise. While this may seem rather obvious, most of the studies to be reviewed in the following sections have not relied upon such a "design strategy." Also, use of a control group in such experimentation should be viewed as a *necessary* not a *sufficient* design consideration. It is equally important, indeed, it is imperative, that a placebo group or sham strategy be routinely employed. Numerous behavioral artifacts are permitted to profoundly influence one's interpretations of results otherwise.

The types of behavioral artifacts referred to are demand characteristics, compliance, "pact of ignorance," response distortion, halo effect, Hawthorne effect, and so on (35, 43). There are various ways in which these behavioral artifacts can be minimized or evaluated, such as use of appropriate experimental designs, sampling procedures, and statistical models; single, double, and/or total blinds; placebo or sham conditions; debriefing; cross-over and counterbalancing procedures; "hold-out" controls where necessary; and so on (35).

The importance of adopting such design strategies is readily reinforced in contemporary literature. For example, it has been demonstrated by Michaels et al. (23) that transcendental meditation (TM) is *associated* with a decrement in circulating plasma catecholamines, which are known to be related to anxiety. Hence, it would be easy to jump to the conclusion that TM *causes* anxiety or catecholamines to decrease. However, the control group experienced a comparable decrement in catecholamine levels. This, of course, raises the classic question of causality and forces one to conclude that while TM may reduce plasma epinephrine and norepinephrine, it is no more effective than simple rest in a quiet room.

The results of Michaels et al. (23) have recently been supported by investigators employing substantially different procedures. de Vries et al. (10), for example, reported that a simple rest break was just as effective as biofeedback in reducing tension. Tension was measured electromyographically by de Vries et al. (10). In a somewhat related experiment, Bahrke and Morgan (1) found that a control group of subjects who rested quietly in a sound-filtered room experienced a decrement in state anxiety comparable to decreases observed following acute physical activity or noncultic meditation. State anxiety was measured with a standardized self-report inventory (STAI) in this study.

These investigations demonstrate that transcendental meditation (23), biofeedback (10), exercise (1), and noncultic meditation (1) are all capable of reducing anxiety. It is also noteworthy that this finding applies to anxiety whether it is defined biochemically (23), neurophysiologically (10), or in a traditional psychometric sense (1). More importantly, however, is the serendipitous observation that a quiet rest is just as effective as more sophisticated procedures.

It has been reported by Kavanagh et al. (21) that post–myocardial infarction patients who participated in a physical activity program experienced significant physiological gains, but these gains did not surpass those of a sedentary group who practiced a form of autohypnosis. In other words, a presumed placebo treatment was just as effective as exercise. The placebo effect, however, can be just as effective as potent pharmacologic agents or even surgery in the reduction of pain (35).

The report by Chien (6) should be regarded as required reading for any investigator contemplating psychological research with older individuals. Chien (6) assigned 40 patients who lived on a geriatric ward to 1 of 4 groups. One group was administered the drug thioridazine, a popular psychotropic drug treatment in geriatric settings, and the remaining three groups received a beverage in a specially designed "pub" situated in the hospital. These groups received either beer, fruit punch, or fruit punch with thioridazine in the pub setting 5 days per week for a 9 week period. Social interaction (sociotherapy) was encouraged in the pub setting, and each session lasted for 1 hour. The greatest psychological improvement resulted from "beer sociotherapy," and while both drug groups improved, their improvement was not as great as the group receiving beer. In other words, "beer sociotherapy" was found to be superior to an already established drug therapy. The "punch-in-the-pub," or placebo, group received the smallest amount of change.

Chien's (6) work might be considered by those exercise scientists who, for reasons not yet specified, imply that physical activity is inherently capable of achieving results not possible by more "traditional" procedures. If one is willing to accept the results presented earlier (3, 54, 58) suggesting improved psychological states in older individuals as a consequence of chronic exercise, a reasonable question would seem to be, "Would these gains equal or exceed those of a sedentary group receiving 'beer sociotherapy' in place of exercise?"

Some of the basic considerations that must be made in evaluating research designed to study the psychological effects of exercise have been identified. The importance of these considerations will become apparent in the next section. While the present discussion has been limited to behavioral artifacts of a self-report nature, it should be emphasized that test subjects can also comply at a biological level. For example, resting and exercise heart rate, blood pressure, oxygen consumption, skin temperature, muscle tension levels, catecholamine levels, and even amine metabolites in the cerebrospinal fluid (1, 10, 21, 23, 42, 53) can be modified by most compliant individuals. In other words, physiologic, as well as psychologic, parameters are subject to artifactual responsivity.

BENEFICIENCE OF PHYSICAL ACTIVITY

The psychological benefits of involvement in physical activity have been studied primarily from the standpoint of long-term or chronic effects. These investigations have typically ranged from 6 weeks to several months, but shorter as well as longer time periods have occasionally been employed. While the immediate or acute physiological effects of exercise have been studied extensively, there has been very little attention paid to the psychological effects of acute physical activity. It may well be that acute or transitory psychological effects occur in the absence of chronic effects. Daily exercise, for example, may have the primary effect of reducing tension states or anxiety in an episodic manner with the result that chronic changes are not observed. If this, in fact, were the case, then the chief psychologic benefit of exercise would reside in its preventive powers. The present review will consider research that has utilized both acute and chronic paradigms.

As mentioned earlier, there have been quite a few investigations involving comparisons of athletes and nonathletes, but this particular research will not be addressed in the present chapter since most of these studies have been cross-sectional in nature. It is noteworthy, however, that athletes have consistently been found to possess more favorable psychological profiles than nonathletes from the standpoint of mental health (20, 36, 38, 40, 43, 46, 47). The issue of causality has seldom, however, been studied in this earlier research. In other words, do athletes and nonathletes differ from the outset, or does involvement in sport produce psychological change? This question has been addressed in earlier papers, but it remains unanswered (36, 40).

Acute Effects

There has been very little research involving the psychological effect of acute physical activity, and the limited existing research has been concerned with anxiety. The prevalence of anxiety states in both the general and psychiatric populations (1, 37, 42, 51, 52) suggests that the effect of exercise on anxiety warrants attention. Also, it has been proposed by Pitts and McClure (51) and Pitts (52) that acute physical activity will produce anxiety symptoms and anxiety attacks in persons suffering from anxiety neurosis, as well as normal individuals under certain circumstances. The fallacy of the Pitts-McClure hypothesis, however, has been challenged in several subsequent publications (8–10, 13, 15, 37, 38, 48, 55, 59).

One of the first investigators to examine the effect of physical activity was Byrd (4) who reported that bowling produced a reduction in tension as measured by a self-report inventory. This particular investigation was characterized by numberous design flaws, and even if bowling did "cause" the reduction in anxiety it was probably due to the *diversional* impact of the activity not exercise per se.

In a series of well-controlled investigations by de Vries and his associates (8, 9) it has been demonstrated that both acute and chronic physical activity of a vigorous nature produces a reduction in tension as measured electromyographically. Furthermore, in one of these studies (9), exercise was found to be superior to a commonly employed tranquilizer (meprobamate) in reducing anxiety (i.e. resting EMG). It is well known, of course, that other seemingly diverse "inactive" therapies involving techniques such as progressive relaxation, biofeedback, meditation, and hypnosis are also capable of reducing anxiety, and this is true whether anxiety is measured electromyographically or psychometrically.

One of the most frequently prescribed exercise therapies employed by physicians has been walking (5). Morgan et al. (34) tested the effect of walking 1 mile at 3.5 mph on the state anxiety of young adult males and females. The subjects were randomly assigned to exercise groups that walked on level grade or 5 percent grade, and their responses were compared with those of a control group consisting of subjects who simply rested quietly in the supine position. The control, 0 percent grade, and 5 percent grade walks resulted in heart rates of 73, 126, and 144 bpm, respectively, for the women, and 69, 111, and 125 for the men. This particular experiment did not demonstrate an exercise effect on anxiety. One possible explanation would be that exercise might need to be more vigorous in order to demonstrate an effect. A second possibility would be that the anxiety scale employed in this investigation, the IPAT 8-Parallel-Anxiety Battery, was not sensitive to changes since it appears to be more of a trait than a state measure. On the other hand, shifts in anxiety consistently have been demonstrated with this instrument under a variety of circumstances (31, 32, 38).

Sime's (57) recent research indicating that light exercise does not modify state anxiety corroborates the earlier work of Morgan et al. (34) reported above. It is also noteworthy that Sime (57) employed a more universally accepted measure of state anxiety, the STAI. These reports (34, 57) seem to suggest that exercise of a light nature does not alter state anxiety.

A series of investigations dealing with exercise performed at 70 to 80 percent of $\dot{V}O_2$max have now been completed, and these investigations reveal that state anxiety is consistently decreased following such exercise (37, 40, 45). In other words, it appears that exercise must be of a fairly high intensity in order to provoke decrements in anxiety. It should be emphasized, however, that meditation, both cultic (23) and noncultic (1), "time out" therapy (1), and simple rest breaks (10) are also capable of reducing circulating catecholamines, electromyographic activity, oxygen consumption, heart rate, and self-report measures of anxiety. These findings have special relevance from an applied standpoint since certain therapies, for a variety of reasons, are often contraindicated in the case of specific individuals.

Partial support for the research described above (37, 40, 45) has recently been presented by Wood (59) who administered the state anxiety scale (STAI) to college males and females before and following a 12 minute run test. The males (n = 62) experienced a significant reduction in state anxiety, whereas the females (n = 44) did not. These results were in disagreement with those of Morgan (37) who reported a significant decrement in state anxiety for both adult males and females following vigorous physical activity. It also appears that Wood's (59) study may have suffered from behavioral and/or statistical artifacts since a subsidiary analysis described in his paper reveals that high and low anxious males and females regressed toward the mean following the exercise treatment.

Exercise has been successfully employed by Orwin (50) to treat agoraphobia, as well as a specific phobia. It appears that the anxiety response is inhibited as a result of the exercise-induced autonomic arousal "competing" with the anxiety reaction. Driscoll (11) has compared the efficacy of systematic desensitization and exercise plus "pleasant fantasies" in their ability to reduce anxiety. The two procedures were found to be comparable. While exercise or fantasy alone produced a decrement in anxiety as well, the decrease was not as great as that produced with exercise and fantasy combined.

None of the investigations reviewed to this point attempted to evaluate the time course of anxiety changes observed following acute physical activity. A recent attempt to clarify this issue has yielded some interesting results. Seemann (55) evaluated the state anxiety of middle-aged men and women before and following aerobic jogging for approximately 45 minutes. Both groups experienced a significant decrement in state anxiety following acute physical activity, which is in agreement with the earlier research described above (37, 40, 45). Seemann (55) also evaluated the state anxiety of these subjects across the following 24 hour period, and it was observed that anxiety gradually returned to the baseline levels within 4 to 6 hours in both groups. In other words, the tension reduction associated with this vigorous exercise was found to last for about 4 to 6 hours on the average. This finding suggests that one of the major benefits of regular exercise may reside in its ability to reduce anxiety on a daily basis and, hence, *prevent* the development of chronic anxiety.

Chronic Effects

There is a great deal of evidence available concerning the physiological effect of chronic physical activity, but there is very little evidence on the psychological consequences (40–42). It is widely reported by investigators who work in this field that individuals report an increased sense of well-being following the adoption of an exercise program (28, 33, 42). The "feeling better" sensation that accompanies regular physical activity is so obvious that it is one of the few universally accepted benefits of exercise. Indeed, individuals who themselves do not exercise will readily admit that exercise "is good for you!"

Despite the absence of a substantial experimental literature supporting the value of physical activity in the prevention and restoration of psychopathologic states, there are a number of indirect and theoretical bases for suggesting that chronic exercise possesses psychologic beneficence. First, if one accepts the totality of mind and body, it is not difficult to accept that psychic or somatic health or disease are likely to influence one another. To the extent that exercise improves physical health, and there is considerable evidence to suggest that it does (7, 8, 14, 21, 49, 61), a concurrent improvement in, or maintenance of, mental health should follow. The unity of mind and body is such, of course, that it is only one's vantage point that permits a distinction between the two.

In addition to the theoretical basis for the belief that chronic exercise possesses psychologic beneficence, there is a substantial amount of correlational evidence in this area (18, 19, 28, 40, 56, 60, 61). While such evidence cannot be offered as causal support, the relationship is consonant with theoretical expectations.

While former athletes and nonathletes appear to be more alike from the standpoint of general health and longevity (24), it is of interest that athletes consistently have been found to possess more desirable mental health profiles than nonathletes (20, 36, 38, 40). These reported differences, while consistent and statistically significant, have not been of a remarkable magnitude. Also, it is of further interest that former athletes have been found to possess more favorable *attitudes* toward physical activity and greater *estimates* of physical ability than nonathletes, but their *actual* levels of physical activity and aerobic power have been reported to be comparable (40, 44).

Psychiatric patients have consistently been found to score low on standard measures of physical fitness (25, 27–29, 33, 39), but there is not a consensus on the issue of whether or not degree of psychopathology is related to physical fitness (25, 27–29). On the other hand, it has been demonstrated that level of physical fitness at the time of admission to a psychiatric facility is inversely related to length of hospitalization (30); that is, the higher the muscular endurance and strength at the outset, the shorter the duration of stay.

There is also evidence that hyperponesis or heightened muscle tension levels increases as a function of psychopathology (26). In other words, hyperponetic states are more common in anxious, neurotic, or depressed patients than in normal individuals or even patients not suffering from these particular problems. Since there is considerable evidence suggesting that either acute or chronic exercise decreases resting muscle tension levels (8, 9), it is reasonable to *predict* that exercise would improve behavioral states such as anxiety and depression.

In addition to the theoretical, correlative, and epidemiologic reports summarized above, there have also been a number of experimental investigations conducted over the past 10 years that addressed the issue of whether or not chronic exercise would produce improvements in psychologic states. These investigations will now be summarized and critiqued.

One of the first experiments was conducted at the University of Missouri, and it involved the influence of various physical activity programs on the level of depression in adult males (33). While approximately 85 percent of the individuals who exercised reported an improved *sense of well-being,* none of the groups differed significantly from the control group on depression as measured by Zung's Self-Rating Depression Scale. It was found, however, that a significant ($p < .01$) reduction in depression occurred for those individuals (n = 11) who were clinically depressed (SDS = 50>) from the outset.

The finding that psychological changes did not occur in those individuals who scored within the normal range on the SDS should not be surprising. This observation was in agreement with an earlier report by Naughton et al. (49) who found that daily exercise for a period of 1 hour did not alter the MMPI profiles of their subjects following 6 months of exercise.

In a more recent report by Kavanagh et al. (22), the MMPI was administered to patients between 16 and 18 months following myocardial infarction, and those with severe depression were studied for 2 to 4 years. Those patients, who took part in a regular running program, experienced a significant improvement in depression as measured by the MMPI scale. The improvement in depression was not accompanied by alterations in other MMPI scores. Therefore, it is quite possible that the decrement in depression represented chance alone, or it may have reflected the course of recovery per se rather than an exercise-induced effect. As with most research in this area, however, adequate controls were not employed.

The psychological effect of participating in a jogging program was evaluated in college students by Folkins et al. (12). The psychological measures were performed at the beginning and conclusion of a semester-long course, and comparisons were made with a control group of subjects enrolled in archery or golf courses. Significant improvements in anxiety and depression accompanied gains in physical fitness for women in the jogging program, but changes were not observed for the men. The changes for the women may have represented statistical regression since they scored significantly higher than the controls from the very outset on the various psychological measures. At any rate, there is no evidence presented to suggest that exercise *caused* the improvement in psychological state.

In a similar investigation Sharp and Reilley (56) administered the MMPI to 65 male students before and after an aerobics conditioning class that met twice a week for 45 minutes per session. The length of the course was not specified, and it is not clear whether or not an actual physiological training effect resulted. However, correlative data were presented relative to change scores, and the authors stated that ". . . changes in aerobic physical fitness are related to score changes on selected scales of the MMPI for college males who participated in an aerobic exercise program" (p. 430). The statistical analysis employed in this study (i.e. 160 bivariate r's) makes it very difficult to interpret the psychologic effect of the aerobics program. However, the present investigation, like most others in this area, did not employ a control or placebo group; therefore, the issue of causality cannot even be entertained.

A frequently cited investigation in this field is the paper by Ismail and Trachtman (16), who reported that middle-aged men who embarked on a regular exercise program experienced an alteration in their personality as measured by the 16 PF. However, it would be hazardous to suggest that exercise *caused* the change in personality since neither a control nor placebo group was employed for comparison purposes. Also, Ismail and Trachtman (16) made no attempt to evaluate response distortion in their study. Deceptive subjects can not only fake behavioral self-report measures such as the 16 PF with ease (43), but it has also been shown that simulation can actually result in biological alterations as mentioned earlier.

The Cattell 16 PF test was administered by Ismail and Young (17) to 56 middle-aged subjects before and following a 4 month physical fitness program. These authors feel that their results "tend to suggest that the physical fitness program helps in stabilizing the factors affecting personality" (p. 56). Employing the phrase "tend to suggest" is certainly appropriate since there were no controls with which to draw comparisons. It might be argued, of course, that these subjects served as their own controls. While such an argument is acceptable for certain experimental designs, it does not appear to be appropriate in the present case. The same criticism can be leveled at subsequent papers (18, 19, 60). These investigations, in the author's opinion, have been characterized by biologic, psychometric, and statistical rigor of what appears to be the highest order. Furthermore, these writers themselves do not argue vigorously that exercise causes personality to change; rather, they suggest that factor structures change following chronic exercise. Nevertheless, the implication has been that exercise causes personality to change, and that has not been possible to convincingly demonstrate with the designs employed in the aforementioned studies (16–19, 60).

Anxiety and depression has been reported by Folkins (13) to decrease significantly in a group of adult males who exercised 3 days per week for 12 weeks. These individuals had previously been judged to be high-risk from a coronary risk factor perspective, and they were matched by age, occupation, and risk factors with a group of nonexercise controls. The control group did not change on any of the psychological variables measured. Also, it is noteworthy that the exercise group only changed on 2 of the 5 measures. Alterations in self-confidence, adjustment, and body image did not occur. These findings suggest that chronic exercise was *associated* with a reduction in anxiety and depression, but there is no way of evaluating whether or not the exercise program *caused* the change. Use of a placebo group, in addition to the control group, would have been preferred.

It has been reported by Buccola and Stone (3) that a group of men ranging in age from 60 to 79 years experienced a change on 2 of the factors of the 16 PF Inventory following a walk-jog program. Exercise was performed 3 days per week for 14 weeks. A group of subjects in the same study participated in a cycling program, and while they experienced physiological changes similar to those of the walk-jog group, they did not experience psychological changes. Therefore, exercise per se must not have been responsible for the changes observed in the walk-jog group. In view of the fact that only 2 of the multiple comparisons were significant, these changes may have been due to chance alone. Also, since appropriate control groups were not employed, it is difficult to evaluate the meaningfulness of these observations. In other words, both groups might have improved significantly on a number of variables, but there would be no way of determining whether this was due to the (i) exercise programs, (ii) special attention effect (35), or (iii) interaction of both of these forces.

A recent investigation has been described by Griest et al. (14) in which a unique experimental design was employed. Thirteen men and 15 women patients who sought treatment for neurotic or reactive depression were randomly assigned to running therapy, time-limited psychotherapy, or time-unlimited psychotherapy. The findings revealed that running was just as effective as psychotherapy in the treatment of moderate depression. In other words, rather than comparing the effect of exercise with a control group (i.e. "any treatment" versus "no treatment" paradigm) or no group at all, an attempt was made to quantify exercise effects within the context of more traditional therapies. Running was found to be just as effective as psychotherapy in the treatment of young men and women with *moderate* depression in this study.

SUMMARY

In the present chapter an attempt has been made to summarize the existing literature dealing with the influence of exercise on personality. Theoretical, correlational, epidemiologic, and experimental evidence have been presented. While most of this literature suggests that exercise, both acute and chronic, is *associated* with an improved psychological state, there has been no attempt to identify the *mechanisms* underlying such improvement. The tacit assumption in most of the experimental research has been that exercise was responsible for, or *caused*, the observed changes. Such an assumption, however, must be regarded as questionable in light of the fact that quasi-experimental designs have been the rule. If, in fact, this research had been conducted with acceptable designs, it would remain rather difficult to address the *why* of the matter. The challenge for future investigators in this area will be to adopt rigorous research designs, and it is suggested that answers to the question of "why exercise improves affect" will be found at a biochemical and neurophysiological level.

312   *Exercise in Health and Disease*

REFERENCES

1. Bahrke, M.S. and Morgan, W.P.: Anxiety reduction following exercise and meditation. *Cognitive Ther Res, 2*:323, 1978.
2. Brown, R.S.; Ramirez, D.E.; and Taub, J.M.: The prescription of exercise for depression. *Phys Sportsmed, 6*:35, 1978.
3. Buccola, V.A. and Stone, W.J.: Effects of jogging and cycling programs on physiological and personality variables in aged men. *Res Q, 46*:134, 1975.
4. Byrd, O.E.: Viewpoints of bowlers in respect to the relief of tension. *Phys Educ, 21*:119, 1964.
5. Byrd, O.E.: The relief of tension by exercise: A survey of medical viewpoints and practices. *J Sch Health, 42*:238, 1963.
6. Chien, C.P.: Psychiatric treatments for geriatric patients: "Pub" or drug? *Am J Psychiatr, 127*:1070, 1971.
7. Clarke, H.H. (Ed.): Exercise and aging. *Phy Fit Res Dig, 7*:1, 1977.
8. deVries, H.A.: Immediate and long term effects of exercise upon resting muscle action potential. *J Sports Med, 8*:1, 1968.
9. deVries, H.A. and Adams, G.M.: Electromyographic comparison of single doses of exercise and meprobamate as to effects on muscular relaxation. *Am J Phys Med, 51*:130, 1972.
10. deVries, H.A.; Burke, R.K.; Hopper, R.T.; and Sloan, J.H.: Efficacy of EMG biofeedback in relaxation training. *Am J Phys Med, 56*:75, 1977.
11. Driscoll, R.: Anxiety reduction using physical exertion and positive images. *Psychol Record, 26*:87, 1976.
12. Folkins, C.H.; Lynch, S.; and Gardner, M.M.: Psychological fitness as a function of physical fitness. *Arch Phys Med Rehabil, 53*:503, 1972.
13. Folkins, C.H.: Effects of physical training on mood. *J Clin Psychol, 32*:385, 1976.
14. Greist, J.H.; Klein, M.H.; Eischens, R.R.; Faris, J.; Gurman, A.S.; and Morgan, W.P.: Running as treatment for depression. *Compr Psychiatry, 20*:41, 1979.
15. Grosz, H.J. and Farmer, B.B.: Blood lactate in the development of anxiety symptoms. *Arch Gen Psychiatry, 21*:611, 1969.
16. Ismail, A.H. and Trachtman, L.E.: Jogging the imagination. *Psychol Today, 6*:78, 1973.
17. Ismail, A.H. and Young, R.J.: The effect of chronic exercise on the personality of middle-aged men by univariate and multivariate approaches. *J Hum Ergol (Tokyo), 2*:47, 1973.
18. Ismail, A.H. and Young, R.J.: Influence of physical fitness on second- and third-order personality factors using orthogonal and oblique rotations. *J Clin Psychol, 32*:268, 1976.
19. Ismail, A.H. and Young, R.J.: Effect of chronic exercise on the multivariate relationships between selected biochemical and personality variables. *Multivariate Behav Res, 12*:49, 1977.
20. Johnson, R.W. and Morgan, W.P.: Personality characteristics of college athletes. (In preparation).
21. Kavanagh, T.; Shephard, R.J.; Pandit, B.; and Doney, H.: Exercise and

hypnotherapy in the rehabilitation of the coronary patient. *Arch Phys Med Rehabil, 51*:578, 1970.

22. Kavanagh, T.; Shephard, R.J.; and Tuck, J.A.: Depression after myocardial infarction. *Can Med Assoc J, 113*:23, 1975.

23. Michaels, R.R.; Huber, M.J.; and McCann, D.S.: Evaluation of transcendental meditation as a method of reducing stress. *Science, 192*:1242, 1976.

24. Montoye, H.J.: Health and longevity of former athletes. In *Science and Medicine of Exercise and Sports,* edited by W.R. Johnson and E.R. Buskirk. New York, Har-Row, 1974.

25. Morgan, W.P.: Selected physiological and psychomotor correlates of depression in psychiatric patients. *Res Q, 39*:1037, 1968.

26. Morgan, W.P.: Hyperponetic states and psychopathology: A review. *Am Correct Ther J, 22*:165, 1968.

27. Morgan, W.P.: A pilot investigation of physical working capacity in depressed and nondepressed psychiatric males. *Res Q, 40*:859, 1969.

28. Morgan, W.P.: Physical fitness and emotional health: A review. *Am Correct Ther J, 23*:124, 1969.

29. Morgan, W.P.: Physical working capacity in depressed and nondepressed psychiatric females. *Am Correct Ther J, 24*:14, 1970.

30. Morgan, W.P.: Physical fitness correlates of psychiatric hospitalization. In *Contemporary Psychology of Sport,* edited by G.S. Kenyon. Chicago, Athletic Inst, 1970.

31. Morgan, W.P.: Psychological effect of weight reduction in the college wrestler. *Med Sci Sports, 2*:24, 1970.

32. Morgan, W.P.: Pre-match anxiety in a group of college wrestlers. *Int J Sport Psy, 1·7,* 1970.

33. Morgan, W.P.; Roberts, J.A.; Brand, F.R.; and Feinerman, A.D.: Psychological effect of chronic physical activity. *Med Sci Sports, 2*:213, 1971.

34. Morgan, W.P.; Roberts, J.A.; and Feinerman, A.D.: Psychologic effect of acute physical activity. *Arch Phys Med Rehabil, 52*:442, 1971.

35. Morgan, W.P.: Basic considerations. In *Ergogenic Aids and Muscular Performance,* edited by W.P. Morgan. New York, Acad Pr, 1972.

36. Morgan, W.P.: Sport psychology. In *Psychomotor Domain: Movement Behavior,* edited by R.N. Singer. Philadelphia, Lea & Febiger, 1972.

37. Morgan, W.P.: Influence of acute physical activity on state anxiety. In *Proceedings of the College Physical Education Association.* Pittsburgh, 1973.

38. Morgan, W.P. and Hammer, W.M.: Influence of competitive wrestling upon state anxiety. *Med Sci Sports, 6*:58, 1974.

39. Morgan, W.P.: Exercise and mental disorders. In *Sport Medicine,* edited by A.J. Ryan and F.L. Allman, Jr. New York, Acad Pr, 1974.

40. Morgan, W.P.: Psychological consequences of vigorous physical activity and sport. In *The Academy Papers,* edited by M.G. Scott. Iowa City, Am Acad Phy Educ, 1976.

41. Morgan, W.P.: *Influence of chronic physical activity on selected psychological states and traits of police officers.* Technical Report. Int Assoc Chiefs Police, Gaithersburg, MD, 1976.

42. Morgan, W.P. and Pollock, M.L.: Physical activity and cardiovascular health:

314 *Exercise in Health and Disease*

Psychological aspects. In *Physical Activity and Human Well-being*, edited by F. Landry and W.A.R. Orban. Miami, Symposia Special, 1978.

43. Morgan, W.P.: Sport personology: The credulous-skeptical argument in perspective. *Proceedings of the 3rd Symposium on Integrative Development*, edited by A.H. Ismail. Indianapolis, Indiana State Board of Health, 1977.

44. Morgan, W.P. Involvement in vigorous physical activity with special reference to adherence. In *Proceedings of the College Physical Education Association*. Orlando, 1977.

45. Morgan, W.P.; Horstman, D.H.; Cymerman, A.; and Stokes, J.: Use of exercise as a relaxation technique. *Prim Cardiol, 6*:48, 1980.

46. Morgan, W.P. and Pollock, M.L.: Psychologic characterization of the elite distance runner. *Ann NY Acad Sci, 301*:382, 1977.

47. Morgan, W.P. and Johnson, R.W.: Psychological characterization of national level oarsmen differing in level of ability. *Int J Sport Psychol, 9*:119, 1978.

48. Morgan, W.P.: Anxiety reduction following acute physical activity. *Psychiatr Ann, 9*:34, 1979.

49. Naughton, J.; Bruhn, J.G.; and Lategola, M.T.: Effects of physical training on physiologic and behavioral characteristics of cardiac patients. *Arch Phys Med Rehabil, 49*:131, 1968.

50. Orwin, A.: Treatment of a situational phobia—a case for running. *Br J Psychiatry, 125*:95, 1974.

51. Pitts, F.N., Jr. and McClure, J.N., Jr.: Lactate metabolism in anxiety neurosis. *N Engl J Med, 277*:1329, 1967.

52. Pitts, F.N., Jr.: Biochemical factors in anxiety neurosis. *Behav Sci, 16*:82, 1971.

53. Post, R.M. and Goodwin, F.K.: Simulated behavior states: An approach to specificity in psychobiological research. *Biol Psychiatry, 7*:237, 1973.

54. Powell, R.R.: Psychological effects of exercise therapy upon institutionalized geriatric mental patients. *J Gerontol, 29*:157, 1974.

55. Seemann, J.C.: *Changes in state anxiety following vigorous exercise.* M. S. Thesis, University of Arizona, 1978.

56. Sharp, M.W. and Reilley, R.R.: The relationship of aerobic physical fitness to selected personality traits. *J Clin Psychol, 31*:428, 1975.

57. Sime, W.E.: A comparison of exercise and meditation in reducing physiological response to stress. *Med Sci Sports, 9*:55, 1977.

58. Stamford, B.A.; Hambacher, W.; and Fallica, A.: Effects of daily physical exercise on the psychiatric state of institutionalized geriatric mental patients. *Res Q, 45*:34, 1974.

59. Wood, D.T.: The relationship between state anxiety and acute physical activity. *Am Correct Ther J, 31*:67, 1977.

60. Young, R.J. and Ismail, A.H.: Personality differences of adult men before and after a physical fitness program. *Res Q, 47*:513, 1976.

61. Young, R.J. and Ismail, A.H.: Relationships between anthropometric, physiological, biochemical and personality variables before and after a four month conditioning program for middle-aged men. *J Sports Med, 16*:267, 1976.

SUMMARY

HENRY J. MONTOYE

Bruno Balke: Physical educator, physician and physiologist. Careful investigator and international authority on sports medicine. Dedicated Fellow and past president of the College who still finds time to set an example of lifelong participation in healthful exercise.

THIS INSCRIPTION from the Honor Award presented to Dr. Balke by the American College of Sports Medicine shows the esteem and respect which Bruno's colleagues hold for him. These proceedings represent another tribute to Dr. Balke because they are examples of the accomplishments of his pupils. The productivity of his students is impressive; even a cursory perusal of the scientific literature will verify the frequency with which their names appear in distinguished scholarly journals.

Part I included chapters that, for the most part, pertain to pulmonary and cardiovascular adjustments to exercise as observed in human beings. It is well known that ventilation increases when sea level residents sojourn at altitude. Hubert Forster presented data and arguments that attempt to explain this phenomenon by changes in excitability of the medullary respiratory neurons. In the next chapter, Michael Sharratt and Morag Bruce investigated the possibility that there exists in muscle a receptor that is activated by the accumulation of fatigue products during exercise. The results of their experiments were consistent with the presence of such a receptor, which in turn could trigger the increase in systolic blood pressure and ventilation that occurs during exercise. Frank Cerney next reported little difference in the pulmonary and circulatory responses to exercise between normal children and children with cystic fibrosis (except those most seriously afflicted). He shared with us his experiences and those of his co-workers in developing an exercise test for use in prescribing exercise programs for cystic fibrosis children. The chapter by Weaver and Thomson contained somatotypic and cardiopulmonary data on prepubertal and pubertal age-group figure skaters.

315

There was little difference in the two groups in somatotype ratings and both groups had low mean percent body fat. Their observations suggest that changes in cardiopulmonary capacity from pre to post puberty of these high performance athletes were the result of growth not training.

A continuing controversy in exercise physiology is the question of whether oxygen transport, metabolic capacity at the cellular level, or some other factor is responsible for limiting muscular work. Norman Gledhill and others attempted to arrive at an answer to this question by reinfusing blood. This approach has been used before but methodological problems vitiated the results. Gledhill and his group were able to avoid these methodological problems to a considerable extent. However, the increase in maximal oxygen uptake was not commensurate with the additional O_2 in arterial blood. This led to the conclusion that metabolism at the muscle cell level cannot be discounted as the site of fatigue. The final chapter of Part I by Jerome Dempsey contained data on arterial hemoglobin saturation during heavy exercise in well-trained athletes. Until recent years, it had been thought that resting levels of arterial saturation (97–98%) are maintained during exercise despite increased tissue oxygen consumption, reduction of oxygen in mixed venous blood, and reduced time for equilibration of alveolar gas and red cells in the pulmonary capillaries. Twelve of seventeen endurance runners during heavy exercise showed decreased hemoglobin saturations, some decreases being sizable. The authors concluded this was due to inadequate alveolar PO_2.

Part 2 of the symposium comprised reports of histochemical and metabolic studies in animals and several experiments with human beings. James Gale presented an extensive review of electron microscopy studies in which acute and chronic effects of exercise were studied. He attempted to explain many of the reported changes at the cellular level on the basis of technical (methodological) effects. He concluded that little cardiac or skeletal muscle failure during exercise has been explained by observable changes at the molecular level. J. Duncan MacDougall reported on biopsies of the vastus lateralis muscle in thirteen preschool children. After comparing the fiber typing in these children with published data on adults, he found that, histochemically and ultrastructurally, skeletal muscle in six-year-old children does not differ from skeletal muscle in adults. The work of Robert Fitts was also concerned with the site of fatigue during strenuous exercise. After a thorough review of his own work and that of others, he became convinced that muscle fatigue in high intensity, short duration exercise is due to elevation of muscle lactate. In prolonged exercise of a high aerobic component, carbohydrate depletion may be responsible for terminating exercise. Increased mitochondria content was seen as an effort of the body to spare glycogen. Another possibility suggested was the decreased capacity of the sarcoplasmic reticulum to regulate cell Ca^{++}. The chapter by Howard Green also involved muscle typing. They investigated the appropriateness of the fiber classification of Peter et al. (*Biochemistry*, *11*:2627, 1972) for selected respiratory muscles (internal and external intercostals and the diaphragm). It was concluded that the utilization of four categories of NADH-TR activity can lead to considerably more information regarding muscle fiber differentiation than the high and low oxidative activity categories proposed by Peter and others.

James Hagberg and colleagues studied the early adjustment to exercise (i.e. from onset until a "steady state" is reached) and recovery immediately after exercise. Their observations led them to believe that the delay in reaching a steady state in oxygen uptake at the start of exercise has an "alactacid" component (i.e. it is due to a reduction in creatine phosphate and ATP stores). However, the second phase of adaptation is thought to be the result of direct and indirect effects of an increase in temperature, not to a "lactacid" component, as commonly believed. These authors agree that the first phase of recovery from exercise is related to repletion of creatine phosphate, ATP, and venous and myoglobin oxygen stores. However, the second phase was attributed primarily to a temperature effect and secondarily to the metabolism of lactate. Jack Daniels measured highly trained pentathletes, competitive canoe paddlers, and untrained college men in arm and leg tests of $\dot{V}O_2$max. He also measured $\dot{V}O_2$ in paddlers on water. Maximal heart rate and $\dot{V}_E$max were lower in arm work. However, differences in arm and leg $\dot{V}O_2$max were thought to be due to the state of training of the particular muscle group.

Edward Howley, in a very thorough presentation, summarized a number of his experiments to test the hypothesis proposed by von Euler that catecholamine secretion as a result of exercise might constitute an "effort index." Total urinary catecholamine was not found to be useful for this purpose. Although epinephrine secretion did not reflect the exercise intensity, norepinephrine did. John Faulkner next reported some interesting observations of the training and performance of three cross country skiers in a Canadian 160 km ski marathon. Because of the extreme cold and wind, the competition in 1979 constituted a natural experiment in hypothermia. Comparisons were also made of this competition with the 1978 ski marathon, which was conducted under normal environmental conditions. The final chapter of this Part was a discussion of so-called senile, or idiopathic, osteoporosis. Everett Smith described his work and that of others in which a substantial case is made for an increase in physical activity in middle-aged and older people to prevent or delay senile osteoporosis.

The third Part included chapters on the programmatic aspects of exercise as well as several presentations of the psychological correlates of physical exercise. Richard Peterson described the health education-physical fitness program at Hope College and the students response to it. Alan Claremont presented oxygen uptake data on various water exercises performed by older men and women. The exercises described are feasible and safe with this population. However, the decrease in body temperature and the decreased heart rate (21 beats per minute) at the same $\dot{V}O_2$ during exercise out of the water has important implications for prescribing water exercise.

John Naughton described the National Exercise and Heart Disease Project. The design includes an exercise and control group, all subjects being survivors of at least one myocardial infarction. The patients have been followed from 2½ to 3 years; however, the results of the exercise program have not been analyzed as yet. Observations about the testing procedure and the feasibility of conducting such trials were discussed.

Glen Porter discussed a treadmill test score for diagnosing coronary artery disease. An imperical point scale was assigned for the presence of inverted T-waves in the resting ECG and for the following responses to treadmill exercise: (a) ST-segment configuration and degree of depression, (b) presence of chest pain, (c) systolic blood pressure response, and (d) presence and frequency of premature beats. Using these criteria, the presence of disease was predicted accurately in 87 percent of the positive tests and the absence of disease was predicted accurately in 83 percent of the negative tests. Neil Oldridge reviewed the various factors that are related to adherence in an exercise cardiac rehabilitation program. He drew heavily from his experience in the Ontario Exercise Heart Collaborative Study. The following features characterize a typical drop-out. He is a blue collar worker, inactive in his leisure, smokes, and has had more than one infarction. Rodney Dishman also discussed adherence to exercise programs. From his retrospective and prospective studies he concluded that the drop-out is more likely to be symptom free, fatter, have a higher metabolic capacity and lower scores on a self-motivation test.

Michael Ross related his experiences in conducting exercise tests with psychiatric patients. Only two patients could not withstand the stress of an exercise test. For the others, their average metabolic capacity was about the same as that of normal subjects. The patients had a lower estimate of their physical ability and were less attracted to physical activity, but effort perception was similar to normals. Michael Bahrke, in the next chapter, reported the results of an experiment with middle-aged subjects. A bout of exercise or a rest period were found to be no different in their effects on anxiety during the subsequent twenty-four hours. The final chapter by William Morgan was a fitting conclusion to a stimulating scientific program. He thoroughly reviewed the literature on the effects of exercise on mental state. Both acute and chronic exercise is associated with improved psychological states but poor research design renders the results questionable from the standpoint of causation.

INDEX